ADVANCES IN
HUMAN GENETICS

6

CONTRIBUTORS TO THIS VOLUME

Laurence Corash
Hematology Service, Clinical Pathology Department
Clinical Center, National Institutes of Health
Bethesda, Maryland

Aldur W. Eriksson
Samfandet Folkhälsans Genetiska Institut
Populationsgenetiska Avdelningen
Helsinki, Finland

Johan Fellman
Samfandet Folkhälsans Genetiska Institut
Populationsgenetiska Avdelningen
Helsinki, Finland

Claude Laberge
Department of Medicine
Laval University Medical Center
Quebec City, Canada

James H. Mielke
Department of Sociology, Anthropology, and Social Work
Wright State University
Dayton, Ohio

Sergio Piomelli
Division of Pediatric Hematology
New York University School of Medicine
New York, New York

Leon E. Rosenberg
Department of Human Genetics
Yale University School of Medicine
New Haven, Connecticut

J. Edwin Seegmiller
Department of Medicine, Division of Rheumatology
University of California, San Diego
La Jolla, California

Peter L. Workman
Department of Anthropology
University of New Mexico
Albuquerque, New Mexico

A Continuation Order Plan is available for this series. A continuation order will bring delivery of each new volume immediately upon publication. Volumes are billed only upon actual shipment. For further information please contact the publisher.

ADVANCES IN HUMAN GENETICS

6

Edited by

Harry Harris

Galton Professor of Human Genetics
University College London
London, England

and

Kurt Hirschhorn

Arthur J. and Nellie Z. Cohen Professor of Genetics and Pediatrics
Mount Sinai School of Medicine of The City University of New York

SPRINGER SCIENCE+BUSINESS MEDIA, LLC

The Library of Congress cataloged the first volume of this title as follows:

Advances in human genetics. 1–
New York, Plenum Press, 1970–

    v. illus. 24 cm.

    Editors: v. 1–   H. Harris and K. Hirschhorn.

    1. Human genetics—Collected works.   i. Harris, Harry, ed.
    ii. Hirschhorn, Kurt, 1926–   joint ed.

QH431.A1A32   573.2'1   77–84583

Library of Congress   70 ₍4₎

Library of Congress Catalog Card Number 77-84583
ISBN 978-1-4615-8266-3   ISBN 978-1-4615-8264-9 (eBook)
DOI 10.1007/978-1-4615-8264-9

© Springer Science+Business Media New York 1976
Originally published by Plenum Press, New York in 1976
Softcover reprint of the hardcover 1st edition 1976

ARTICLES PLANNED FOR FUTURE VOLUMES:

CONTENTS OF EARLIER VOLUMES:

Preface to Volume 1

During the last few years the science of human genetics has been expanding almost explosively. Original papers dealing with different aspects of the subject are appearing at an increasingly rapid rate in a very wide range of journals, and it becomes more and more difficult for the geneticist and virtually impossible for the nongeneticist to keep track of the developments. Furthermore, new observations and discoveries relevant to an overall understanding of the subject result from investigations using very diverse techniques and methodologies and originating in a variety of different disciplines. Thus, investigations in such various fields as enzymology, immunology, protein chemistry, cytology, pediatrics, neurology, internal medicine, anthropology, and mathematical and statistical genetics, to name but a few, have each contributed results and ideas of general significance to the study of human genetics. Not surprisingly it is often difficult for workers in one branch of the subject to assess and assimilate findings made in another. This can be a serious limiting factor on the rate of progress.

Thus, there appears to be a real need for critical review articles which summarize the positions reached in different areas, and it is hoped that "Advances in Human Genetics" will help to meet this requirement.

Each of the contributors has been asked to write an account of the position that has been reached in the investigations of a specific topic in one of the branches of human genetics. The reviews are intended to be critical and to deal with the topic in depth from the writer's own point of view. It is hoped that the articles will provide workers in other branches of the subject, and in related disciplines, with a detailed account of the results so far obtained in the particular area, and help them to assess the relevance of these discoveries to aspects of their own work, as well as to the science as a whole. The reviews are also intended to give the reader some idea of the nature of the technical and methodological problems involved, and to indicate new directions stemming from recent advances.

The contributors have not been restricted in the arrangement or organization of their material or in the manner of its presentation, so that the reader should be able to appreciate something of the individuality of approach which goes to make up the subject of human genetics, and which, indeed, gives it much of its fascination.

JANUARY 1, 1970

HARRY HARRIS
The Galton Laboratory
University College London

KURT HIRSCHHORN
Division of Medical Genetics
Department of Pediatrics
Mount Sinai School of Medicine

Contents

Chapter 2

Inherited Deficiency of Hypoxanthine-Guanine Phosphoribosyltransferase in X-Linked Uric Aciduria (the Lesch–Nyhan Syndrome and Its Variants)

J. Edwin Seegmiller

Chapter 3

**Hereditary Hemolytic Anemia Due to Enzyme
Defects of Glycolysis**

Sergio Piomelli and Laurence Corash

Chapter 4

Population Structure of the Åland Islands, Finland

*James H. Mielke, Peter L. Workman, Johan Fellman, and
Aldur W. Eriksson*

Chapter 5

**Population Genetics and Health Care Delivery:
The Quebec Experience**

Claude Laberge

Erratum to Volume 2

The sentence beginning in line 5 of page 36 in Chapter 1 now reads:

Some subcultures revealed the electrophoretically fast band; others revealed the electrophoretically slow band; but one of the subcultures from single cells had both electrophoretic bands of G-6-PD.

The final portion should read:

but *none* of the subcultures from single cells had both electrophoretic bands of G-6-PD.

Chapter 1

Vitamin-Responsive Inherited Metabolic Disorders

Leon E. Rosenberg

Department of Human Genetics
Yale University School of Medicine
New Haven, Connecticut

INTRODUCTION

We now recognize 25 different metabolic disorders which meet the three essential criteria for inclusion in this review: a genetic etiology, a characteristic clinical or biochemical aberration, and an unequivocal biochemical and/or clinical response to a supraphysiological amount or an extraphysiological route of administration of a single vitamin. Most of these vitamin-responsive or, as they have often been called, "vitamin-dependent" conditions have been described in the past decade. Yet their discovery can be traced to the logical interaction of two older scientific disciplines which date back to the early years of this century. One, human biochemical genetics, stems from Archibald Garrod's descriptions of four "inborn errors of metabolism."[39] The other, concerned with the structure and function of vitamins, was founded by Frederick G. Hopkins[105] during his investigations of "accessory food substances."

Progress in both fields was very slow at first but has accelerated dramatically during the past three decades. While Garrod's disciples characterized and catalogued literally hundreds of human phenotypes resulting from single gene mutations, Hopkins' followers conducted the inquiries which led to the recognition that vitamins are organic compounds which must be ingested in minute amounts for normal

1

human growth, homeostasis, and reproduction. Just as endogenously synthesized building blocks and macromolecules differ markedly in structure and function, so do the vitamins. Some are obtained from animal sources; others from vegetables. Some are water soluble; others fat soluble. Some, such as vitamin D, function as hormones in target tissues, while others (the B complex) act as coenzymes for one or more enzymatic reactions.

Although quite separate initially, the fields of biochemical genetics and vitaminology have been drawn together by the expanding knowledge in each. For instance, the demonstration that pyridoxal-5'-phosphate, the active form of pyridoxine (vitamin B_6), functions as a coenzyme in a large number of enzymatic decarboxylation, transamination, and condensation reactions for amino acids culminated in the discovery that this vitamin was of therapeutic value in several inherited disorders of amino acid metabolism. Similarly, only after elucidation of the biochemical pathways for the stepwise conversion of vitamin D (cholecalciferol) to 25-hydroxycholecalciferol and 1, 25-dihydroxycholecaldiferol could the pathobiology of patients with vitamin D dependent rickets be understood.

Although each of the known vitamin-responsive inborn errors appears to be rare, some having been described in only a single pedigree, their impact has already been consequential. First, because they epitomize that class of inherited diseases that clinicians are most interested in—those in which early detection and appropriate therapy can prevent acute illness, chronic disability, or death. Second, because they prove that assimilation and utilization of ingested vitamins by the human organism depend on precisely the same kind of genetic determinants which regulate all other phases of intermediary metabolism. Third, because they offer unusual testimony to the biochemical and genetic heterogeneity which abounds in human mutations. And, fourth, because they underscore the primitive state of our knowledge about such processes as vitamin transport into and within cells, coenzyme synthesis from vitamin precursors, regulation of apoenzyme content by coenzyme supply, and the dichotomy between holoenzyme activity *in vitro* and metabolic capacity *in vivo*.

During the past 5 years, several progress reports on the vitamin-responsive inborn errors have been published, and these reports have been used liberally throughout this review.[92,98,123−125,130,136,141]

VITAMIN DEFICIENCY: HISTORICAL PERSPECTIVE

Although the term "vitamine" was not coined by Funk until 1912 in his description of the beriberi-curing substance,[38] there is considerable evidence for a very long period of informal awareness about these accessory substances.[105]

A text entitled *Medical Experiences of a Frontier Official* had appeared in China in the eighth century AD wherein conditions resembling deficiency of vitamin A and vitamin D were described. In the fourteenth century, and again from China, the book *Principles of Correct Diet* described a condition resembling beriberi. Two hundred years later, the French explorer Cartier (1545) described in a report to his king how the drinking of the liquor from boiled spruce needles, prepared for him by the Indians of the St. Lawrence Valley region, cured the scurvy of his crew members.[17]

This anecdotal approach to vitamins and vitamin deficiencies continued until the end of the nineteenth century, when certain diseases, presumed to be infectious, were linked unequivocally to a deficiency of specific food factors.

During the next 50 years, the chemical nature of the vitamins was defined and the human nutritional requirements for these substances were investigated. Two general approaches have been used to assess such nutritional requirements. The first uses dietary surveys in regions of endemic deficiency and compares intake in such locales with that in regions free of deficiency. The second titrates intake of a single vitamin against the physiologial and biochemical process which depend on its presence. Since both approaches are fraught with problems of control and interpretation, it is not surprising that considerable controversy still exists regarding exact quantitative requirements.[104,108,118,119] Nonetheless, both "minimum requirements" and "recommended dietary allowances" have been defined which prevent deficiency and toxicity in the vast bulk of the population. In Table I, the age-dependent, recommended dietary allowances for most of the fat- and water-soluble vitamins are presented.

If the intake of a specific vitamin is consistently less than the minimum age-dependent requirement, a deficiency state characteristic for that vitamin will ensue. The clinical and chemical manifestations of

TABLE I. Recommended Dietary Allowances for Several Vitamins (amount/day)[a]

Vitamin	Unit	Infant (<12 months)	Child (1–8 years)	Youth (9–17 years)	Adult
Thiamine (B₁)	mg	0.4	0.8	1.4	1.2
Riboflavin (B₂)	mg	0.6	1.3	2.0	1.7
Pyridoxine (B₆)	mg	0.4	1	2	2
Cobalamin (B₁₂)	μg	2.5	2.5	5	5
Folic acid	mg	0.05	0.05	0.1	0.1
Niacin[b]	mg	6	14	22	19
Ascorbic acid (C)	mg	30–100[c]	60	80	70
Vitamin A	units	1500	3500	5000	5000
Vitamin D[d]	units	400	400	100–400	100

[a] From Scriver.[136] The recommended dietary allowances are intended to serve as a guide in planning food supplies and for the interpretation of food consumption of groups of people.[104,118,119] Minimum and maximum allowable intakes are another concept.[30]
[b] L-Tryptophan 60 mg is equivalent to 1 mg niacin.
[c] Higher allowance recommended for premature infants or full-term infants with postnatal tyrosinemia.
[d] 100 units of vitamin D = 2.5 μg cholecalciferol.

such deficiency can be corrected simply by supplementing the diet up to the recommended intake of the vitamin. Thus deficiency of any given vitamin in man is typified by a nutritional deficit, a particular group of clinical and chemical aberrations, and complete correction following intake of physiological amounts of the vitamin in question.

Not all vitamin deficiency is explained in these simple terms. Gastrointestinal malabsorption of many etiologies can impair absorption of water- or fat-soluble vitamins and lead to vitamin deficiency despite an adequate oral intake. Pharmacological agents may interfere with vitamin metabolism in many ways and lead to signs or symptoms of vitamin deficiency. For example, isoniazid competitively inhibits the kinase which converts pyridoxine to pyridoxal phosphate, thereby interfering with the many enzymatic reactions which depend on this coenzyme.[164] Similarly, such anticonvulsant medications as phenobarbital and dilantin stimulate nonspecific microsomal enzymes which inactivate vitamin D, thereby occasionally producing frank rickets or osteomalacia.[27,51]

Age, too, has a bearing on vitamin requirements (Table I) which is highlighted by the entity called neonatal tyrosinemia.[136] When the ascorbic acid requirement in premature and full-term infants is assessed in terms of its ability to maintain efficient oxidation of the tyrosine catabolite p-hydroxyphenylpyruvic acid, it is found to be increased in about one-third of prematures and one in 200 full-term infants. This transient exaggeration of the requirement for vitamin C depends on a unique set of interactions between ascorbate, in its reduced form, and the enzyme p-hydroxyphenylpyruvic acid oxidase. In the absence of reduced ascorbate, activity of this enzyme is very susceptible to inhibition by its ketoacid substrate. The relationships among the amount of apoenzyme in the hepatic cells of the neonate, the fraction of apoenzyme present as holoenzyme, and the tyrosine intake in the diet are such as to predispose to such inhibition of enzyme activity. Dietary supplementation with ascorbate prevents neonatal typrosinemia in nearly all cases, the quantitativᵉ requirement to achieve this goal being about 25 mg/kg of ascorbate compared to a requirement of about 1 mg/kg in the older child or adult In this setting, we recognize a transient, physiological elevation of the ascorbate requirement in the young infant which reflects a particular developmental schedule.

VITAMIN RESPONSIVENESS OR DEPENDENCY

Vitamin deficiency, then, can be produced by nutritional, absorptive, pharmacological, or developmental interferences with vitamin utilization in all humans. In contrast, we now know that some few individuals have a constant, specific requirement for a particular vitamin that differs from normal in one of two ways: either the *route* of vitamin administration must be changed from oral to parenteral or the *quantity* of the vitamin must be increased to 10–1000 times that usually recommended. The prevention of disease in such individuals is, in fact, dependent on such altered administration. This group of patients with *vitamin-dependent* or *vitamin-responsive* conditions can be contrasted to those with vitamin-deficient states in several ways. First, vitamin-responsive states have a genetic etiology, whereas typical vitamin deficiencies are acquired. Second, if the inherited abnormality impairs intestinal absorption of the vitamin, then its clinical and biochemical manifestations will be identical to those of an acquired deficiency, but the mode of vitamin administration needed to correct these manifestations will differ. Third, vitamin-responsive disorders usually reflect an underlying biochemical abnormality in only a single reaction, while vitamin deficiency states commonly lead to interference with several reactions. Fourth, most vitamin-responsive conditions improve only after a pharmacological dose of a specific vitamin, not a physiological one.

These features of vitamin-responsive disorders can best be illustrated by referring to the two classical papers in this field. In 1937, Albright et al.[1] reported a 16-year-old boy with intractable rickets and hypophosphatemia from his earliest years who healed his bones dramatically when he was given 1000 times the usually required dose of vitamin D, but failed to respond to physiological or even 100 times the physiological intake of this sterol. Intestinal malabsorption of the vitamin was excluded by appropriate trials of parenteral vitamin administration. Although not appreciated at the time, this boy unquestionably suffered from familial hypophosphatemic rickets, a disorder now reknowned for its X-linked dominant inheritance and its resistance to huge doses of vitamin D.[169] Seventeen years later, in 1954, inherited responsiveness to the water-soluble vitamin pyridoxine was discovered in a very different clinical setting by Hunt et al.[68] They described female sibs with a previously unrecognized disorder. The first child began to have convulsions at 2 days of age and died of uncontrollable seizures on day 3. Postmortem findings were unremarkable. Her younger sister, jittery at birth, also began having major motor seizures on day 5. Routine laboratory evaluation was unrevealing and no response to such anticonvulsants as barbiturates, magnesium sulfate, or calcium gluconate was noted. As part of general supportive care, she was given a multivitamin preparation (Berocca C) parenterally. Almost immediately the seizures stopped, only to reappear promptly when the vitamin preparation was discontinued. Repeated administration and cessation of this multivitamin during the next few weeks demonstrated convincingly that the vitamin preparation was controlling the seizure disorder. Individual vitamins were then tried sequentially and pyridoxine was found to be the specific protective agent. Significantly, seizures were not controlled by pyridoxine doses in the physiological range (0.3 mg/day) but only when approximately ten times this amount was given orally or parenterally. These observations led Hunt and his colleagues to propose that this child was "dependent" on larger than normal quantities of pyridoxine, the term "dependency" being coined to contrast with pyridoxine deficiency. It is somewhat ironic that the two conditions which ushered in the field of inborn errors responsive to vitamin supplements remain two of the least well understood entities among a fast-growing list of related disorders. Before discussing in detail the clinical, genetic, and chemical findings in these conditions, I will turn to a discussion of the biochemical genetics of vitamins *per se*.

Genetic Control of Vitamin Metabolism

The very fact that all of the compounds we call vitamins must be supplied in the diet is *prima facie* evidence that, in the course of evolution, the human species has lost the genetic information required to synthesize these compounds. But it does not follow therefrom that man's genes play no part in vitamin metabolism. On the contrary, it is clear that a number of proteins and therefore a number of genes regulate all facets of vitamin metabolism once ingestion has occurred. These proteins are of two general types: those concerned with vitamin transport and those required for intracellular vitamin utilization (Table II). For example, at least nine proteins are needed if ingested vitamin B_{12} is to function as a coenzyme: gastric intrinsic factor, which binds B_{12} in the stomach and carries it to the small bowel; specific receptors in the ileal mucosa, which facilitate absorption of B_{12} to and from tissue cells; two plasma binding proteins; at least three intracellular enzymes which convert the vitamin to its active coenzyme forms; and finally two apoenzymes which require B_{12} coenzymes for catalytic activity. Even this extensive array of proteins specifically concerned

TABLE II. Classes of Proteins
Participating in Vitamin-Dependent
Reactions

Transport proteins
1. Intestinal receptor
2. Plasma binding
3. Tissue receptor
          Intracellular proteins
4. Activating enzyme
5. Intracellular binding
6. Holoenzyme synthetase
7. Apoenzyme

with the use of this vitamin may be incomplete. There may also be specific lysosomal or mitochondrial binding proteins for B_{12}[114,115] and perhaps, as has been shown for biotin, holoenzyme synthetases which act to catalyze the binding of coenzyme to apoenzyme.[19] Although not all of the vitamins appear to require as intricate a set of regulatory reactions as B_{12} does, there is a large body of data which shows that, with the exception of ascorbate and biotin, each of the other vitamins is modified by one or more enzyme-catalyzed steps prior to carrying out its unique intracellular function. Thus, there is a large array of vitamin-regulating proteins whose structure and function could be altered by specific mutations in their respective genomes.

Biochemical Role of Vitamins

As mentioned earlier, there is great diversity of vitamin source and structure. Not surprisingly, this diversity is also apparent as one examines the biochemical and physiological role of these accessory substances. Classically the vitamins are divided into two groups: fat soluble and water soluble.

The fat-soluble vitamins (A, E, K, and D) share one feature in addition to their common extractability into organic solvents, their ultimate derivation from isoprenoid building blocks.[81] Such isoprene units are most easily seen in vitamins A, E, and K (see vitamin A structure in Fig. 1). Functionally, however, the fat-soluble vitamins differ greatly (Table III). Vitamin A (retinol), which exists in animal tissues in two major chemical forms (or vitamers) called A_1 and A_2, is required for epithelial integrity and visual excitation. In the latter

TABLE III. Role of Fat-Soluble Vitamins

Vitamin	Generic name	Function
A	Retinol	Rhodopsin synthesis, epithelial surface integrity
D	Calciferol	Bone mineral metabolism, intestinal calcium absorption
E	Tocopherol	Antioxidant (?)
K	Naphthoquinone	Prothrombin synthesis

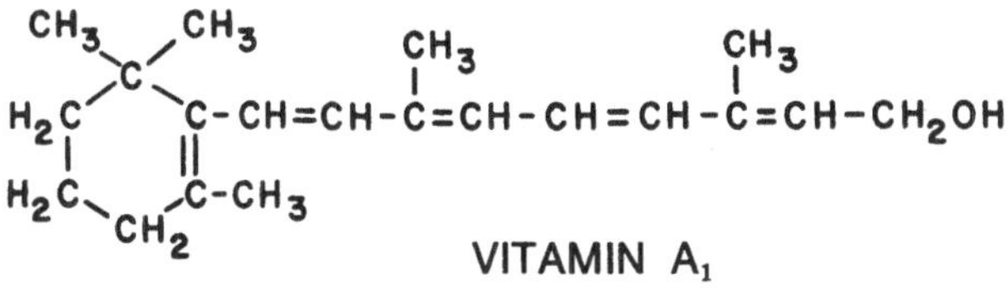

VITAMIN A₁

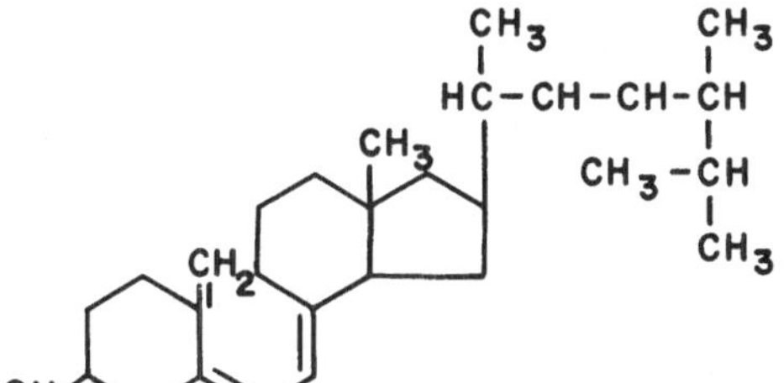

VITAMIN D₃

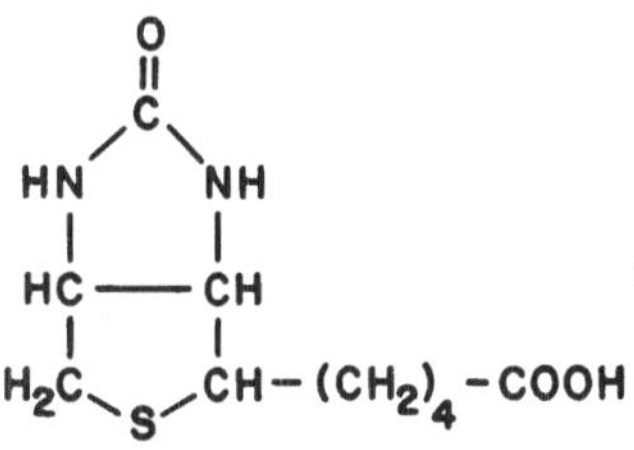

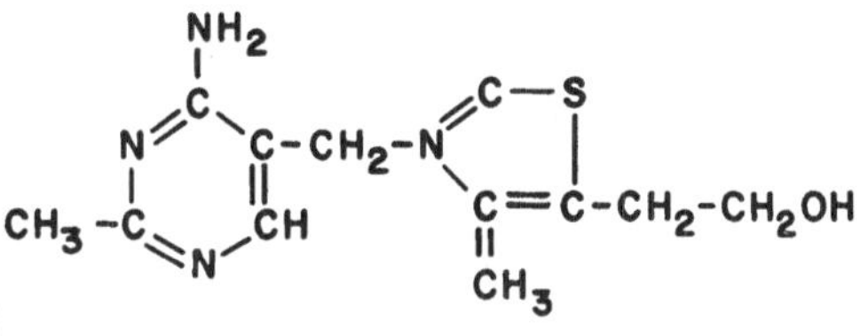

BIOTIN   THIAMINE

Fig. 1. Chemical structures of selected fat- and water-soluble vitamins. Note the isoprenoid structure of vitamin A₁ and the steroid conformation of vitamin D₃. Biotin is unique among the water-soluble vitamins in that it binds to apoenzymes covalently via a peptide bond between its carboxyl group and an ε-amino group of a lysine residue on the apoprotein. The active coenzyme form of thiamine is thiamine pyrophosphate, the pyrophosphate group attaching to the terminal oxygen atom of the hydroxyl group.

case, it must first be oxidized to vitamin A aldehyde (retinal), which then combines with a protein in the rod cells, opsin, to yield rhodopsin. When rhodopsin absorbs light energy, the vitamin A component dissociates from opsin and undergoes a conformational change which excites the nerve cells of the rods. Simply stated, vitamin A is a key structural component of the visual cycle. Vitamin E, composed of several closely related vitamins found in vegetable oils, is also called tocopherol. Although the specific molecular mechanisms which underlie this vitamin's role are not known, there is growing evidence that tocopherols prevent the destructive attack of molecular oxygen on the polyunsaturated fatty acids of tissue lipids, and therefore they are referred to as "antioxidants." Vitamin K, widely distributed in plants as two vitamins (K_1 and K_2), is a naphthoquinone required for the synthesis of the blood-clotting protein, prothrombin. Vitamin D differs from the other fat-soluble vitamins in that it is a steroid derivative (Fig. 1). It, too, has multiple chemical forms (to be discussed in greater detail subsequently) which act to preserve normal bone mineral metabolism by stimulating intestinal calcium absorption and bone calcium resorption. Since the target organ for this vitamin (the gut) differs from those responsible for its sequential chemical activation (liver and kidney), vitamin D metabolism has been likened to an endocrine system, with the ingested vitamin being referred to as a prohormone and its ultimately active form as a hormone.[26]

In contrast to this lack of a common functional thread among the fat-soluble vitamins, the water-soluble vitamins all act as cocatalysts in enzymatic reactions.[88] Some enzymes depend for activity only on their structure as proteins, while others require one or more nonprotein cofactors for activity. Some cofactors are simple cations; others are more complex, heat-stable organic compounds called coenzymes. Each of the known water-soluble vitamins acts as a coenzyme or a coenzyme precursor (Table IV). The coenzyme binds to its appropriate protein species, called the apoenzyme, to form a holoenzyme. Coenzyme-dependent apoenzymes bind their cofactors in different ways and with different degrees of affinity. Biotin (Fig. 1), for instance, is covalently and tightly bound to its apoenzymes via peptide linkage and cannot be removed by dialysis or other gentle treatments. Most of the other coenzymes share weaker hydrogen or hydrophobic bonds with their apoenzymes and can be dissociated by dialysis or other means. Some apoenzyme–coenzyme interactions follow typical Michaelis–Menten kinetics whereas others are considerably more complex.[98,107]

Once formed, the holoenzyme combines with its substrate(s) and catalyzes the formation of a product(s). Although each coenzyme has a unique mechanism in its preferred reactions, it is generally true that coenzymes function as intermediary carriers of electrons, specific atoms, or functional groups which are transferred during the overall enzymatic reaction. Thiamine pyrophosphate, for example, participates in the enzymatic decarboxylation of α-keto acids by carrying free

TABLE IV. Coenzyme Role of Water-Soluble Vitamins

Vitamin	Coenzyme form	Function
Thiamine (B_1)	Thiamine pyrophosphate	Activation of carboxyl derivatives, aldehyde transfer
Riboflavin (B_2)	Flavin mononucleotide and flavin adenine dinucleotide	Hydrogen atom (electron) transfer
Pyridoxine (B_6)	Pyridoxal-5'-phosphate	Amino group transfer, amino acid decarboxylation, etc.
Cobalamin (B_{12})	Methylcobalamin	Methyl group transfer for N^5-methyltetrahydrofolate-homocysteine methyltransferase
	5'-Deoxyadenosylcobalamin	Hydrogen transfer in isomerization of L-methylmalonyl-CoA to succinyl-CoA
Folic acid	Tetrahydrofolate	One-carbon fragment activation and transfer
Niacin	Nicotinamide adenine dinucleotide (phosphate)	Hydrogen atom (electron) transfer
Ascorbic acid (C)	L-Ascorbic acid	Reducing agent
Pantothenic acid	Coenzyme A	Acyl transfer
Biotin	Biotin	CO_2 activation and transfer

aldehyde groups, while pyridoxal phosphate transfers amino groups in many enzymatic transaminations. Similarly, cobalamin coenzymes transfer alkyl or methyl groups, biotin carries carboxyl groups, and the folate coenzymes participate in one-carbon fragment transfers. Just as the structure of the coenzyme defines the nature of the functions it can participate in, so the primary sequence and conformation of the apoenzyme regulate substrate specificity and reaction rate.

Coenzymes have another important role which is not directly related to their chemical participation in catalysis. The steady-state concentration of certain apoenzymes can be regulated by their coenzymes. Apoenzymes normally undergo a cycle of synthesis and degradation within the cell, and the balance between the two phases of the cycle is an important focal point for regulation of the amount and activity of the enzyme in higher organisms.[171] The rate of inactivation is probably the more important site of enzyme regulation in diploid cells.[9] Some apoenzymes are induced by exposure to their coenzyme. In this way, the effective concentration of holoenzyme as well as the absolute amount of apoenzyme can be increased. Such induction has been well documented for certain amino transferases and for tryptophan pyrrolase.[83] Binding of coenzyme to apoenzyme may also slow apoenzyme degradation. Litwack and Rosenfield,[85] using pyridoxal phosphate dependent reactions, pointed out an impressive correlation between ease of dissociation of coenzyme from apoenzyme *in vitro* and the observed turnover rate of the enzyme *in vivo*: the tighter the binding between apoenzyme and coenzyme, the longer the half-life. Thus coenzymes may modulate enzyme activity in three important ways: by determining what fraction of total cellular apoenzyme is in its catalytically active form, by regulating the rate of synthesis of apoenzyme, and by controlling the rate of apoenzyme degradation.

Effect of Mutation on Vitamin Function: Theoretical Possibilities

From the foregoing discussion, it is clear that a wide variety of different mutations could theoretically interfere with the activity of a vitamin (Fig. 2). The mutant allele could impair vitamin transport at one of several points: the intestine, the plasma, the tissue cells, or within intracellular organelles. The mutant allele could block any one of the reactions by which the vitamin is converted intracellularly to coenzyme or hormone. The mutant allele could alter a specific apoenzyme in such a way that its normal interaction with coenzyme is disturbed. Finally, the mutant allele could lead to the synthesis of an altered apoenzyme whose turnover rate in the presence of normal amounts of coenzyme is distinctly increased. The very fact that any such mutation would demonstrate vitamin responsiveness implies that the mutation is partial or "leaky."

The clinical and biochemical specificity of such mutations could also be predicted to vary considerably. Mutations interfering with intestinal absorption of a vitamin or its transport in the blood might be expected to produce a clinical disorder similar or identical to the disorder observed in acquired deficiency of that vitamin: reduced tissue stores or generalized pathophysiological disturbance. At the other extreme, mutations involving a single coenzyme-dependent apoenzyme

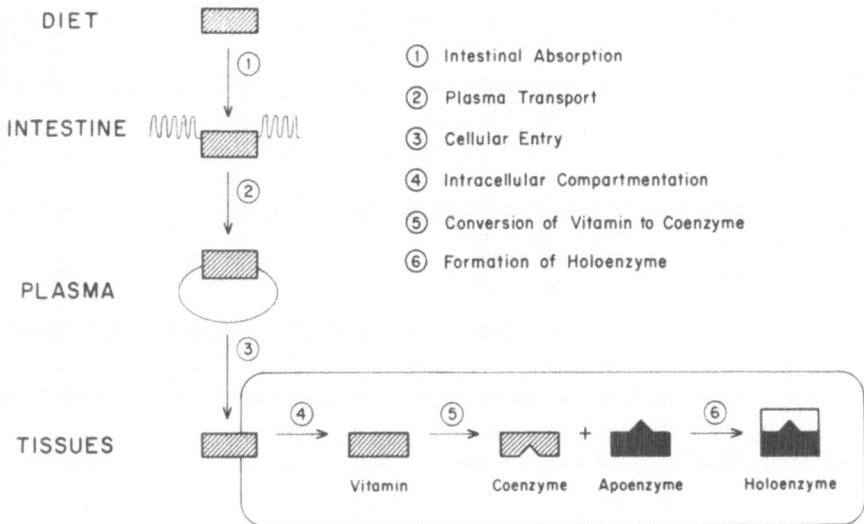

Fig. 2. Schematic representation of sites at which mutations could interfere with vitamin metabolism and vitamin-catalyzed reactions. See text for additional details.

might be expected to alter only that enzymatic function and leave unimpaired all of the other enzymatic reactions whose function depends on the same coenzyme. In this instance, tissue vitamin content would, of course, be normal. The effect of mutations altering conversion of inactive vitamin to active coenzyme or hormone would depend on the metabolic pathway for the particular vitamin in question. This can be illustrated by contrasting pyridoxine (B_6) with cobalamin (B_{12}). Pyridoxine has only one active coenzyme form (pyridoxal phosphate), whose synthesis is catalyzed by a single enzyme, pyridoxal kinase. A defect of this kinase would very likely reduce pyridoxal phosphate concentrations in tissues and interfere with all pyridoxal phosphate dependent reactions despite normal tissue pyridoxine concentrations. Conversely, there are two different coenzymes derived from vitamin B_{12}, each catalyzing a single different reaction and each being synthesized by distinct reaction sequences. Hence, a single mutation could alter the synthesis of one cobalamin coenzyme while leaving the other unaltered, and thereby impair one cobalamin-dependent apoenzyme but not another. It is apparent then that the specificity of the biochemical alterations, the cellular stores of vitamin and coenzyme, and the effective route of vitamin replacement thereapy will depend on the site of the mutations diagrammed in Fig. 2. Let us now examine the known vitamin-responsive inborn errors to see how these theoretical considerations relate to observed phenomena.

DEFECTS OF VITAMIN TRANSPORT AND COENZYME SYNTHESIS

Before any vitamin-derived coenzyme (or hormone) can function biochemically, three general processes must be satisfied: the vitamin must be absorbed from the intestinal tract; it must be transported to the tissues; and, in most instances, the inactive vitamin must be converted to its active coenzyme form. With some notable exceptions, transport of vitamins across cell membranes has not been investigated extensively. In ascites tumor cells, the nonphosphorylated forms of vitamin B_6 cross the plasma membrane much more readily than do their phosphorylated counterparts,[110] but these events have not been examined in mammalian gut. Likewise, ascorbic acid is reabsorbed from the renal tubule by a mediated process,[148] but again no intestinal transport studies have been carried out. Riboflavin is absorbed from the jejunum by a specific, saturable system also present in the renal tubule.[72] Almost nothing is known about the intestinal absorption of niacin, but malabsorption of the amino acid precursor of this vitamin, tryptophan, presents us with a unique example of a vitamin-responsive disorder. Patients with Hartnup disease, an autosomal recessive trait characterized by defective intestinal and renal transport of tryptophan and a number of other neutral aliphatic and aromatic amino acids, often develop a pellagra-like skin rash and cerebellar ataxia which respond dramatically to nicotinamide supplements.[71] Since a portion of the human requirement for niacin is met by converting tryptophan to nicotinamide intracellularly, it appears likely that patients with this disease are prone to nicotinamide deficiency consequent to their tryptophan malabsorption. In this instance, the physiological requirement for a vitamin is increased because its precursor is available in insufficient amount. None of the other known vitamin-responsive disorders is caused by such a disturbance.

In contrast to this paucity of information about the mechanism of

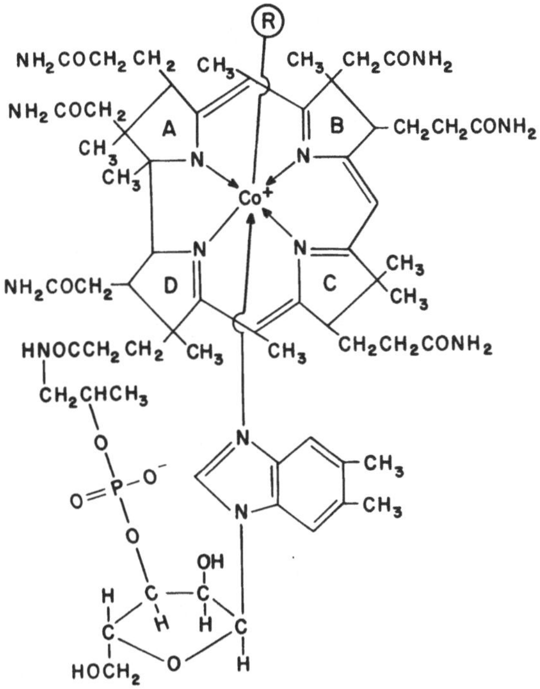

Fig. 3. Chemical structure of cobalamin (vitamin B_{12}). The planar corrin ring system is composed of four pyrrole rings designated A, B, C, D. Ⓡ refers to several different radicals, e.g., CN^- or OH^-, which are coordinately linked to the cobalt nucleus above the plane of the corrin ring. Such radicals provide the following cobalamins with their chemical and biological specificity: CN^-, cyanocobalamin; OH^-, hydroxocobalamin; CH_3, methylcobalamin; 5'-deoxyadenosyl, 5'-deoxyadenosylcobalamin.

absorption of most of the vitamins, a great deal is known about the processes by which vitamin B_{12} and folate are absorbed. It is therefore not surprising that only for these two vitamins do well-documented examples of inherited defects of transport exist. I shall discuss absorption and activation of these vitamins in detail to illustrate the principles alluded to previously and to emphasize what we are likely to learn about other vitamins when their metabolism is investigated as thoroughly as has been that of B_{12} and folate.

Cobalamin (Vitamin B₁₂)

The structure and function of vitamin B_{12} have fascinated biologists of all stripes since Minot and Murphy demonstrated in 1926 that crude liver extract was effective in the treatment of pernicious anemia.[95] By 1948, this "anti-pernicious anemia factor" had been isolated from several animal sources and renamed vitamin B_{12} or cobalamin.[120,147] Cobalamin is synthesized almost exclusively by microorganisms in soil, water, and the rumen and intestine of animals. Although the exact human requirement has not been defined, less than 1 μg daily is sufficient to prevent signs or symptoms of deficiency.

Chemistry

The chemical structure of cobalamin is complex (Fig. 3). It has two characteristic components. The first, and most characteristic, is a planar corrin ring system containing four pyrrole rings each coordinated through its nitrogen atom to a central cobalt nucleus. The second is a dimethylbenzimidazole ribotide portion extending down from the plane of the corrin ring.[57] The molecule is completed by coordinate linkage of one of several different radicals to the cobalt atom. This radical extends up from the corrin plane. Thus cyanocobalamin (CN-Cbl), the commercial form of vitamin B_{12}, is formed by attachment of a cyanide radical to the cobalt atom. This compound, however, is an artifact of the chemical procedures used to isolate cobalamins and does not occur naturally in bacteria or animal tissues. Three other cobalamins have been isolated from mammalian sources and appear to be the biologically important forms of this vitamin. Hydroxocobalamin (OH-Cbl) is the major form of B_{12} in the blood, and is very likely the precursor of the two active coenzyme forms of B_{12}: methylcobalamin (Me-Cbl); and 5'-deoxyadenosylcobalamin (Ado-Cbl). Each coenzyme is known in man to participate in only a single reaction. Me-Cbl acts with homocysteine-methyltetrahydrofolate methyltransferase in the methylation of homocysteine to methionine; Ado-Cbl acts with methylmalonyl-CoA mutase in the isomerization of L-methylmalonyl-CoA to succinyl-CoA (Fig. 4).

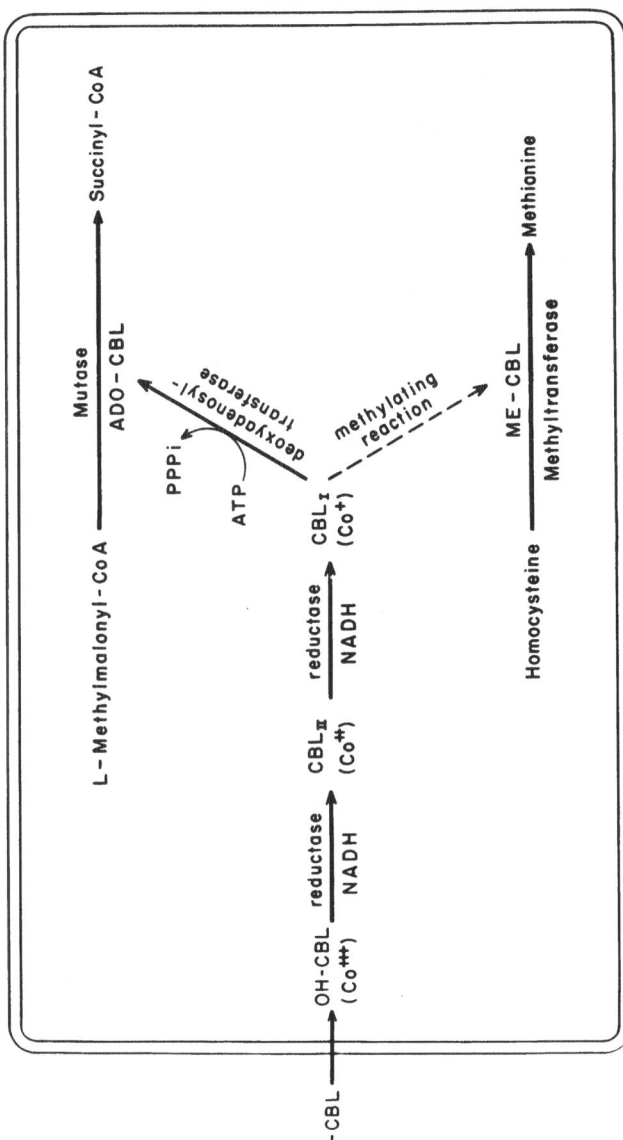

Fig. 4. Pathway of intracellular cobalamin metabolism. The centered scheme depicts the sequence of enzymatic reactions required for conversion of the vitamin hydroxocobalamin (OH-CBL) to its active coenzymes, 5'-deoxyadenosylcobalamin (ADO-CBL) and methylcobalamin (ME-CBL). The broken line leading to ME-CBL reflects uncertainty concerning the point of divergence of its biosynthetic pathway from that leading to ADO-CBL formation. At the top and bottom, the two enzymatic reactions dependent on cobalamin coenzymes are also shown: methylmalonyl-CoA mutase and N^5-methyltetrahydrofolate-homocysteine methyltransferase. The methyltransferase reaction requires S-adenosylmethionine and N^5-methyltetrahydrofolate as cofactors in addition to ME-CBL. These reactions are discussed in detail in the text.

Absorption and Activation

Vitamin B_{12} has a unique and highly specialized mechanism of intestinal absorption which requires both gastric and ileal components. The gastric substance is "intrinsic factor," a glycoprotein which binds B_{12} in the intestinal lumen by forming an intrinsic factor–B_{12} (IF-B_{12}) complex.[18] This complex then moves down the intestinal tract and interacts through its protein moiety with specific receptor sites in the ileum. During this process, the IF-B_{12} complex dissociates and free B_{12} is transported across the ileal wall into the portal blood. Once in the bloodstream, free B_{12} is tightly bound to two different globulin proteins called transcobalamins I and II.[53] Transcobalamin I (TC I) is an α-globulin which carries the majority of B_{12} found in plasma. TC II, a β-globulin, carries less total B_{12}, but is almost certainly the transport protein for B_{12} newly absorbed from the intestinal tract.[53,59] When labeled CN-Cbl was administered intravenously or orally, most of the cobalamin was immediately bound to TC II and disappeared from the plasma in a few hours. Only a small fraction associated with TC I and this component turned over very slowly.

TC II also facilitates uptake of B_{12} by mammalian tissues. Finkler and Hall[30] showed that CN-Cbl bound to TC II was accumulated by HeLa cells in culture much more rapidly than was free CN-Cbl or CN-Cbl bound to TC I, intrinsic factor, or other binding proteins. TC II mediated uptake was inhibited by cyanide, iodoacetamide, and dithiothreitol, thereby demonstrating that the process involved depended on aerobic metabolism and sulfhydryl group reactivity.[54] These results were confirmed by Rosenberg et al.[126] working with cultured human diploid fibroblasts. In this system, TC II mediated uptake of CN-Cbl was concentrative, sulfhydryl dependent, and saturable. These findings, coupled with the observations that TC II disappeared from plasma as TC II-Cbl was absorbed,[161] have generated the notion that TC II mediates rapid cobalamin uptake by cells throughout the body and that this TC II mediated uptake process has two phases: first, adsorption of TC II–Cbl to a surface recognition site on the cell membrane and, second, intracellular entry of the TC II–Cbl complex by an endocytotic process.

Once in tissue cells, cobalamin is converted to its coenzyme forms by a series of enzymatic reactions which were examined first in microbial systems.[165,166] As shown in Fig. 4, hydroxocobalamin (OH-

Cbl) is the precursor vitamin and exists with its cobalt atom oxidized to a trivalent state (Co^{3+}). OH-Cbl is reduced successively to Cbl II (Co^{2+}) and Cbl I (Co^+) by reductase enzymes, which are flavoproteins requiring NAD as a cofactor. Cbl I is then converted enzymatically to Ado-Cbl by a third enzyme called ATP:Cbl I 5'-deoxyadenosyltransferase. The precise chemical reactions involved in Me-Cbl synthesis have not been defined but are presumed to follow those shown for Ado-Cbl during the reductase steps.

Evidence is accumulating which indicates that mammalian cell metabolism of cobalamin may proceed by a similar set of reactions. In 1964, Pawalkiewicz et al.[112] showed that human liver and kidney homogenates could convert CN-Cbl to Ado-Cbl. Several years later, Ado-Cbl synthesis from OH-Cbl was observed in HeLa cell extracts incubated with ATP and a powerful reducing system which bypassed the enzymatic reduction of OH-Cbl to Cbl II.[76] Subsequently, Mahoney and Rosenberg[91] demonstrated the synthesis of both Ado-Cbl and Me-Cbl by intact human skin fibroblasts growing in a tissue culture medium containing [57]Co-OH-Cbl and have characterized this system in cell extracts. As with the HeLa cell system, chemical reductants were employed to carry out the first reduction of OH-Cbl. In this system, fibroblast extracts synthesized Ado-Cbl, leading to the conclusion that the second reductase and the adenosylating enzymes found in bacteria (Fig. 4) also exist in these normal human cells.[89]

Since methylmalonyl-CoA mutase, the apoenzyme which requires Ado-Cbl for activity, is thought to be a mitochondrial protein,[55] whereas the methyltransferase apoenzyme appears to be cytoplasmic,[168] it is obvious that complete understanding of intracellular cobalamin metabolism must also include knowledge of the subcellular transport and órganellar localization of the vitamin and its coenzyme forms. Based on timed cell fractionation studies after intravenous administration of free [57]Co-CN-Cbl, two groups[106,114,115] have proposed that cobalamin bound to TC II enters cells by a series of steps which include adsorption to membrane receptors, endocytosis of intact TC II-Cbl, formation of a secondary lysosomal vacuole in which the Cbl is split from TC II, and entry of Cbl into the mitochondrion (Fig. 5). There is limited information which relates this anatomical model to its chemical counterpart shown in Fig. 4. The data of Mahoney et al.[89] suggest that the second cobalamin reductase and the adenosylating enzyme are mitochondrial proteins, but the first reductase has not been

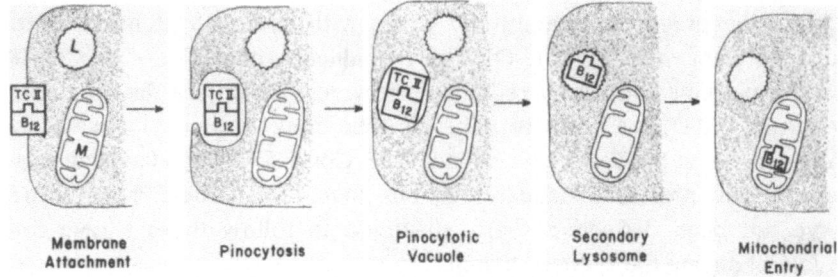

Membrane
Attachment

Pinocytosis

Pinocytotic
Vacuole

Secondary
Lysosome

Mitochondrial
Entry

Fig. 5. Proposed subcellular localization of cobalamin (B_{12}) in mammalian cells. The vitamin, bound to transcobalamin II (TC II), binds to the cell membrane and then enters the cytoplasm via a pinocytotic process. TC II is split off in lysosomes (L), presumably by a hydrolytic enzyme, and the B_{12} then enters the mitochondrion (M). Subcellular localization of the first cobalamin reductase shown in Fig. 4 has not been accomplished, but the second reductase and the deoxyadenosyltransferase are very likely mitochondrial enzymes, as is methylmalonyl-CoA mutase. The methyltransferase, however, is probably cytoplasmic. This scheme is based on reports from several laboratories.[89,106,114,115]

localized. If the sequences shown in Figs. 4 and 5 are correct, however, it is likely that intracellular cobalamin metabolism is controlled by proteins which modulate its intracellular transport as well as by the specific enzymes which catalyze its chemical modification.

Acquired B_{12} Deficiency and Inherited Defects of B_{12} Metabolism

Regardless of etiology, acquired deficiency of vitamin B_{12} leads to a characteristic set of clinical and chemical abnormalities which include megaloblastic changes in bone marrow cells and elsewhere, macrocytic anemia, spinocerebellar neurological dysfunction, reduced content of B_{12} in serum and tissues, and increased excretion of methylmalonate and homocystine. All of these pathological findings disappear rapidly when tissue B_{12} stores are returned to normal by treatment with physiological amounts of B_{12} (1–5 µg/day). Thus we may conclude that the reversible methylmalonicaciduria and homocystinuria seen in B_{12}-deficient patients reflect acquired metabolic blocks due to reduced activity of the B_{12}-dependent mutase and methyltransferase enzymes shown in Fig. 4. The hematological and neurological abnormalities are assumed to be secondary manifestations of these biochemical dysfunctions, although, as will become evident, such chemical–clinical correlations are far from clear. As noted in Table V, each of the clinical and chemical

TABLE V. Inborn Errors of Vitamin B_{12} Metabolism[a]

Phase of metabolism affected	Nature of defect	Manifestation of defect				
		Serum B_{12} concentration	Megaloblastic anemia	Methylmalonic-aciduria	Homo-cystinuria	Quantitative B_{12} requirement *in vivo*
Intestinal absorption	IF deficiency	Low	Yes	Yes	Yes	Normal
	Inactive IF	Low	Yes	NR	NR	Normal
	Defective ileal transport	Low	Yes	NR	NR	Normal
Plasma transport	TC I deficiency	Low	No	NR	NR	Normal
	TC II deficiency	Normal	Yes	No	No	Increased
Tissue utilization	Defective Ado-Cbl synthesis (*cbl A* and *cbl B*)[b]	Normal	No	Yes	No	Increased
	Defective Ado-Cbl and Me-Cbl synthesis (*cbl C*)[b]	Normal	Variable	Yes	Yes	Increased

[a] Abbreviations: IF, gastric intrinsic factor; TC, plasma transcobalamin; Ado-Cbl, 5'-deoxyadenosylcobalamin; Me-Cbl, methylcobalamin; NR, not reported.

[b] *cbl A, B, C* designate discrete mutations which are defined further in the text and in Table VI.

abnormalities seen in B_{12}-deficient patients has now been reported in individuals with inherited disorders of vitamin B_{12} metabolism, but the specific combination of observed pathological findings and their responsiveness to replacement therapy with B_{12} have differed dramatically depending on which phase of B_{12} metabolism is altered: intestinal absorption, plasma transport, or tissue utilization. Eight different human mutations have been identified—three of intestinal absorption, two of plasma transport, and three of tissue utilization.

Defective Intestinal Absorption

Three distinct inherited disorders lead to a syndrome which has been called "juvenile pernicious anemia." Each has occurred in both male and female sibs, suggesting autosomal recessive inheritance. Children with this syndrome demonstrate megaloblastic anemia and reduced serum B_{12} concentrations early in life. No measurements of methylmalonate or homocystine excretion have been reported. Such children all respond dramatically to physiological amounts of B_{12} administered parenterally but not orally. Detailed studies of gastric intrinsic factor (IF), B_{12} binding to IF, and ileal absorption of IF-B_{12} have been responsible for separating this syndrome into three distinct entities. In one, no chemically or immunologically identifiable IF is synthesized.[96,152] In the second, an altered IF is produced which retains normal immunochemical activity and the ability to bind B_{12} but which has a much reduced affinity for the ileal receptor site which binds IF-B_{12}.[74,75] In both of these disorders, patients absorb B_{12} bound to normal IF normally. The third disorder is caused by an as yet undefined lesion in the ileal transport system for B_{12}.[45] In this condition, B_{12} bound to the patient's IF or to exogenous IF is absorbed poorly, thereby distinguishing it from the other causes of "juvenile pernicious anemia." Regardless of specific etiology, each of these disorders is an excellent example of a vitamin-responsive condition in which the route, not the amount, of specific vitamin administration must be altered.

Defective Plasma Transport

Infantile megaloblastic anemia was also the presenting finding in two sisters with an almost complete deficiency of the plasma B_{12}

binding protein, TC II.[52] These sisters presented at 3 and 5 weeks of age, respectively, with failure to gain weight and infections in addition to their severe anemia, leukopenia, and thrombocytopenia. Serum B_{12} content was normal. Hematological remission and growth restoration followed parenteral B_{12} administration, but in this instance only after treatment with 500 μg of B_{12} every second day and only as long as these huge doses of B_{12} were continued. When vitamin supplements were stopped for 6 weeks, hematological relapse occurred but no methylmalonicaciduria or homocystinuria was noted.[133] Since intestinal absorption of IF-B_{12} was also markedly impaired in these children, their findings provide dramatic confirmation of the thesis that TC II is required for the transport of newly absorbed B_{12} and for uptake of B_{12} by body cells. Presumably, the patients' cobalamin requirements can be met only by maintaining serum cobalamin content at such elevated values that uptake by cells occurs via passive diffusion or some other alternate means unrelated to TC II. If, as is widely held, the megaloblastic anemia of B_{12} deficiency is caused by a primary disturbance of methyltetrahydrofolate homocysteine methyltransferase activity, it is curious that megaloblastic anemia in these patients with TC II deficiency occurred without homocystinuria or hypomethioninemia. Although transferase activity was not measured in cells directly, the findings suggest that megaloblastic changes preceded prominent reduction in holomethyltransferase stores. This paradox bears additional scrutiny.

In contrast to these prominent effects of TC II deficiency are the results in a family with reduced TC I content. Carmel and Herbert[16] described two brothers with much reduced serum B_{12} concentrations who were otherwise well. Plasma TC I values in both brothers were about 35% of the control mean, and TC II concentrations were unremarkable. Thus TC I deficiency of moderate severity can lower serum B_{12} content significantly without causing any demonstrable hematopoietic disturbance. Whether total TC I deficiency would be equally innocuous is entirely speculative.

Defective Tissue Utilization: The Methylmalonicacidurias

At least three other mutations lead to B_{12}-responsive disorders (Table V), not because B_{12} absorption or transport is impaired but

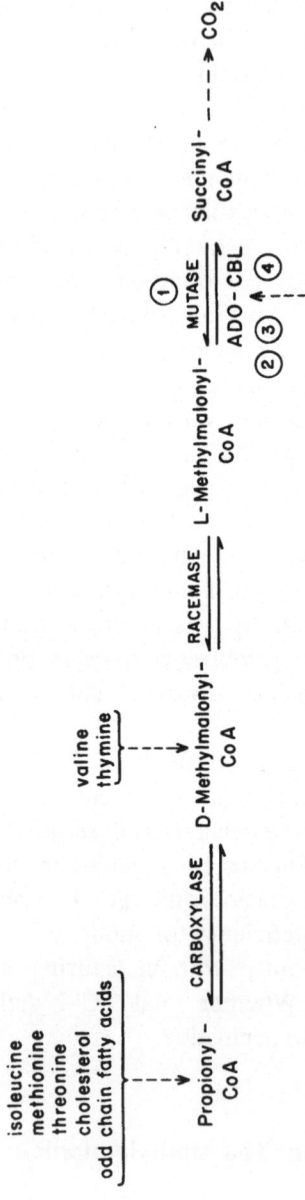

Fig. 6. Pathway of methylmalonyl-CoA formation and utilization. Its precursor, propionyl-CoA, derives from the several sources shown. Its products, succinyl-CoA, has numerous metabolic fates of importance. The encircled numbers surrounding the mutase reaction depict the four known inherited defects leading to methylmalonicaciduria: ① of the mutase apoenzyme, ② and ③ of 5'-deoxyadenosylcobalamin (ADO-CBL) synthesis only, and ④ of synthesis of both cobalamin coenzymes. See text for details.

because coenzyme synthesis in tissue cells is blocked. The phenotype in these conditions differs markedly from that of the disorders of B_{12} metabolism discussed above and focuses on the enzymatic isomerization of L-methylmalonyl-CoA to succinyl-CoA by the Ado-Cbl dependent enzyme methylmalonyl-CoA mutase. As mentioned earlier, methylmalonicaciduria due to reversible impairment of this enzyme activity had been demonstrated in acquired B_{12} deficiency in 1962, and this chemical abnormality was proposed as an early diagnostic test for pernicious anemia.[24] In 1967, Oberholzer et al.[109] and Stokke et al.[154] described critically ill infants with profound metabolic acidosis and developmental retardation who accumulated huge amounts of methylmalonate in blood and urine. These children had none of the other hematological or neurological stigmata of B_{12} deficiency and failed to respond to B_{12} supplements. They were presumed to have a congenital defect of the mutase apoenzyme or of the preceding racemase which catalyzes the conversion of D-methylmalonyl-CoA to L-methylmalonyl-CoA (Fig. 6). Although direct support for this thesis was to come somewhat later,[73,97] these descriptions focused attention on the metabolic significance of the propionate pathway which leads from propionate to succinate via methylmalonate. Although it was known that several amino acids, odd chain fatty acids, the side chain of cholesterol, and thymine all fed their carbon skeletons into the citric acid cycle via propionate and methylmalonate, the significance of this pathway to human health had not been appreciated until these critically ill infants with inherited blocks in it were identified.

Rosenberg et al.[127] and Lindblad et al.[84] described similar children with acidosis and methylmalonicaciduria who responded to pharmacological (1000 μg/day) but not physiological (1 μg/day) or even supraphysiological (200 μg/day) doses of B_{12} with a marked fall in methylmalonate excretion (Fig. 7) and clinical improvement, this response being noted only as long as the B_{12} supplements were continued.[65] Leukocytes and cultured fibroblasts from the boy reported by Rosenberg et al. failed to oxidize ^{14}C-propionate or ^{14}C-methylmalonate to $^{14}CO_2$, thus demonstrating a block in methylmalonate metabolism and providing a convenient tissue source for additional biochemical investigation.[128] Fibroblasts from this boy contained less than 10% of normal Ado-Cbl content, suggesting a defect in Ado-Cbl synthesis from precursor vitamin. His fibroblasts, too, were B_{12} responsive (Fig. 7) in that addition of very large amounts of OH-Cbl to the culture medium

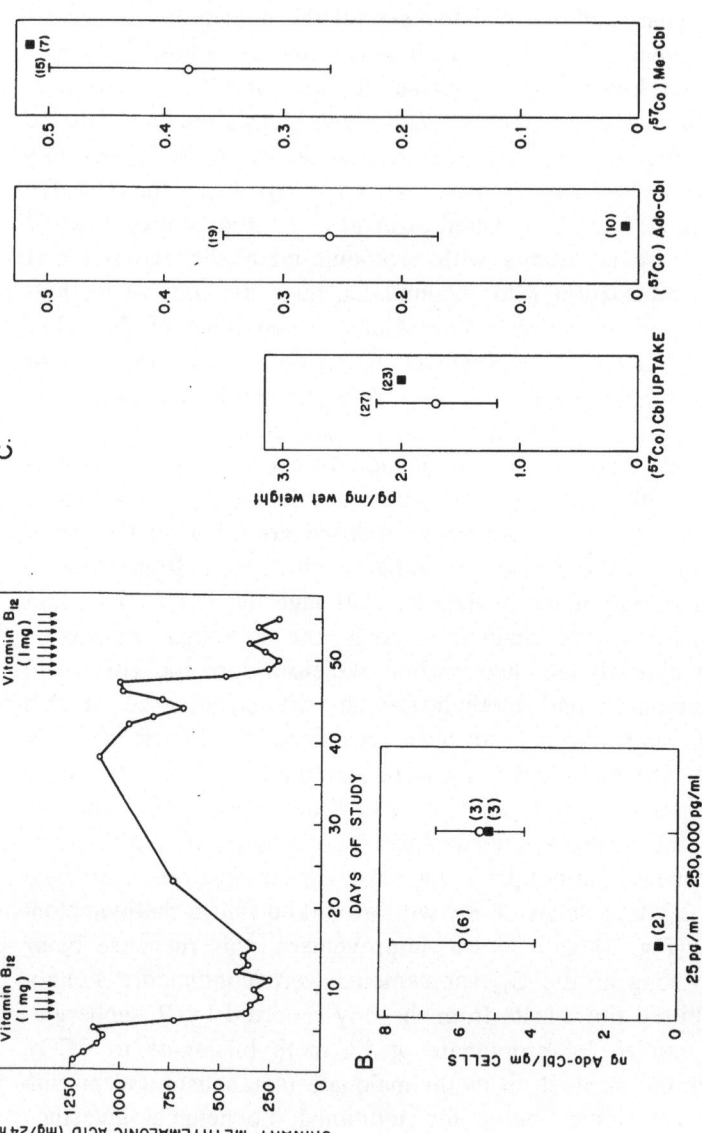

Fig. 7. The trail of evidence in the first boy reported with B₁₂-responsive methylmalonicaciduria. A: Fall in urinary methylmalonate excretion upon intramuscular administration of 1 mg CN-Cbl daily. Treatment with smaller quantities of CN-Cbl (50–250 μg daily) produced no fall in methylmalonate excretion. B: Reduced content of 5'-deoxyadenosylcobalamin (Ado-Cbl) in his cultured skin fibroblasts (■) compared to controls (o) when propagated in medium containing 25 pg/ml of B₁₂, and restoration of normal Ado-Cbl content in cells grown in medium containing 10,000 times as much B₁₂ (250,000 pg/ml). C: Defective accumulation of ⁵⁷Co-Ado-Cbl by his intact fibroblasts (■) grown in medium containing ⁵⁷Co-OH-Cbl. Note that uptake of ⁵⁷Co-Cbl and conversion to ⁵⁷Co-Me-Cbl are in normal range (o). Figures taken from reports of Rosenberg et al.[128,129] and Mahoney et al.[93] with permission of the authors and publishers.

restored propionate oxidation toward normal and raised Ado-Cbl content to the normal range.[129]

In 1969, still another variant of congenital methylmalonicaciduria was described by Mudd et al.[101] They reported a male infant with developmental arrest and methylmalonicaciduria who, unlike any of the preceding cases, had homocystinuria and reduced plasma methionine concentrations as well. His liver contained only a tiny fraction of the Ado-Cbl content found in normal liver and his fibroblasts revealed a B_{12}-responsive defect in propionate oxidation. This constellation suggested a block in both B_{12} dependent reactions due to an abnormality in the synthesis of both B_{12} coenzymes.[103] Two male sibs with these same biochemical abnormalities were described subsequently by Goodman et al.[44]

Subsequent collaborative studies reported by Mahoney et al.[89,93] have been conducted with cultured fibroblasts from these and more than ten other patients with the several variants of inherited methylmalonicaciduria. These studies, which have included analysis of propionate oxidation, cobalamin metabolism, and mutase holoenzyme activity in whole fibroblasts or cell free-extracts thereof, have led to the identification of four distinct phenotypes enumerated in Fig. 6 and

TABLE VI. Contrasting Features of Mutase Apoenzyme and Cobalamin Mutants in Cultured Fibroblasts

Tissue preparation	Parameter	Mutant[a]			
		Mutase apoenzyme	cbl A	cbl B	cbl C
Whole cells	Propionate oxidation[b]	−	−	−	−
	Ado-Cbl accumulation[c]	+	−	−	−
	Me-Cbl accumulation[c]	+	+	+	−
Cell-free extracts	Mutase activity[d]	−	+	+	+
	Ado-Cbl synthesis[e]	+	+	−	+

[a] Symbols: +, normal phenotype; −, abnormal phenotype.
[b] Evolution of $^{14}CO_2$ from ^{14}C-propionate. See Rosenberg et al.[128]
[c] Conversion of ^{57}Co-OH-Cbl to ^{57}Co-coenzymes. See Mahoney et al.[93]
[d] Isomerization of ^3H-methylmalonyl-CoA to ^3H-succinyl-CoA with added Ado-Cbl (10^{-5} M). See Rosenberg et al.[129]
[e] Conversion of ^{57}Co-OH-Cbl to ^{57}Co-Ado-Cbl under anaerobic conditions in presence of dithiothreitol, FAD, Mg^{2+}, and ATP. See Mahoney et al.[89]

summarized in Table VI. Each mutant shows impaired propionate (and presumably methylmalonate) oxidation but differs in one or more of the other parameters measured. The first, representative of the patients with B_{12}-unresponsive methylmalonicaciduria, converts OH-Cbl to Ado-Cbl and Me-Cbl normally, but has minimal holomutase activity in cell extracts. These cells have a primary defect in their mutase apoenzyme. The second and third phenotypes, typical of patients with B_{12}-responsive methylmalonicaciduria, are unable to convert OH-Cbl to Ado-Cbl in whole cells while making Me-Cbl normally (Fig. 7). Their holomutase activity in cell-free extracts is normal. They are distinguished from one another by assays of Ado-Cbl synthesis in cell-free extracts. That class of mutant (designated *cbl B*) in which Ado-Cbl formation is blocked in both intact and broken cells is presumed to have a defect either in the second cobalamin reductase or in the adenosyltransferase enzyme noted in Fig. 4. In contrast, that class which is unable to synthesize Ado-Cbl in whole cells but which can synthesize this coenzyme normally in cell-free extracts (*cbl A*) very likely has an abnormality of the first cobalamin reductase or of some as yet undefined intracellular transport step required for Ado-Cbl synthesis. The fourth mutant phenotype (designated *cbl C*), representative of patients with both methylmalonicaciduria and disordered sulfur amino acid metabolism, has the following hallmarks: defective accumulation of both Ado-Cbl and Me-Cbl in whole fibroblasts, normal Ado-Cbl synthesis in cell extracts, and normal holomutase activity in cell extracts. These cells have no defect in initial TC II–B_{12} uptake,[126] thereby focusing attention on some other early step in cobalamin metabolism common to the synthesis of both coenzymes. Such steps may include lysosomal accumulation of TC II–B_{12}, hydrolysis of the TC II–B_{12} complex, or attachment of B_{12} to an intracellular binding protein. Preliminary experiments from our laboratory, in fact, suggest that these cells functionally lack a high molecular weight protein which normally binds B_{12} sometime after the vitamin has entered the cell.[131]

Experiments currently in progress in our laboratory provide genetic evidence in support of the existence of these four biochemically distinct phenotypes. Using an autoradiographic assay which measures ^{14}C-propionate incorporation into TCA-precipitable material in intact fibroblasts *in situ*,[56] Gravel *et al.*[46] have examined 12 mutant cell lines and have shown that each of the four mutant phenotypes described above incorporates negligible amounts of radioactivity when compared to control cells. Activity is likewise negligible when the different mutants are mixed without Sendai virus or when homokaryons are produced by self-fusion. Heterokaryons produced by fusing members of each of the four mutant classes with representations of any other class recover the ability to incorporate ^{14}C-propionate to levels comparable to those in control lines. Heterokaryons produced between members of the same class, however, fail to complement in all cases.

In conclusion, there now exists both biochemical and genetic evidence for at least three distinct complementation groups identified by mutations of B_{12} metabolism which impair coenzyme synthesis primarily and holoenzyme activity secondarily. Although the molecular basis of none of these mutations is known, it is clear that patients with each of them require far more than physiological amounts of B_{12} if they are to synthesize sufficient quantities of B_{12} coenzymes for normal growth or, in some cases, for prolonged viability.

Folic Acid

Clinicians have often considered cobalamin and folic acid in tandem because megaloblastic anemia is the hallmark of deficiency of both vitamins. These two vitamins have other prominent similarities pertinent to this discussion: both have complex systems of intestinal absorption and coenzyme synthesis and both demonstrate a panorama of vitamin-responsive mutations in these transport and synthetic processes.

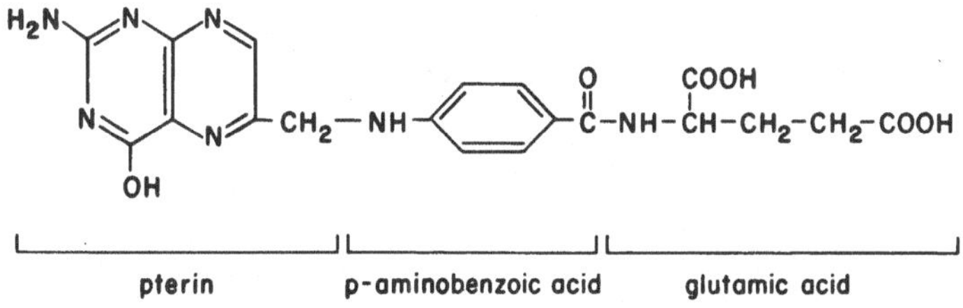

Fig. 8. Chemical structure of folic acid (pteroylglutamic acid). The molecule is composed of a pterin ring, p-aminobenzoic acid, and glutamic acid. The most common form of folate in foods is the polyglutamate, in which several additional glutamate residues are joined to the parent glutamate in γ-glutamyl linkage. The active folate coenzymes are formed by enzymatic reduction of the nitrogen atoms in the pterin ring.

Like cobalamin, folic acid has a complex chemical structure (Fig. 8). It is composed of three moieties: a pterin ring, p-aminobenzoic acid, and glutamic acid. Humans require about 50 μg of folate daily and can satisfy this requirement by ingesting a large number of vegetables, fruits, and meats rich in folic acid. There are no fewer than five coenzyme forms of folate, all of which participate in the transfer of one-carbon units vital for the synthesis of DNA, RNA, methionine, glutamate, and serine.

Absorption and Coenzyme Synthesis

The principle dietary form of folate is not the monoglutamate form shown in Fig. 8 but rather folic acid polyglutamate, in which one to six glutamic acid residues are linked to the parent molecule by γ-peptide formation. The polyglutamyl form of folate cannot be absorbed intact but must be converted in the intestinal tract to its monoglutamate form.[11] This conversion is catalyzed by a conjugase enzyme found in intestinal mucosa, stomach, and pancreas. Once folic acid monoglutamate is formed, it is absorbed by active transport processes in the duodenum and jejunum. Free folate is then carried to the tissues, where a series of complex reactions convert the inactive vitamin to its active coenzyme forms.[81] First, the pterin ring of folate must be reduced to its dihydro- and then tetrahydrofolate form (Fig. 9). Tetrahydrofolate (THF) has two principal fates. It serves as the acceptor of the β-carbon of serine when the latter is cleaved to glycine. This carbon atom forms a methylene bridge between nitrogen atoms 5 and 10 of THF to yield N^5, N^{10}-methyleneTHF, which is reduced enzymatically to N^5-methylTHF. N^5-MethylTHF then acts as the principal methyl group donor in the methyltransferase-catalyzed synthesis of methionine from homocysteine. Alternatively, THF may be converted to N^5,N^{10}-methenylTHF, the precursor of the formyl and formimino coenzyme forms of THF. These formyl and formimino coenzymes are required for several one-carbon transfer reactions principally concerned with purine and pyrimidine synthesis, histidine metabolism, and cyclic interconversion of the various folate compounds. It should be emphasized that several other coenzymes participate in these "folate cycles": pyridoxal phospate in the decar-

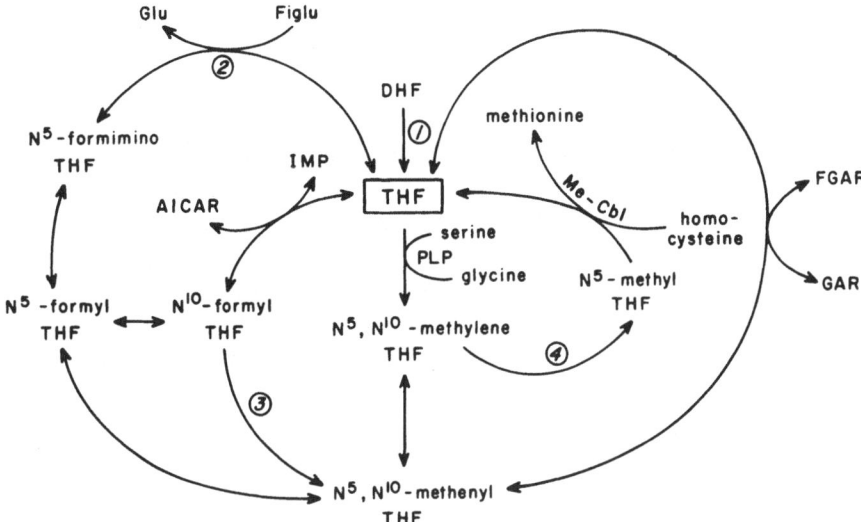

Fig. 9. Some principal interconversions of folate coenzymes. Numbered reactions refer to enzyme systems for which inherited defects have been proposed: ① dihydrofolate reductase, ② formiminotransferase, ③ cyclohydrolase, and ④ N^5,N^{10}-methylenetetrahydrofolate reductase. Abbreviations: DHF, dihydrofolate; THF, tetrahydrofolate; PLP, pyridoxal-5'-phosphate; Figlu, formiminoglutamic acid; AICAR, 5'-aminoimidazole-4-carboxamide ribonucleotide; IMP, inosinic acid; GAR, β-glycinamide ribonucleotide; FGAR, N-formylglycinamide ribonucleotide; Me-Cbl, methylcobalamin.

boxylation of serine, Me-Cbl in the methylation of homocystine to methionine, and NAD and ascorbic acid in several of the oxidation–reduction steps.

Folate Deficiency

Natural and experimental folic acid deficiency have been produced by dietary restriction and intestinal malabsorption. The cardinal manifestations of folate deficiency are reduced serum and tissue folate concentrations and hematopoietic dysfunction (megaloblastic anemia, hypersegmented polymorphonuclear leukocytes, and thrombocytopenia). Sleeplessness, irritability, and even a peripheral neuropathy or myelopathy have been reported in extreme cases. In these situations, oral or parenteral administration of physiological doses of folic acid leads to prompt correction.

Folate-Responsive Errors of Absorption and Coenzyme Synthesis

It is now apparent that several inherited defects of folate absorption or coenzyme formation may also interfere with normal folate utilization (Table VII). Luhby et al.[87] described mentally retarded siblings with a relapsing form of megaloblastic anemia beginning in infancy. Folic acid absorption was impaired, but no other evidence of intestinal malabsorption was apparent. Anemia was corrected by oral administration of 10 mg of folate daily, more than 100 times the normal requirement. In 1970, Lanzkowsky et al.[80] described another girl with megaloblastic anemia, mental retardation, and severe neurological dysfunction dating to the first months of life. She also had selective folate malabsorption. Oral administration of $250\mu g$ of folic acid was of no therapeutic value, but this same dose given intramuscularly produced prompt but transient hematological remission. Folate absorption was not enhanced by the oral administration of normal duodenal mucosa, lyophilized jejunum, or lyophilized pancreas. The specific nature of the mutation remains obscure.

The first enzymatic defect in folate coenzyme synthesis was described in 1963 by Arakawa et al.[5] Between 1963 and 1968, they reported four children, including two sibs, with physical and mental retardation, cerebral cortical atrophy, and abnormal electroencephalograms whose urinary excretion of formiminoglutamic acid (Figlu) after a histidine load was markedly increased despite higher than normal serum folate values. No consistent hematological abnormalities were noted, but one of these children had a megaloblastic anemia which responded, in part, to folate supplements. Hepatic assays of folate cycle enzymes revealed selective reduction in formiminotransferase activity (see Fig. 9). Subsequently, this group of investigators[3,4] reported single children with marked central nervous system dysfunction and hyperfolicacidemia who had different, seemingly specific deficiencies in two other enzymatic activities involving folate coenzyme utilization: N^5-methylTHF-homocysteine methyltransferase and cyclohydrolase (required for converting N^5,N^{10}-methanylTHF to N^{10}-formylTHF). These reports contain no mention of attempted treatment with large amounts of folate. Confirmation of these observations in other laboratories has, thus far, not been reported.

In 1967, Walters[167] described an infant with megaloblastic anemia and a normal serum folate content who responded hematologically to

TABLE VII. Inborn Errors of Folic Acid Metabolism

Phase of metabolism affected	Nature of defect	Serum folate concentration	Manifestation of defect			Quantitative folate requirement *in vivo*
			Megaloblastic anemia	CNS dysfunction[a]		
Intestinal absorption	Undefined	Low	Yes	Yes		Normal
Tissue utilization	Formininotransferase deficiency	High	No	Yes		Increased
	Cyclohydrolase deficiency	High	No	Yes		NR[b]
	Dihydrofolate reductase deficiency	Normal	Yes	No		Increased
	N^5,N^{10}- Methylenetetrahydrofolate reductase deficiency	Low-normal	No	Yes		Increased

[a] Includes mental retardation, psychotic behavior, seizures, EEG abnormalities, cerebral cortical atrophy.
[b] Not reported.

parenteral administration of 100 μg of N^5-formylTHF but not to the same dose of folic acid. Hepatic enzyme assays showed a distinct reduction in dihydrofolate reductase activity compared to that in control liver.

Finally, three teenage children have been described with a folate-responsive form of homocystinuria. Two of these patients were sibs—a 15-year-old black girl with catatonic schizophrenia and mental retardation and her mildly retarded but nonpsychotic younger sister.[35] The third was a boy, age 16, who presented with muscle weakness, seizures, and an abnormal EEG.[144] None of these patients had anemia or excess methylmalonate in their urine. All had normal activity of cystathionine synthase and N^5-methylTHF-homocysteine methyltransferase in extracts of cultured fibroblasts. Their cells, however, were markedly deficient in N^5,N^{10}-methyleneTHF reductase activity, the enzyme which converts N^5,N^{10}-methyleneTHF to N^5-methylTHF.[102] Each of these children has been treated with more than 10 mg of folic acid daily, with prompt reduction in homocystine excretion. Significantly, folate therapy was also associated with marked behavioral improvement in the psychotic girl mentioned above, with relapse occurring after folate supplements were discontinued. Presumably the homocystinuria in these patients results from reduced N^5-methylTHF-homocysteine methyltransferase activity secondary to impaired synthesis of N^5-methylTHF.

Thus, although the number of affected patients is too small to be conclusive, it appears that five different mutations of folate transport and coenzyme synthesis may have been identified: one involving intestinal absorption and four concerned with coenzyme formation and interconversion. It is noteworthy that most of these patients, regardless of the site of the defect, have suffered major central nervous system dysfunction. No other reproducible clinical findings have emerged thus far, nor have any of these patients been treated early enough to determine if their CNS disease could be prevented by appropriate folate supplements.

Calciferol (Vitamin D)

As of this writing, only one fat-soluble vitamin, vitamin D, can be included in this discussion of vitamin-responsive inherited disorders.

As pointed out earlier, the concept that some few humans require far greater amounts of a particular vitamin than do most other people can rightfully be said to have been introduced by the description of a boy with vitamin D resistant rickets in 1937.[1] Although that entity, now called X-linked hypophosphatemic rickets, has not yet yielded its etiological secret, it remains one of the important landmarks in the study of genetic control of vitamin metabolism and now stand as one of two distinct inherited disorders which respond to supraphysiological amounts of vitamin D.

Structure and Function

Vitamin D is a steroid derivative (Fig. 10). It actually consists of a group of vitamins which are formed from provitamin steroid precursors by the opening of the "b" ring. Vitamin D_2 (ergocalciferol) is derived by ultraviolet radiation from the plant sterol ergosterol; its congener, vitamin D_3 (cholecalciferol), is formed in the liver of various fishes and in mammalian skin from 7-dehydrocholesterol. In the presence of adequate sunlight, no vitamin D is required in the diet since adequate amounts of vitamin D_3 will be made in skin. Because civilized man

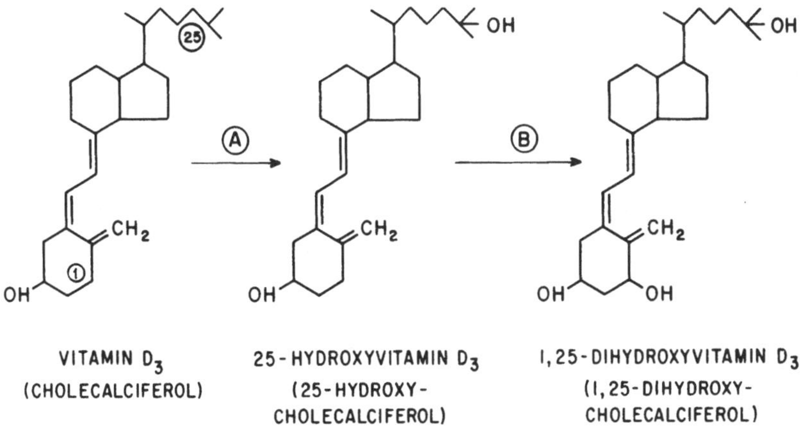

VITAMIN D_3 | 25-HYDROXYVITAMIN D_3 | 1,25-DIHYDROXYVITAMIN D_3
(CHOLECALCIFEROL) | (25-HYDROXY-CHOLECALCIFEROL) | (1,25-DIHYDROXY-CHOLECALCIFEROL)

Fig. 10. Steps in enzymatic conversion of vitamin D_3 (cholecalciferol) to active calcium-mobilizing "hormone," 1,25-dihydroxycholecalciferol. Reaction Ⓐ is catalyzed by cholecalciferol-25-hydroxylase found in liver; reaction Ⓑ is catalyzed by 25-hydroxycholecalciferol-1-hydroxylase found in kidney. The active "hormone" then acts on gut and bone.

effectively shields himself from sunlight, however, the vitamin must usually be provided exogenously, its recommended daily allowance being about 400 International Units (10 μg cholecalciferol).

The classic effect of vitamin D is to bring about calcification of bone. This it accomplishes by supplying calcium and phosphate to the calcification sites in the skeleton. Two major mechanisms appear to act in concert in explaining this effect of vitamin D on skeletal calcification. The first involves stimulation of intestinal absorption of calcium and phosphorus, the second mobilization of calcium from previously formed bone to blood. In these ways (and perhaps by acting on renal tubular reabsorption of calcium and phosphate), vitamin D elevates plasma calcium and phosphate to concentrations needed for normal mineralization. Parathyroid hormone normally acts in concert with vitamin D, but the details of this orchestration are beyond the scope of this article (see Potts and Deftos[116]).

Absorption and Activation

During the past decade, increases in our knowledge of vitamin D metabolism have been enormous.[25] The fundamental theme of this inquiry is, however, familiar—that the ingested vitamin is metabolically inert and must undergo chemical modification before assuming its biological role. Like so many other lipid-soluble compounds, vitamin D is absorbed from the jejunum and ileum into the intestinal lymphatics by processes facilitated by bile salts. In the lymph and blood it circulates bound primarily to α_2-globulins, with smaller amounts carried by albumin and α_1-globulin. Circulating vitamin D is rapidly taken up by the liver, where the first of its chemical modifications takes place. DeLuca and his colleagues[13,64] demonstrated that a microsomal hydroxylating enzyme exists in hepatocytes which converts cholecalciferol to 25-hydroxycholecalciferol (Fig. 10). This compound, more polar than the parent vitamin, may have some biological activity but it is not the final active principle. 25-Hydroxycholecalciferol leaves the liver, again bound to α_2-globulin, and is carried to the kidney, where a second hydroxylating enzyme adds an additional hydroxyl group at the 1-position, yielding 1, 25-dihydroxycholecalciferol.[26] It is now believed that this compound, formed by two sequential hydroxylations in two different organs, then circulates to gut and skeleton, where it enhances calcium absorption and mobilization, respectively.

Acquired and Inherited Rickets

The skeletal disorder known as rickets was described in the seventeenth century, long before any appreciation of the existence of vitamin D or its effect on bone mineral metabolism.[116] In the eighteenth century, cod liver oil was being prescribed for rachitic patients, but 200 years were to elapse before it was learned that sunlight and fish liver oil were both acting to restore the normal tissue content of a sterol which we now recognize as vitamin D. Currently, rickets is usually acquired in civilized humans who shield thenselves from sunlight and who ingest insufficient vitamin D to meet the body's needs. In this setting, blood calcium and phosphorus fall and skeletal calcification is impaired, leading to the typical radiological findings of rickets in children or ostomalacia in adults. This disorder responds promptly to small amounts of vitamin D.

We now recognize two inherited disorders in which the typical radiological appearance of rickets or osteomalacia occurs but does not respond to physiological vitamin D replacement. The first has had many names since its original description by Albright (vitamin D resistant rickets, vitamin D refractory rickets) but is now called X-linked hypophosphatemic rickets (XHR) or familial hypophosphatemic rickets (FHR). A reduced serum concentration of inorganic phospate is the most constant biochemical feature of this X-linked dominant trait.[169] Hemizygous affected males exhibit hypophosphatemia and severe rickets; heterozygous females tend to have a higher serum phosphate concentration and less severe bone disease. Hyperphosphaturia and reduced intestinal absorption of calcium and phosphate complete the chemical picture.

Two conflicting theories of pathogenesis have evolved. One view holds that a primary defect in endogenous conversion of vitamin D to its active metabolite(s) is responsible for intestinal malabsorption of calcium. This in turn leads to secondary hyperparathyroidism, resulting in decreased renal tubular reabsorption of phospate, hypophospha-temia, and rickets. The following recent evidence has tended to weaken this argument: serum concentration of 25-hydroxycholecalci-ferol in patients with FHR is normal[50]; serum parathyroid hormone concentrations have been variable reported as normal, reduced, and modestly elevated[6,82,122]; and treatment with physiological doses of 1, 25-dihydroxycholecalciferol produces unimpressive results.[14] The alternate view proposes a primary membrane transport defect for inorganic phosphate in the proximal renal tubule and intestine which results secondarily in calcium malabsorption and renal phosphate diabetes.[41, 145]

Despite this lack of consensus concerning etiology, there is widespread agreement that the bone disease in FHR can be treated effectively with huge doses of vitamin D (more than 1000 times the physiological requirement), large amounts of inorganic phosphate by mouth, or a combination thereof. Depending on which pathogenetic mechanism is confirmed, vitamin D responsiveness can be thought of either as pharmacological therapy for a primary phosphate transport defect or a massive substrate loading for a partial, but severe, abnormality in synthesis of the active hormone from the parent vitamin.

The second vitamin D responsive condition appears to be less common and less complicated than FHR. It has been called "vitamin D dependent rickets" or "hereditary pseudo vitamin D deficiency rickets," respectively, by the two groups which described the entity originally.[34,117] Despite intakes of vitamin D that would ordinarily prevent rickets, affected patients have all of the clinical and biochemical features of advanced deficiency of vitamin D: hypocalcemia, hypophosphatemia, secondary hyperparathyroidism, and severe rachitic bone lesions. Treatment with 100 times the usual daily requirement of vitamin D corrects the features of this condition, which affects males and females equally and appears to be inherited as an autosomal recessive trait. Fraser et al.[33] have reported recently an impressive study which indicates that this vitamin D dependent disorder is due to a block in the conversion of 25-hydroxycholecalciferol to 1, 25-dihydroxycholecalciferol (Fig. 10). They showed that massive doses of ergocalciferol, cholecalciferol, or 25-hydroxycholecalciferol were required to heal the rachitic lesions whereas physiological doses of 1, 25-dihydroxycholecalciferol promptly initiated healing. These results, although as yet unsupported by in vitro observations, suggest a defect in the renal hydroxylating enzyme which catalyzes the final conversion of 25-hydroxycholecalciferol to its dihydroxy form. This postulate would place vitamin D dependent rickets in precisely the same category of illness as noted earlier for certain cobalamin- and folate-responsive conditions—namely one in which a specific block in vitamin activation leads to failed synthesis of coenzyme or, in the case of vitamin D, of active hormone.

DEFECTS OF COENZYME-DEPENDENT APOENZYMES

In the preceding pages, I have discussed those processes, normal and abnormal, which regulate vitamin transport and coenzyme synthesis. But these processes only prepare the vitamin or coenzyme for its definitive cellular role. That role for all of the water-soluble vitamins is to act as a cofactor for one, several, or a large number of apoenzyme proteins. Such apoenzyme–coenzyme interaction depends, of course, not only on the availability of coenzyme but also on the quality and quantity of the apoenzyme. It follows that mutations which alter apoenzyme structure or content might interfere with such apoenzyme–coenzyme interaction and thereby reduce holoenzyme activity. Depending on the precise molecular pathology of such apoenzyme mutations, holoenzyme function may be altered considerably, little, or not at all by increasing the supply of the coenzyme. A growing list of inherited enzymopathies responsive to supraphysiological amounts of pyridoxine, biotin, or thiamine argues for such coenzyme-enhanced holoenzyme activity. I shall concentrate on the pyridoxine-responsive disorders because they were the first such apoenzyme mutations described and because they have been most thoroughly investigated to date.

Pyridoxine (Vitamin B$_6$)

Pyridoxine was discovered in 1934 by Gyorgy[49] during his exhaustive studies of the nutritional effects of B complex vitamins in rats. The vitamin is widely distributed, being found in abundance in yeast, seeds, grains, egg yolk, muscle meats, and liver. Human requirements vary with protein intake and age: infants needing up to 0.5 mg per day, adults requiring approximately 1–2 mg daily. The biochemistry and metabolism of vitamin B$_6$ have been studied extensively by Snell[150,151] and many others.

Activation, Metabolism, and Function

The vitamin is a substituted pyridine ring which occurs in several natural forms (Fig. 11). Pyridoxal, pyridoxamine, and pyridoxine have

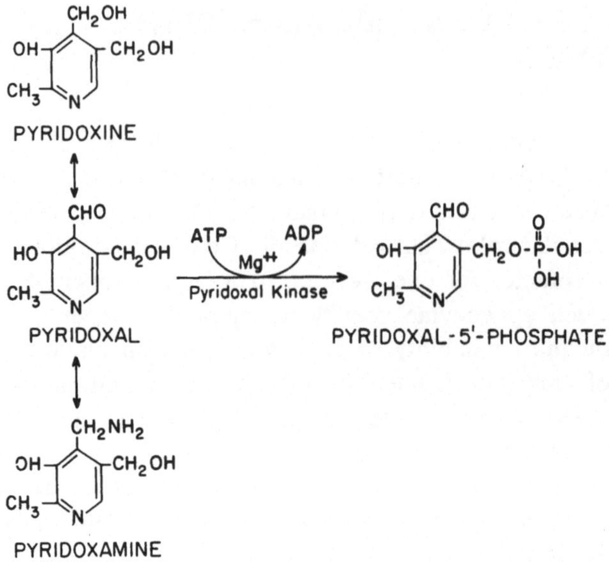

Fig. 11. Chemical structures of the B_6 vitamers (pyridoxine, pyridoxal, pyridoxamine) and coenzyme (pyridoxal-5'-phosphate). The coenzyme attaches to its apoenzymes by formation of a Schiff base between the aldehyde group of pyridoxal-5'-phosphate and an ε-amino nitrogen group of a lysine residue on the apoenzyme.

been isolated from foods and extracellular fluid, but none of these is the active coenzyme form. In the cell, these chemically interconvertible precursors are phosphorylated to pyridoxal-5'-phosphate (PLP) or pyridoxamine-5'-phosphate by a specific kinase which requires magnesium and ATP. The phosphorylated compound PLP acts as the coenzyme for a large number of different apoenzymes which regulate the catabolism of amino acids, glycogen, and short-chain fatty acids. The turnover of PLP in the cell is rapid. It is oxidized in the liver to 4-pyridoxic acid, which is then excreted in the urine. PLP functions as a coenzyme in such diverse reactions as racemization, transamination, decarboxylation, deamination, alcohol formation, α-β elimination, α-β addition, and amine oxidation. Snell and his colleagues showed that PLP reacts with amino acids under appropriate conditions to form Schiff bases which promote electron shifts and subsequent metabolic rearrangements. In fact, such Schiff base formation can take place in a protein-free chemically defined system. However, the *rate* and the *specificity* of such rearrangements have been shown to depend on the interaction between PLP and a specific apoenzyme. Presumable, a modified Schiff base is formed between the phosphate and aldehyde groups of PLP and moieties on the apoenzyme surface. In this configuration, specific holoenzyme functions are carried out. PLP has been shown to have a much greater affinity for some apoenzymes than others. Thus its affinity for transaminases far exceeds that for decarboxylases or kynureninase. These differences in affinity are reflected in the enzymatic dysfunctions seen in pyridoxine deficiency states.

Pyridoxine Deficiency

Pyridoxine deficiency is rare but has been observed in several settings in which the total tissue pool of PLP and its precursors is reduced.[135] Dietary insufficiency has been reported in infants after prolonged breast feeding by malnourished mothers, and in children and adults with inadequate general nutrition. An "epidemic" of pyridoxine deficiency was produced in 1953 by the marketing of a milk preparation unusually low in this vitamin.[94] Other causes of deficiency include gastrointestinal malabsorption and the use of drugs such as isoniazid or penicillamine, which act, respectively, by competitive inhibition of PLP kinase[164] and by the formation of a stable thiazolidine complex.[70]

The diagnosis of pyridoxine deficiency rests on the demonstration of reduced cellular or extracellular concentrations of the vitamin, its active coenzyme, or its catabolite. It is possible to measure serum and tissue concentrations of pyridoxine and PLP by microbiological or chemical means, and quantitation of urinary 4-pyridoxic acid also provides a useful measure of tissue stores.[137] Alternatively, indirect means have been used to estimate the adequacy of tissue pyridoxine content. Assay of PLP-requiring enzymes in serum or tissue has been proposed as a measure of deficiency, but the usefulness of this approach has been compromised by variability either in the affinity of specific apoenzymes for PLP or in the rate of turnover of particular apoprotein species. Until recently, an even more indirect approach has depended on the metabolic response to tryptophan loading. Pyridoxine-deficient patients excrete increased amounts of kynurenine, hydroxy-kynurenine, and xanthurenic acid because the PLP-requiring steps which catalyze the further breakdown of these tryptophan metabolites are partially blocked. We shall point out subsequently that this test can no longer be considered in any way specific for pyridoxine deficiency.

The clinical manifestations of pyridosine deficiency vary considerably with age. In infants, a potentially lethal convulsive disorder dominates the clinical scene. The precise mechanism of such cerebral dysfunction is not clear but may be related to reduced activity of glutamic acid decarboxylase, a PLP-cocatalyzed reaction which converts glutamic acid to the inhibitory neurotransmitter, γ-aminobutyric acid (GABA). A deficiency of GABA is then proposed to predispose the brain to hyperirritability and seizures. Adults with confirmed deficiency may present a vague symptom complex of lassitude, weakness, and anorexia along with an iron-resistant microcytic, hypochromic anemia. Why pyridoxine-deficient infants have such different clinical manifestations than adults has not been determined.

Pyridoxine-Responsive Inborn Errors

The six inherited disorders shown to demonstrate pyridoxine responsiveness are listed in Table VIII. None has been associated with any suggestion of pyridoxine deficiency, and all require 5–50 times the usual physiological dose of pyridoxine for biochemical and/or clinical improvement. The mutant apoenzyme responsible for these disorders has been defined with the single exception of pyridoxine-responsive anemia. However, the biochemical basis for the beneficial role of

TABLE VIII. Inherited Disorders Demonstrating Pyridoxine Responsiveness

Disorder	Biochemical hallmarks	Mutant enzyme
Infantile convulsions	None described	Glutamic acid decarboxylase (?)
Anemia	None described	Undefined
Cystathioninuria	Increased urinary cystathionine	Cystathionase
Xanthurenic aciduria	Increased urinary xanthurenic acid	Kynureninase
Homocystinuria	Increased plasma and urinary methionine and homocystine	Cystathionine synthase
Hyperoxaluria	Increased urinary oxalate and glyoxylate	Glyoxylate: α-ketoglutarate carboligase

pyridoxine has been explored in only four of the five conditions where a specific apoenzyme defect is known or suspected (infantile convulsions, cystathioninuria, xanthurenic aciduria, and homocystinuria). No studies have been reported on the mechanism by which large doses of pyridoxine lower urinary oxalate excretion in some patients with hyperoxaluria.[149]

In 1954, Hunt and his associates first described two infant sibs with seizures uncontrolled by anticonvulsants or physiological doses of B_6. These children responded dramatically to parenteral administration of 5–25 mg of pyridoxine, as have more than 40 similar patients described subsequently. Ten years later, it was proposed that this classic form of "pyridoxine dependency" was caused by a mutation in glutamate decarboxylase such that its interaction with PLP was impaired.[134] Following the demonstration that this enzyme existed in kidney tissue as well as brain,[142] a defect in renal glutamate decarboxylase was reported by Yoshida et al.[173] in a single patient with pyridoxine-responsive seizures. These workers showed that addition of large concentrations of PLP in vitro led to full correction of decarboxylase activity in the tissue of the affected patient.

Very similar results have been reported in two other pyridoxine-responsive disorders: cystathioninuria and xanthurenic aciduria. In cystathioninuria, administration of large amounts of pyridoxine leads to marked reduction in urinary excretion of cystathionine,[37] a similar response being observed for excretion of xanthurenic acid and other tryptophan metabolites in patients with xanthurenic aciduria.[159] These in vivo observations were paired with interesting data in vitro (Fig. 12). Frimpter[36] demonstrated that the liver homogenate from one patient with cystathioninuria had distinctly reduced cystathionase activity and that addition of pyridoxal phosphate to the incubation medium enhanced enzyme activity markedly. Likewise, Tada et al.[158,159] showed that the defective kynureninase activity found in liver of patients with pyridoxine-responsive xanthurenic aciduria was restored to nearly normal values with in vitro addition of saturating amounts of PLP. These results indicate that such patients synthesize a mutant apoenzyme whose interaction with coenzyme is impaired either because the apoprotein has a reduced affinity for coenzyme or because its rate of binding to coenzyme is slowed.[98] The fact that nearly full holoenzyme activity is restored by PLP in vitro, however, implies that the intracellular content of apoenzyme is not significantly less than that found in normal cells.

Other studies indicate that such full correction of holoenzyme activity is not seen in all patients with pyridoxine-responsive disorders. In two other patients with pyridoxine-responsive cystathioninuria, activity of cystathionase was increased only modestly by PLP addition.[31,36] Another disorder of sulfur amino acid metabolism has yielded similar observations. In homocystinuria due to cystathionine synthase deficiency,[100] plasma and urine concentrations of homocystine and methionine are markedly increased in association with dislocated optic lenses, osteoporosis, and a high incidence of thrombotic vascular disease and central nervous system dysfunction.[140] Barber and Spaeth[8] first reported that such patients responded to large supplements of pyridoxine with a prompt return of plasma and urine concentrations of methionine and homocystine to normal (Fig. 13). This observation has been confirmed by several groups of investigators in some, but not all,

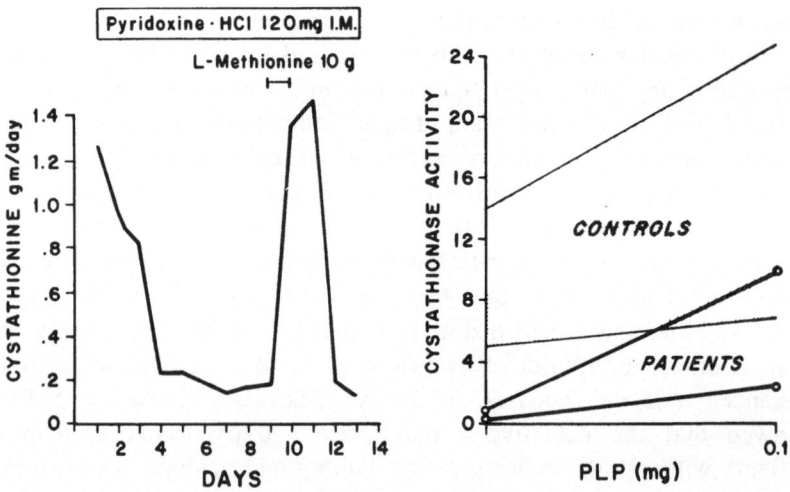

Fig. 12. Pyridoxine responsiveness in cystathioninuria due to cystathionase deficiency. The left panel shows the marked reduction in urinary cystathionine excretion which followed administration of pyridoxine hydrochloride and the transient increase in cystathionine excretion occasioned by a loading dose of Y-methionine. Redrawn from Frimpter et al.[37] with permission of the author and publisher. The right panel shows that hepatic cystathionase activity, much reduced in two patients in the absence of added pyridoxal-5'-phosphate (PLP), increased markedly when PLP was added in vitro. From Frimpter.[36]

patients with cystathionine synthase deficiency.[140] The enzymatic findings in these patients have been of particular interest. Some pyridoxine-responsive patients show very small increases in synthase activity in hepatic or cultured fibroblast extracts when saturating concentrations of PLP are added[99,143,174] while other patients seem to have no demonstrable enhancement of enzyme activity *in vitro*.[40,58] Furthermore, Uhlendorf *et al.*[163] studied fibroblast extracts from 38 patients with cystathionine synthase deficiency and reported that those with pyridoxine responsiveness *in vivo* had detectable basal levels of synthase activity *in vitro* which were not stimulated appreciably by PLP whereas pyridoxine-unresponsive patients had no demonstrable activity with or without added PLP. Based on these observations, Mudd[98] argues convincingly that a very small increase in cystathionine synthase activity (from 1% of normal without pyridoxine to 3–4% of normal with pyridoxine) may be sufficient to normalize sulfur amino acid metabolism *in vivo* to an extent compatible with the striking improvement in plasma and urine findings observed. He furthermore proposes that, as originally suggested by Rosenberg,[123] PLP may be acting to stabilize a mutant synthase apoenzyme which is otherwise labile. Additional support for such a thesis has come from the work of Kim and Rosenberg.[77] They prepared partially purified cystathionine synthase from skin fibroblasts of normals and pyridoxine-responsive homocystinuria patients and found much reduced activity in their mutant lines which was increased only modestly by PLP (Fig. 13), much reduced affinity of mutant enzyme for PLP, and much increased thermolability of the mutant enzyme which was increased toward normal by the addition of PLP during the heat step. These findings, taken in conjuction with previous studies which suggest that a PLP-dependent holoenzyme is more slowly degraded than its "naked" apoenzyme,[85] suggest the following formulation.[77] Patients with pyridoxine-responsive homocystinuria bear a mutation which alters the cystathionine synthase apoenzyme in such a way that its affinity for coenzyme is markedly reduced. This primary defect has two important consequences. First, it leads to reduced holoenzyme activity; second, it leads to reduced apoenzyme content because the mutant apoenzyme turns over more rapidly than does normal apoenzyme. In this setting, addition of saturating concentrations of PLP *in vitro* leads to only modest increase in enzyme activity because there is only a very small amount of apoenzyme which can be converted to active holoenzyme.

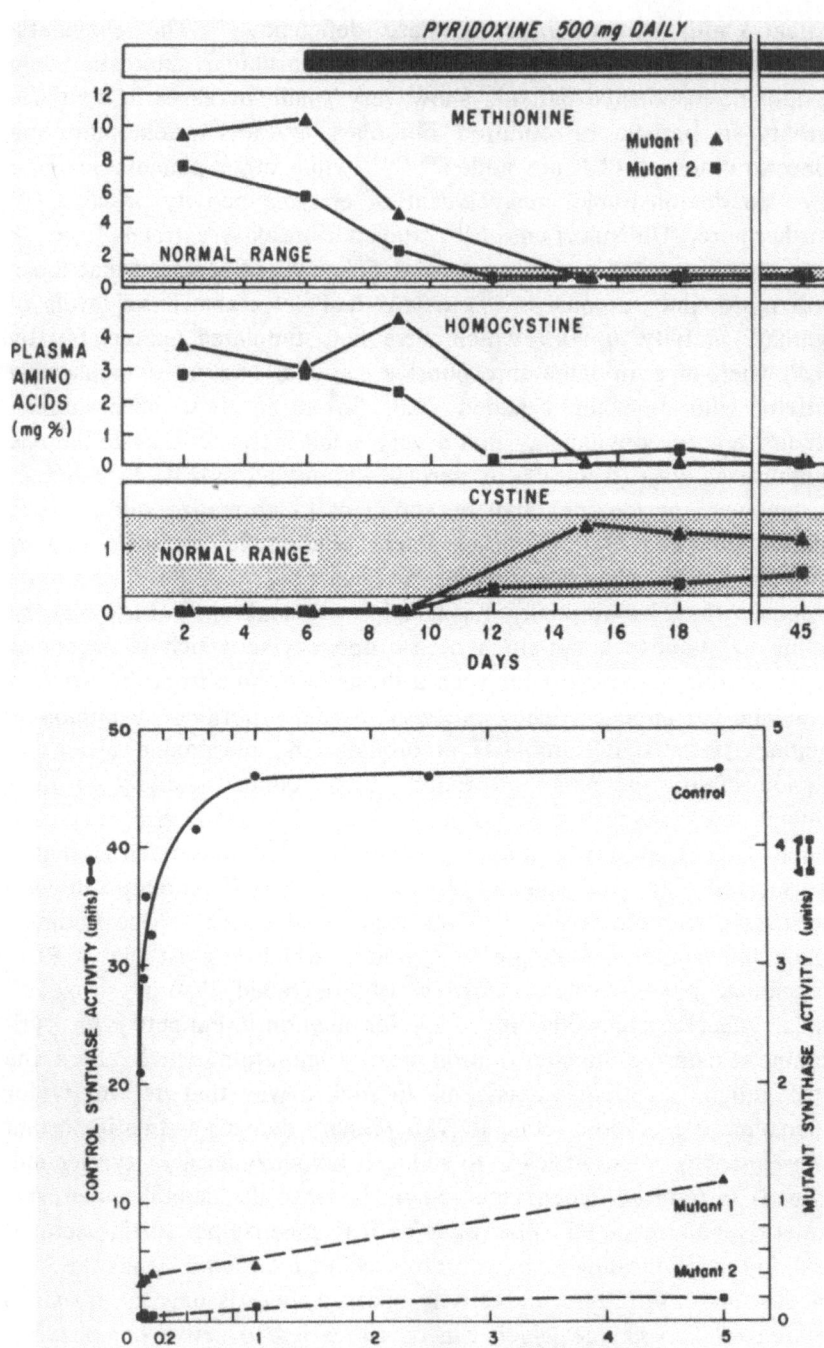

Proof of this hypothesis will require actual quantitation of apoenzyme content—not activity. This conjecture is described in some detail because it is consistent with all of the known data for pyridoxine-responsive homocystinuria and because it may be applicable to other vitamin-responsive disorders in which only limited correction is observed when enzyme activities are measured *in vitro*.

To complete this perusal of pyridoxine-responsive disorders, we must mention a unique infant described in 1963 by Scriver and Hutchison.[138] On a normal intake of pyridoxine, this child grew slowly, had repeated convulsions, was cystathioninuric, and responded to an oral tryptophan load with an exaggerated increase in xanthurenic acid output. Activity of glutamic-oxalacetic and glutamic-pyruvic transaminases in serum was normal. The child responded impressively when his diet was supplemented with 2.5 mg pyridoxine per day—only four to five times the normal infant dose. Since several PLP-requiring enzymes were defective in this child, it is possible that he suffered from a derangement in vitamin absorption or coenzyme formation analogous to that discussed previously for B_{12} and folic acid. Studies of serum and tissue vitamin and coenzyme content would be of great interest in such children.

Biotin

Biotin is a water-soluble vitamin required by higher animals and yeast. It is composed of a heterocyclic ring structure containing nitrogen, carbon, and sulfur atoms to which is attached an aliphatic side chain terminating in a carboxyl group (Fig. 1). Biotin is widely distributed in plant and animal tissues and is readily synthesized by a variety of bacteria. Spontaneous deficiency of this vitamin has not been

←───

Fig. 13. Pyridoxine responsiveness in homocystinuria due to cystathionine synthase deficiency. The upper panel shows correction of plasma amino acid abnormalities by oral administration of pyridoxine in two patients (mutants 1 and 2). The lower panel shows that cystathionine synthase activity increases in fibroblast extracts from controls and mutants 1 and 2 when saturating concentrations of pyridoxal-5′-phosphate are added *in vitro* but that mutant activity (right ordinate) is less than 5% of control (left ordinate) with and without cofactor. Note the tenfold difference in scale of the two ordinates. Data in the upper panel are reproduced from Seashore *et al*.[143] with permission of the author and publisher. The lower panel is based on data from Kim and Rosenberg.[77]

reported in man, probably because intestinal microorganisms synthesize sufficient quantities of biotin to meet human needs, even in the absence of a nutritional source. Experimental biotin deficiency has been produced in animals or man by ingestion of large amounts of egg white, which contains avidin, a protein known to bind and inactivate biotin.[32] Under these conditions, the experimental subjects developed cutaneous pallor, dermatitis, depression, lassitude, muscle pains, hyperesthesia, and finally anemia and electrocardiographic changes.[156] All these manifestations were reversed rapidly by administration of 150–300 μg of biotin daily for a few days. Although the precise human requirement for a biotin is unknown, studies in animals suggest that humans require approximately 10 μg daily.

Coenzyme Function

Biotin serves as a coenzyme in a number of ATP-dependent carboxylations. Typical examples of biotin-dependent enzymes include propionyl-CoA carboxylase, which converts propionyl-CoA to D-methylmalonyl-CoA, and β-methylcrotonyl-CoA carboxylase, which catalyzes the formation of β-methylglutaconyl-CoA from β-methylcrotonyl-CoA. The reaction mechanism of these biotin-dependent carboxylations is particularly well understood.[79] First, biotin is joined covalently to its apoenzyme via a peptide bond between the carboxyl group of biotin and an ϵ-amino nitrogen moiety on the apoenzyme. This covalent attachment between apoenzyme and coenzyme is catalyzed enzymatically by another enzyme called apocarboxylase-biotin ligase.[19,146] Then bicarbonate is attached to the ureido nitrogen of the biotin ring, forming a carboxybiotin–apoenzyme intermediate. Finally, this complex reacts in turn with the substrate (i.e., propionyl-CoA) and transfers the carboxyl group from biotin to it, thereby forming the new product (i.e., D-methylmalonyl-CoA). Among the water-soluble vitamins which concern us in this discussion of vitamin-responsive disorders, biotin is unique in the following ways: its dietary form is identical to its coenzyme form, i.e., no chemical modification of the vitamin is necessary prior to assuming its coenzyme function; it is covalently linked to its apoenzyme(s) and is nondialyzable once attached; and it requires a specific ligase enzyme to bind it to its apoenzyme. These features may assume great importance as we learn more about the biotin-responsive inborn errors.

Biotin-Responsive Propionicacidemia and
β-Methylcrotonylglycinuria

Since 1968, it has become apparent that a number of infants and children accumulate large amounts of propionate in blood and urine due to a primary defect in the activity of propionyl-CoA carboxylase.[42, 61, 66, 67] The clinical course of these patients has often been devastating: neonatal ketosis and acidosis, failure to thrive, protein intolerance, and early demise. Several of these children have had enzyme assays performed on fibroblast extracts[67] or hepatic mitochondria,[42] and in both tissue preparations striking reduction of propionyl-CoA carboxylase activity has been observed in the absence of an abnormality of other biotin-dependent carboxylases. Well-documented biotin responsiveness has now been reported in two such patients. In the first, reported by Barnes et al.,[10] administration of 10 mg of biotin daily modified the metabolic response to a test dose of the propionate precursor, isoleucine. Without biotin, isoleucine caused a marked rise in plasma propionate that was sustained for 12 hr and was associated with prominent ketonuria. When this test was repeated during biotin therapy, the rise in plasma propionate was much diminished, it returned to normal within 4 hr, and no ketonuria was observed. Very similar findings were obtained by Mahoney et al.[90] in a second girl. Despite her apparent response to biotin in vivo, neither addition of large amounts of biotin to the growth medium nor massive supplementation of the enzyme assay mix produced any significant increase in the much reduced activity of propionyl-CoA carboxylase in fibroblast extracts from this child. Thus there is at present no in vitro confirmation of biotin responsiveness which would be so useful in defining its mechanism further.

More recent reports of two unrelated children suggest an inherited defect of another biotin-dependent enzyme, β-methylcrotonyl-CoA carboxylase. Although both of these children excreted large amounts of β-methylcrotonyl-glycine in their urine, they were otherwise dissimilar. One had retarded motor development, muscular atrophy, and hypotonia. She was given 250 μg of biotin daily without effect on her urinary metabolites.[155] The second child's illness was characterized by vomiting, acidosis, and a severe skin rash.[43] When he was given 10 mg of biotin daily, the effect was dramatic. The vomiting ceased, the acidosis was corrected, the skin rash cleared, and the β-methylcrotonylglycine disappeared from the urine. Although it seems most likely that the latter child has a biotin-responsive form of β-methylcrotonyl-CoA carboxylase deficiency, this conclusion must remain tentative until *in vitro* confirmation has appeared, until some rectification of the striking clinical differences between these two children is provided, and until it is certain that he was not suffering from biotin deficiency, as so many of his signs and symptoms suggest.

Thiamine (Vitamin B₁)

Following the classic experiments of Eijkman[28] and Grijns[48] on human and animal beriberi, Jansen and Donath isolated a crystalline substance with potent antineuritic activity. This substance was thiamine (vitamin B_1), whose structure is shown in Fig. 1. Thiamine consists of a substituted pyrimidine ring linked by a methylene group to a substituted thiazole. It is water soluble and unstable to heating, particularly at pHs above 7. Thiamine is widely distributed in cereal grains, meat, fish, and poultry. In cereals it is found largely in the free form, while in meat products it is present as thiamine pyrophosphate (TPP). It is this pyrophosphoric acid ester of thiamine, not the free compound, which is the active intracellular coenzyme.

Metabolism, Activation, and Coenzyme Function

Only free thiamine is absorbed from the intestinal tract, where it circulates in plasma bound to α- and β-globulins. In the tissues, thiamine is converted to TPP by an ATP-dependent kinase. TPP participates as a coenzyme in several enzymatic reactions involving oxidative and nonoxidative decarboxylation of α-keto acids. The details of the organic reaction mechanisms of such TPP-dependent systems are beyond the scope of this review, but it should be pointed out that the thiazole ring of TPP acts as the carrier for the substrate (i. e., pyruvate or α-ketoglutarate) during its subsequent enzymatic attack and decarboxylation.[88] A TPP-dependent enzyme, such as pyruvate decarboxylase, constitues one of several enzymes and cofactors organized in a very large multienzyme complex. For instance, the pyruvate dehydrogenase complex which is responsible for converting pyruvate to acetyl-CoA contains three apoenzymes (pyruvate decarboxylase, dihydrolipoyl transacetylase, and hydrolipoyl dehydrogenase) and five coenzymes (TPP, lipoic acid, FAD, NAD, and CoA) with a total molecular weight of 4 million. A similar complex catalyzes the decarboxylation of branched-chain keto acids formed during catabolism of the branched-chain amino acids (leucine, isoleucine, and valine).

Although TPP is the only thiamine derivative with demonstrable coenzyme function, studies during the past decade have begun to focus attention on a closely related compound, thiamine triphosphate (TTP). This substance is widely distributed in animal and microbial cells and appears to be formed enzymatically by a phosphotransferase which reacts TPP with ATP to yield TTP and ADP.[69] Cooper and his colleagues have argued that TTP plays a role in nerve conduction independent of any coenzyme function and have reported that TTP constitutes 5–15% of the total thiamine content in brain and spinal cord.[22]

Requirements and Deficiency

Children and adults require about 1 mg of thiamine daily. In the absence of this additive, a well-defined deficiency picture has been produced experimentally and clinically. Thiamine deficiency is still an important public health problem in Asia, where rice is the staple foodstuff and polished rice the preferred table food. Cardiovascular and neurological findings are the hallmarks of the thiamine deficiency syndrome called beriberi. Congestive heart failure is often seen, with involvement of both the left and right ventricles. Peripheral neuropathy and central neurological dysfunction can lead, in the full-blown cases to parasthesias, foot drop, ataxia, confusion, extraocular muscle palsies, psychosis, coma, and, eventually, death. These clinical findings are associated with demyelination of peripheral nerves and capillary damage producing pinpoint hemorrhage in various areas of the central nervous system. Significantly, blood pyruvate and lactate concentrations are often elevated in thiamine deficiency, these elevations plus reduced erythrocyte activity of the TPP-dependent enzyme transketolase being used as the most reliable chemical indices of thiamine deficiency. It should also be emphasized that the cardiac, neurological, and chemical aberrations seen in beriberi respond fully to thiamine replacement, with chemical improvement often appearing within hours.

Thiamine-Responsive Metabolic Diseases

Within the past 5 years, a number of patients with diverse signs
and symptoms have been reported to demonstrate clinical or biochemical improvement on supraphysiological doses of thiamine (Table IX).
The first of these patients was an 11-year-old girl with a refractory
form of megaloblastic anemia.[121] This child's anemia responded dramatically when she was treated with 20 mg of thiamine daily. Her serum
thiamine content was normal, as were activities of several TPP-
dependent enzymes. The biochemical basis for this form of thiamine
responsiveness is totally obscure and, to my knowledge, no other
similar patients have been reported.

Well-documented thiamine responsiveness was also reported in a
single patient with a variant form of branched-chain ketoaciduria.[139]
This disorder is characterized chemically by accumulation of the
branched-chain amino acids (leucine, isoleucine, and valine) and
enzymatically by deficiency of the enzyme complex which catalyzes
branched-chain keto acid decarboxylation. The child in question
appears to have a mild variant of branched-chain ketoaciduria as
evidenced by her appearance at a relatively advanced age—11 months.
When she was given 10 mg of thiamine daily, her elevated branched
chain plasma amino acid concentration normalized but rose again
when the thiamine was discontinued. Since TPP is the coenzyme for
the involved branched-chain keto acid decarboxylase, it seems likely
that, in this setting, thiamine supplements acted to increase the activity
of a partially defective enzyme, but no such stimulation was observed
in vitro.

TABLE IX. Thiamine-Responsive Metabolic Disorders

Disorder	Biochemical hallmarks	Mutant apoenzymes
Anemia	None described	Undefined
Branched-chain ketoaciduria	Increased plasma concentrations of branched-chain amino and keto acids	Branched-chain decarboxylase
Pyruvicacidemia	Increased blood pyruvate, lactate, and alanine	Pyruvate decarboxylase
Subacute necrotizing encephalomyelopathy	Increased blood pyruvate and lactate	Pyruvate carboxylase (?)

A third child, and a third clinical picture, shifts the setting of thiamine responsiveness to pyruvate metabolism, where a number of interesting, provocative, and conflicting observations appear. Lonsdale et al.[86] described a boy with intermittent ataxia, choreoathetosis, and ocular incoordination whose serum and urinary pyruvate and alanine concentrations were abnormally elevated during clinical attacks. Thiamine in huge doses (600 mg/day) appeared to ameliorate the clinical and biochemical abnormalities, but it is not clear that such supplements modified the cause of the disease. No data on pyruvate decarboxylase activity in this patient have been reported, but a patient with very similar clinical and chemical findings has been described with a significant reduction in pyruvate decarboxylase activity in extracts of leukocytes and fibroblasts.[12] This child, however, did not respond to thiamine. The clinical resemblance of these patients with presumed primary pyruvate decarboxylase deficiency to subjects with neurological manifestations of thiamine deficiency is of note.

Finally, we can complete the panorama of thiamine-responsive disorders by exploring the findings in patients with reported pyruvate carboxylase deficiency and those with subacute necrotizing encephalomyelopathy (SNE), or Leigh's disease. SNE was the term used by Leigh to describe a 7-month-old boy who died with a clinical picture characterized by increasing lethargy and spasticity. At autopsy, symmetrical necrotic lesions in the brain stem and medulla were seen— these lesions subsequently being said to resemble strikingly those found in patients dying of thiamine deficiency. Nearly 100 patients with a similar clinical and neuropathological picture have been reported subsequently, and the disease appears to be inherited as an autosomal recessive trait. In the past few years, hyperpyruvicacidemia, lactic acidosis, and hyperalaninemia have been observed in patients with presumed SNE, thus leading to an examination of the enzymes of pyruvate metabolism in this disorder. In 1968, Hommes et al.[62] pointed out that an infant with typical SNE and elevations of serum lactate and pyruvate had less than 0.1% of the normal hepatic pyruvate carboxylase activity whereas pyruvate decarboxylase activity was normal. Subsequently, several other children with presumed or possible SNE have also had low pyruvate carboxylase activities measured in their liver.[15,60,157,160] In each case, the TPP-dependent decarboxylase system was normal. Nonetheless, two of these children were reported to respond to large doses of thiamine with impressive biochemical improvement.[15,60] Since pyruvate carboxylase is a biotin-dependent enzyme and has no requirement for TPP, it appears likely that the thiamine supplements are acting to stimulate pyruvate decarboxylase activity and thereby provide an increased rate of removal of pyruvate and lactate which accumulate because of the blocked carboxylation system. The notion of vitamin responsiveness due to activation of an alternate pathway of metabolism rather than partial correction of the primary lesion is, if correct, unique to this form of thiamine responsiveness. To complete this discussion, I will refer to the interesting observations of Cooper and Pincus.[22] They have studied a number of patients with SNE and find two things unreported by others: first, a marked reduction is brain content of TTP (the triphosphate ester) but normal amounts of total thiamine[21] and, second, a heat-labile, nondialyzable inhibitor of the brain enzyme which catalyzes the synthesis of TTP in the serum and urine of untreated patients with SNE.[23,113] Some of their patients also respond to thiamine supplements with impressive clinical improvement.[22] It is impossible at this time to reconcile these observations with those suggesting a primary defect of pyruvate carboxylase in SNE, but it is interesting that the presence of an inhibitor of TTP synthesis in urine and reduced hepatic pyruvate carboxylase activity have been reported together in rare patients.[162] I will offer a scheme which could explain most of the observations: a primary defect in pyruvate carboxylase produces elevated pyruvate concentrations; this in turn augments pyruvate decarboxylase activity, thereby increasing the demand for TPP; in the face of increased need for TPP, synthesis of TTP in the brain is inhibited; this fall in TTP content ultimately leads to brain dysfunction and cell damage. Alternatively, of course, a primary defect in TTP synthesis ultimately leading to secondary pyruvate carboxylase impairment could be proposed, but this seems even more stretched than the thesis just offered. Additional characterization of the putative inhibitor and additional paired enzymatic and chemical studies in affected patients should resolve the controversy.

GENETIC HETEROGENEITY

It has become almost axiomatic that any abnormal human phenotype has more than a single genotype—that, in other words, genetic heterogeneity abounds. Using vitamin responsiveness as a probe, such genetic heterogeneity is clearly apparent among the disorders that we have been discussing. This genetic diversity is noteworthy because it has very real clinical implications in addition to obvious chemical and genetic ones. For instance, the fact that some patients with methylmalonicaciduria respond to B_{12} while others do not is of crucial importance in the management of affected children. At the same time, it provided the clue to contrasting mutations affecting mutase apoenzyme structure on the one hand and B_{12} coenzyme synthesis on the other. Comparable situations exist for many of the vitamin-responsive disorders. Thus the existence of *vitamin-resistant* and *vitamin-responsive* forms of branched-chain ketoaciduria, cysta-thioninuria, homocystinuria, and propionicacidemia means both that more than a single mutant gene produce the biochemical abnormalities observed and that a therapeutic trial of vitamin supplementation will be necessary to distinguish resistant patients from their vitamin-responsive counterparts.

The genetic heterogeneity extant among these vitamin-responsive disorders takes another form, namely that a single mutant phenotype may respond to several different vitamins depending on the nature of the biochemical aberrations. This situation is typified by the different vitamin-responsive "homocystinurias." As shown in Fig. 14, pyridox-ine-responsive homocystinuria is observed in patients with cystathion-

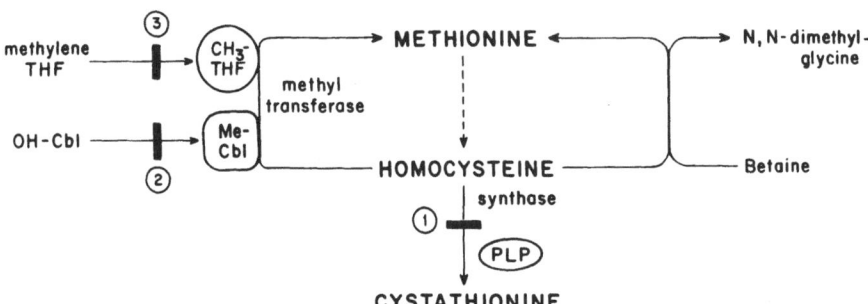

Fig. 14. Enzymatic localization of the three vitamin-responsive "homocystinurias": ① pyridoxine-responsive cystathionine synthase deficiency, ② cobalamin-responsive defect in methylcobalamin synthesis, and ③ folate-responsive N^5,N^{10}-methylenetetrahydrofol-ate reductase deficiency. Abbreviations: CH_3-THF, N^5-methyltetrahydrofolate; OH-Cbl, hydroxocobalamin; Me-Cbl, methylcobalamin; PLP, pyridoxal-5'-phosphate. Redrawn from Scriver and Rosenberg[141] with permission of the authors and publisher.

ine synthase deficiency; cobalamin-responsive homocystinuria reflects a primary abnormality in methylcobalamin synthesis which secondarily impairs the enzymatic methylation of homocysteine to methionine; and folate-responsive homocystinuria depends on a secondary block in methionine synthesis produced by a primary defect in N^5-methyltetra-hydrofolate formation. To the clinician this heterogeneity is important, for he or she must not only know that patients with homocystinuria deserve a trial of vitamin therapy. Now the physician must also know which biochemical constellation calls for which vitamin.

A less well-defined kind of genetic heterogeneity is suggested by differences in the quantitative requirement for a specific vitamin in a single disorder. Pyridoxine-responsive homocystinuria due to cysta-thionine synthase deficiency again serves as the best example. Some patients respond *in vivo* to 25 mg of pyridoxine whereas others require several times that amount.[143] It seems likely that such quantitative differences reflect different mutations of the synthase apoenzyme, and the limited amount of available data *in vitro* support this thesis. It is safe to predict that as more information about the molecular details of these disorders appears additional forms of biochemical and genetic heterogeneity will be uncovered.

CLINICAL PANORAMA

As shown in Table X, we now recognize 25 different vitamin-responsive metabolic disorders, and the list is growing rapidly. Clinical manifestations vary from none (as is probably true for cystathioninuria) to lethal (as in subacute necrotizing encephalomyelopathy, untreated pyridoxine-responsive seizures, and propionicacidemia). Many organ systems have been involved, but neurological and hematological dysfunction are particularly prominent. No less than 14 of these disorders, involving six different water-soluble vitamins, produce neurological abnormalities which may appear almost at birth or be delayed considerably.[125] Such early manifestations as lethargy and coma have been described in branched-chain ketoaciduria, methylma-lonicaciduria, and propionicacidemia. The early onset of seizures, so prominent in the pyridoxine-responsive convulsion disorder, has also been noted in pyruvate carboxylase deficiency and in subacute

TABLE X. Vitamin-Responsive Inherited Metabolic Disorders

Vitamin	Disorder	Therapeutic dose (per day)	Biochemical defect	Clinical hallmarks	Mendelian inheritance	References
Thiamine (B$_1$)	Anemia	20 mg	Unknown	Megaloblastic anemia	Unknown	121
	Branched-chain ketoaciduria	5–20 mg	Branched-chain ketoacid decarboxylase	Episodic ketoacidosis	AR	139
	Pyruvicacidemia	5–20 mg	Pyruvate decarboxylase	Intermittent cerebellar ataxia	Unknown	12, 86
	Subacute necrotizing encephalomyelopathy	>10 mg	Pyruvate carboxylase (?)	Psychomotor retardation, seizures	AR	15, 22, 62
Pyridoxine (B$_6$)	Infantile convulsions	10–50 mg	Glutamate decarboxylase (?)	Seizures	AR	68, 142, 173
	Anemia	>10 mg	Unknown	Hypochromic anemia	XR	63
	Cystathioninuria	>25 mg	Cystathionase	Probably none	AR	36, 37
	Xanthurenic aciduria	5–10 mg	Kynureninase	Mental retardation (?)	Unknown	78, 158, 159
	Homocystinuria	>25 mg	Cystathionine synthase	Dislocated optic lenses, thrombotic vascular disease, CNS dysfunction	AR	8, 77, 99, 143
	Hyperoxaluria	>100 mg	Glyoxylate: α-ketoglutarate carboligase	Nephrolithiasis, renal insufficiency	AR	149

TABLE X. (Continued)

Vitamin	Disorder	Therapeutic dose (per day)	Biochemical defect	Clinical hallmarks	Mendelian inheritance	References
Cobalamin (B_{12})	Anemia	<5 µg	IF deficiency	Megaloblastic anemia	AR	96, 152
	Anemia	<5 µg	Inactive IF	Megaloblastic anemia	AR	74, 75
	Anemia	<5 µg	Ileal transport	Megaloblastic anemia	AR	45
	Transcobalamin II deficiency	>100 µg	TC II deficiency	Megaloblastic anemia	AR	52, 133
	Methylmalonicaciduria	>250 µg	Ado-Cbl synthesis	Ketoacidosis, protein intolerance	AR	89, 93, 128, 129
	Methylmalonicaciduria and homocystinuria	>500 µg	AdoCbl and Me-Cbl synthesis	Developmental retardation, anemia	AR	44, 93, 101
Folic acid	Anemia	<0.05 mg	Intestinal folate absorption	Megaloblastic anemia	Unknown	80, 87
	Forminotransferase deficiency	>5 mg	Forminiotransferase	Mental retardation	AR	3, 5

Vitamin	Disorder	Dose	Enzyme/transport defect	Clinical features	Inheritance	References
	Anemia	>0.1 mg	Dihydrofolate reductase	Megaloblastic anemia	Unknown	167
	Homocystinuria and hypomethioninemia	>10 mg	N^5,N^{10}-Methylenetetrahydrofolate reductase	Mental retardation, schizophrenic psychosis	AR	35, 102, 144
Biotin	Propionicacidemia	10 mg	Propionyl-CoA carboxylase	Ketoacidosis, developmental retardation	AR	10, 42
	β-Methylcrotonylglycinuria	10 mg	β-Methylcrotonyl-CoA carboxylase	Ketoacidosis, skin rash	Unknown	43, 155
Niacin	Hartnup disease	>40 mg	Intestinal and renal transport of tryptophan	Intermittent cerebellar ataxia	AR	71
Calciferol (D)	Hypophosphatemic rickets	>100,000 units	Unknown	Rickets	XD	1, 169
	Vitamin D dependent rickets	>25,000 units	1,25-Dihydroxycholecalciferol synthesis	Rickets	AR	33, 34, 117

necrotizing encephalopathy. A variety of late neurological aberrations have also been documented: cerebellar ataxia in pyruvate decarboxylase deficiency and in Hartnup disease; mental retardation in xanthurenic aciduria, homocystinuria, several disorders of cobalamin and folate metabolism, propionicacidemia, and β-methylcrotonylglycinuria; and marked behavioral abnormalities and frank psychoses in pyridoxine-responsive homocystinuria and in folate-responsive homocystinuria with hypomethioninemia.

In eight of these disorders, anemia has been the presenting finding. Megaloblastic anemia has been observed in seven conditions responding to thiamine, folate, and cobalamin. Among the folate- and cobalamin-responsive conditions, hematological improvement may require either physiological or supraphysiological doses depending on the nature of the specific defect. Only in pyridoxine-responsive anemia have the erythrocytes been microcytic and hypochromic.

Disturbed acid–base balance constitutes another prominent finding among these disorders. Acidosis or ketoacidosis has been seen in five conditions responding to thiamine (branched-chain ketoaciduria, pyruvate carboxylase deficiency), cobalamin (methylmalonicaciduria), and biotin (propionicacidemia and β-methylcrotonylglycinuria). Such acidosis has been severe enough to cause permanent brain damage or death.

This clinical panorama is presented because it emphasizes one of the major themes of this review, namely that prevention or amelioration of clinical sequellae should be possible in most and perhaps all of these conditions provided that they are detected early and managed appropriately.

MENDELIAN INHERITANCE

With the exception of pyridoxine-responsive anemia, inherited as an X-linked recessive, and familial hypophosphatemic rickets, transmitted as an X-linked dominant, all of the other vitamin-responsive disorders for which there is sufficient data appear to be inherited as autosomal recessive traits (Table X). Such a conclusion is based, in the main, on pedigree data. Where sufficient numbers of affected patients of both sexes have been reported, this presumption of autosomal recessive inheritance seems strong. Confirmation of autosomal recessive inheritance by heterozygote detection, however, has been accomplished only rarely (branched-chain ketoaciduria, cystathionine synthase deficiency, transcobalamin II deficiency, and propionicacidemia). Finally, five of these conditions have been described in only one or a few patients, making it impossible to be certain that these disorders are even genetic in etiology. Additional reports should resolve these uncertainties.

PRENATAL DETECTION AND TREATMENT

In the past several years, a large number of inherited metabolic diseases have been detected *in utero*. In the main, such prenatal diagnosis has depended on enzymatic studies in cultured amniotic fluid cells. Only one of the vitamin-responsive disorders has been diagnosed prenatally thus far, and then only in a single patient. Ampola *et al.*[2] have detected cobalamin-responsive methylmalonicaciduria in a fetus whose older sib had died of methylmalonicaciduria of undefined type. Amniotic fluid cells from this high-risk pregnancy failed to oxidize propionate, had normal activity of methylmalonyl-CoA mutase apoenzyme, but were unable to synthesize the needed cobalamin coenzyme, 5'-deoxyadenosylcobalamin. These cellular findings were strengthened by accumulation of methylmalonate in the mother's urine and in amniotic fluid. When large amounts of vitamin B_{12} were administered to this mother (Fig. 15), her methylmalonate excretion fell, suggesting that the B_{12} was crossing the placenta and was being utilized by the affected fetus to correct his abnormal cobalamin metabolism. Following delivery, this infant was shown to have a cobalamin-responsive form of methylmalonicaciduria, thereby confirming the prenatal studies. This report is particularly interesting for several reasons: first, because it demonstrates convincingly that disorders of vitamin metabolism can be diagnosed *in utero*; second, because it asks which other conditions listed in Table X might be so detected; and, third, because it raises the question of prenatal therapy. The results show unequivocally that such treatment was biochemically effective but do not of course answer the more fundamental question which relates to the need for such treatment. Are inborn errors of small molecule metabolism harmless to

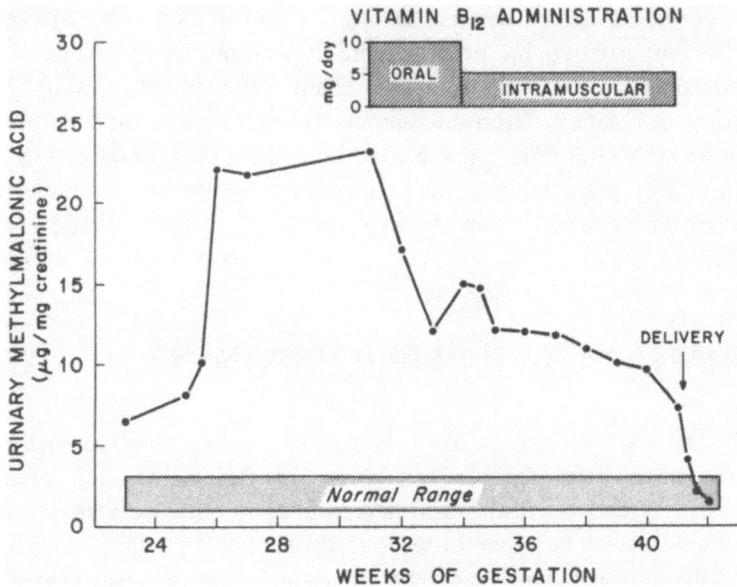

Fig. 15. Prenatal therapy of B_{12}-responsive methylmalonicaciduria. Note significant fall in maternal urinary methylmalonate excretion (ordinate) when oral and parenteral vitamin B_{12} were administered during pregnancy (abscissa) to a woman carrying an affected fetus. The diagnosis of B_{12}-responsive methylmalonicaciduria, made initially in the fetus by studies of cultured amniotic fluid cells, was confirmed in the infant during the neonatal period. From Ampola et al.[2] with permission.

the fetus as we have always supposed? Does the maternal circulation protect effectively the fetus with a disorder of diffusible metabolites? Such questions can now be answered by appropriate study and may open an entire new area to the student of these vitamin-responsive disorders.

PROBLEMS AND PERSPECTIVES

A few general conclusions emerge from the preceding discussion: that a growing list of inherited metabolic disorders respond to single vitamins; that the mutations responsible for these vitamin-responsive disorders alter the metabolism of either the vitamin *per se* or the apoenzymes to which vitamins or their activated coenzymes bind; and that the route and amount of the specific vitamin required for chemical or clinical improvement depend on knowledge of the biochemical basis of any given disorder. These conclusions, while being signposts of some past progress, are as much reflectors of present problems and future perspectives.

The current problems in this field depend on one's vantage. For the biochemist or geneticist, questions abound. Although we have some information about the nature of the mutant gene products responsible for these conditions, we do not even begin to understand them in molecular terms. In no instance have mutant apoenzymes been purified to such an extent that detailed structure–function relationships between apoprotein and coenzyme can be conducted. In no instance have the enzymes necessary for vitamin conversion to coenzyme even been identified thoroughly, much less characterized. In no instance have the intestinal transport systems for vitamins been examined sufficiently to account for inherited abnormalities thereof. In no instance do we understand how administration of ten or a hundred times as much of a particular vitamin leads to sufficient correction of a blocked enzymatic reactions to allow near normal flow of metabolites. In no instance have pedigree analyses or somatic cell hybridization techniques been used to link any of the autosomal loci involved to a specific chromosome.

Equally difficult problems confront the clinician interested in these disorders. Without doubt, some of the vitamin-responsive disorders must be detected in the newborn period if lethal or debilitating consequences are to be prevented, but others seem to produce chemical sequellae only years later. Which, then, of these disorders should be screened for at birth and which can be safely managed by waiting for overt clinical pathology? As vexing as the question of when to diagnose is that concerned with how long to treat. It appears that some inborn errors such as phenylketonuria or galactosemia require treatment for only the first few years of life while vital organs or systems are being formed. This may also be true for some vitamin-responsive disorders. The original proband with B_{12}-responsive methylmalonicaciduria, for instance, received vitamin supplements from age 1 year to age 6 years, at which point his parents discontinued treatment. Two years later, he continues to thrive and shows neither the intolerance to dietary protein nor the developmental retardation which characterized his early months. In contrast, patients with homocystinuria due to cystathionine synthase deficiency usually develop arterial or venous thrombotic disease in their second or third decade, suggesting that pyridoxine therapy in those who respond may have to be continued for many years—perhaps throughout life.

Next we must comment on the hazards of prolonged administration of supraphysiological amounts of a vitamin. We know that certain vitamins are toxic when given to excess: vitamin D can cause permanent renal damage due to calcium deposition,[153] vitamin A causes serious neurological disease,[172] nicotinic acid provokes tachycardia and cutaneous pigment changes,[7,170] and pyridoxine has been reported to cause liver enlargement in rats[20] and seizures in humans.[132] Additional animal and human studies are needed to exclude the possibility that the other water- and fat-soluble vitamins may not also cause toxic manifestations. This information may be of particular importance in titrating a given patient's needs against the possible side effects of overdosage. The second hazard related to vitamin therapy concerns its indiscriminate use. Because some few individuals have specific mutations which render them in need of supplements of a single vitamin, it does not follow at all that many individuals benefit from excesses of several vitamins.[111] The indiscriminate use of "megavitamin" supplements to patients with Down's syndrome, childhood autism, schizophrenia, and even cancer is an ill-advised and potentially very harmful extrapolation of the data obtained from patients with vitamin-responsive inborn errors. Not only may such a "shotgun" approach lead to toxic manifestations, it may also extend false hopes to patients and families trying to cope with complex medical problems. I am sympathetic to the idea that a short course of vitamin therapy may be warranted in patients with neurological, psychiatric, or hematological problems of undefined nature. This, after all, is the way that the known vitamin-responsive metabolic disorders were discovered. But I am much opposed to the long-term, uncritical use of pharmacological amounts of vitamins because of the medical and emotional mischief that such "therapy" may produce.

Finally, given the rapidity with which new vitamin-responsive conditions are being described, it seems safe to predict that many more such conditions will be identified in the near future. Understanding these experiments of nature will both enhance our knowledge of the mechanisms by which the human genome regulates vitamin-dependent functions and offer additional evidence for the view that science can modify the impact of genetic change even if it cannot, and perhaps should not, prevent the change itself.

ACKNOWLEDGMENTS

I am grateful to Robbie Pokora, who initiated my interest in this field, and to Mr. and Mrs. Robert Pokora for their sustained cooperation during our investigations. My work in this area, supported by research and training grants from the John A. Hartford Foundation and the National Institutes of Health (AM-09527, AM-12579, HD-00198), has been accomplished with the invaluable participation of many colleagues: Lalit Ambani, Joseph Durant, Wayne Fenton, Roy Gravel, Anita Hart, Y. Edward Hsia, Young Jin Kim, Anne Lilljeqvist, Maurice Mahoney, Lekha Patel, Margretta Seashore, Katherine Scully, and Kay Tanaka. Preparation of the manuscript was aided immeasurably by the efforts of Marilyn Feldman and Virginia Simon. Finally, I want to thank Dr. Charles Scriver for numerous discussions and personal contributions during the years that we have been occupied, and sometimes preoccupied, with this subject.

BIBLIOGRAPHY

1. Albright, F., Butler, A. M., and Bloomberg, E., Rickets resistant to vitamin D therapy, *Am. J. Dis. Child.* **54:**529 (1937).
2. Ampola, M. G., Mahoney, M. J., Nakamura, E., and Tanaka, K., Prenatal therapy of a patient with vitamin B_{12} responsive methylmalonicacidemia, *New Engl. J. Med.* **293:** 313(1975).
3. Arakawa, T., Congenital defects in folate utilization, *Am. J. Med.* **48:**594 (1970).
4. Arakawa, T., Narisawa, K., Tanno, K., Ohara, K., Higashi, O., Honda, Y., Tamura, T., Wada, Y., Mizuno, T., Hayashi, T., Hirooka, Y., Ohno, T., and Ikeda, M., Megaloblastic anemia and mental retardation associated with hyperfolic acidemia: Probably due to N^5-methytetrahydrofolate transferase deficiency, *Tohoku J. Exp. Med.* **93:**1 (1967).
5. Arakawa, T., Ohara, K., Kudo, K., Tada, K., Hayashi, T., and Mizuno, T., Hyperfolicacidemia with formiminoglutamic aciduria following histidine loading, *Tohoku J. Exp. Med.* **80:**370 (1963).
6. Arnaud, C., Glorieux, F., and Scriver, C. R., Serum parathyroid hormone in X-linked hypophosphatemia, *Science* **173:**845 (1971).
7. Ban, T. A., and Lehmann, H. E., Nicotinic acid in the treatment of schizophrenia, in: *Canadian Mental Health Association Collaborative Study: Progress Report I,* Canadian Mental Health Association, Toronto (1970).

8. Barber, G. W., and Spaeth, G. L., Pyridoxine therapy in homocystinuria, *Lancet* **1**:337 (1967).
9. Barber, K. L., Lee, K. L., and Kenney, F. I., Turnover of tyrosine transaminase in cultured hepatoma cells after inhibition of protein synthesis, *Biochem. Biophys. Res. Commun.* **43**:1132 (1971).
10. Barnes, N. D., Hull, D., Balgobin, L., and Gompertz, D., Biotin-responsive propionicacidaemia, *Lancet* **2**:244 (1970).
11. Bernstein, L. H., Gutstein, S., Weiner, S., and Efron, G., The absorption and malabsorption of folic acid and its polyglutamates, *Am. J. Med.* **48**:570 (1970).
12. Blass, J. P., Avigan, J., and Uhlendorf, B. W., A defect in pyruvate decarboxylase in a child with an intermittent movement disorder, *J. Clin. Invest.* **49**:423 (1970).
13. Blunt, J. W., DeLuca, H. F., and Schnoes, H. C., 25-Hydroxycholecalciferol: A biologically active metabolite of vitamin D_3, *Biochemistry* **7**:3317 (1968).
14. Brickman, A., Coburn, J. W., Kurokawa, K., Bethune, J. E., Harrison, H. E., and Norman, A. W., Actions of 1, 25-dihydroxycholecalciferol in patients, with hypophosphatemic, vitamin D-resistant rickets, *New Engl. J. Med.* **289**:495 (1973).
15. Brunette, M. G., Delvin, E., Hazel, B., and Scriver, C. R., Thiamine-responsive lactic acidosis in a patient with deficient low-K_m pyruvate carboxylase activity in liver, *Pediatrics* **50**:702 (1972).
16. Carmel, R., and Herbert, V., Deficiency of vitamin B_{12}-binding alpha globulin in two brothers, *Blood* **33**:1 (1969).
17. Cartier, J., Brief recit and succincte narration de la navigation faicte as ysles de Canada, Hochelage et Saguenay et autres, avec particuliers mews, langaige et cerimonies des habitans dicelles; fort delectable a veoir (Section subtitled "d'une grosse maladie . . ."), 1545, from facsimile copy of original in British Museum, Ronald Printing Co., Montreal (1953).
18. Castle, W. B., Current concepts of pernicious anemia, *Am. J. Med.* **48**:541 (1970).
19. Cazzulo, J. J., Sundaram, T. K., and Kornberg, H. L., Mechanism of pyruvate carboxylase formation from the apoenzyme and biotin in a thermophilic bacillus, *Nature (London)* **227**:1103 (1970).
20. Cohen, P. A., Schneidman, K., Ginsberg-Fellner, F., Sturman, J. A., Knittle, J., and Gaull, G. E., High pyridoxine diet in the rat: Possible implications for megavitamin therapy, *J. Nutr.* **103**:143 (1972).
21. Cooper, J. R., Itokawa, Y., and Pincus, J. H., Thiamine triphosphate deficiency in subacute necrotizing encephalomyelopathy, *Science* **164**:74 (1969).
22. Cooper, J. R., and Pincus, J. H., Thiamine triphosphate deficiency in Leigh's disease in: *Inborn Errors of Metabolism* (F. A. Hommes and C. J. Van Den Berg, eds.), pp. 119–132, Academic Press, London (1973).
23. Cooper, J. R., Pincus, J. H., Itodawa, Y., and Piros, K., Experience with phosphoryl transferase inhibition in subacute necrotizing encephalomyelopathy, *New Engl. J. Med.* **283**:793 (1970).
24. Cox, E. V., and White, A. M., Methylmalonic acid excretion: Index of vitamin B_{12} deficiency, *Lancet* **2**:853 (1962).
25. DeLuca, H. F., Current concepts: Vitamin D, *New Engl. J. Med.* **281**:1103 (1969).
26. DeLuca, H., The kidney as an endocrine organ for the production of 1, 25-dihydroxy-vitamin D_3, a calcium mobilizing hormone, *New Engl. J. Med.* **289**:359 (1973).
27. Dent, C. E., Richens, A., Rowe, D. J. F., and Stamp, T. C. B., Osteomalacia with long-term anticonvulsant therapy in epilepsy, *Br. Med. J.* **4**:69 (1970).

28. Eijkman, C., Füre beri-beri-ähnlicke Krankheit de Hübner, *Virchows Arch. (Pathol. Anat.)* **148**:523 (1897).
29. *Federal Register*, Washington, D.C., 31FR 15746, December (1966).
30. Finkler, A. E., and Hall, C. A., Nature of the relationship between vitamin B_{12} binding and cell uptake, *Arch. Biochem. Biophys.* **120**:79 (1967).
31. Finkelstein, J. D., Mudd, S. H., Irreverre, F., and Laster L., Deficiencies of cystathionase and homoserine dehydratase activities in cystathioninuria, *Proc. Natl. Acac. Sci. U. S. A.* **55**:865 (1966).
32. Frankel-Conrat, H., Snell, N. S., and Ducay, E. D., Avidin. I. Isolation and characterization of the protein and nucleic acid, *Arch. Biochem. Biophys.* **39**:80 (1952).
33. Fraser, D., Kooh, S. W., Kind, H. P., Holick, M. F., Tanaka, Y., and DeLuca, H. F., Pathogenesis of hereditary vitamin D-dependent rickets, *New Engl. J. Med.* **289**:817 (1973).
34. Fraser, D., and Salter, R. B., The diagnosis and management of the various types of rickets, *Pediat. Clin. N. Am.* **5**:417 (1958).
35. Freeman, J. M., Finkelstein, J. D., Mudd, S. H., and Uhlendorf, B. W., Homocystinuria presenting as reversible "schizophrenia": A new defect in methionine metabolism with reduced methylene-tetrahydrofolate-reductase activity (abst.), *Pediat. Res.* **6**:163 (1972).
36. Frimpter, G. W., Cystathioninuria: Nature of the defect, *Science* **149**:1095 (1965).
37. Frimpter, G., Haymovitz, A., and Horwith, M., Cystathioninuria, *New Engl. J. Med.* **268**:333 (1963).
38. Funk, C., *The Vitamins*, Williams and Wilkins, Baltimore (1922).
39. Garrod, A. E., Inborn errors of metabolism (Croonian Lectures), *Lancet* **2**:1-7, 73-79, 142-148, 214-220 (1908).
40. Gaull, G. E., Rassin, D. K., and Sturman, J. A., Enzymatic and metabolic studies of homocystinuria: Effects of pyridoxine, *Neuropediatrie* **1**:199 (1969).
41. Glorieux, F., and Scriver, C. R., Loss of a parathyroid hormone-sensitive component of phosphate transport in X-linked hypophosphatemia, *Science* **175**:997 (1972).
42. Gompertz, D., Propionic acidaemia in: *Inborn Errors of Metabolism* (F. A. Hommes and C. J. Van Den Berg, eds.), pp. 241-303, Academic Press, London (1973).
43. Gompertz, D., Draffan, G. H., Watts, J. L., and Hull, D., Biotin-responsive β-methylcrotnoylglycinuria, *Lancet* **2**:22 (1971).
44. Goodman, S. I., Moe, P. G., Hammond, K. B., Mudd, S. H., and Uhlendorf, B. W., Homocystinuria with methylmalonic aciduria: Two cases in a sibship, *Biochem. Med.* **4**:500 (1970).
45. Grasbeck, R., Gordin, R., and Kantero, I., Selective vitamin B_{12} malabsorption and proteinuria in young people: A syndrome, *Acta Med. Scand.* **167**:289 (1960).
46. Gravel, R. A., Mahoney, M. J., Ruddle, F. H., and Rosenberg, L. E., Genetic complementation in heterokaryons of human fibroblasts defective in cobalamin metabolism, *Proc. Natl. Aca. Sci. USA*, (August 1975).
47. Greengard, O., The role of coenzyme, cortisone and RNA in the control of liver enzyme levels, *Advan. Enzyme Reg.* **1**:61 (1963).
48. Grijns, G., Overpolyneuritis gallinarum, *Geneeskd. Tijdschr. Ned.-Ind.* **41**:3 (1901).
49. Gyorgy, P., Vitamin B_2 and pellagra-like dermatitis in rats, *Nature (London)* **133**:498 (1934).

50. Haddad, J. G., Chyu, K. J., Hahn, T. J., and Stamp, T. C. B., Serum concentration of 25-hydroxyvitamin D in sex-linked hypophosphatemic vitamin D-resistant rickets, *J. Lab. Clin. Med.* **81:**22 (1973).
51. Hahn, T. J., Hendin, B. A., Scharp, C. R., and Haddad, J. G., Jr., Effect of chronic anticonvulsant therapy on serum 25-hydroxycalciferol levels in adults, *New Engl. J. Med.* **287:**900 (1972).
52. Hakami, N., Neiman, P. E., Canellos, G. P., and Lazerson, J., Neonatal megaloblastic anemia due to inherited transcobalamin II deficiency in two siblings, *New Engl. J. Med.* **285:**1163 (1971).
53. Hall, C. A., and Finkler, A. E., The dynamics of transcobalamin II: A vitamin B_{12} binding substance in plasma, *J. Lab. Clin. Med.* **65:**459 (1965).
54. Hall, C. A., and Finkler, A. E., Protein-mediated uptake of vitamin B_{12} by cells in tissue culture, in: *The Cobalamins* (H. R. V. Arnstein and R. J. Wrighton, eds.), p. 49, Churchill-Livingstone, London (1971).
55. Hegre, C. S., Miller, S. J., and Lane, M. D., Studies on methylmalonyl isomerase, *Biochim. Biophys. Acta* **56:**538 (1962).
56. Hill, H. Z., and Goodman, S. I., Detection of inborn errors of metabolism. II. Defects in propionic acid metabolism, *Clin. Gen.* **6:**73 (1974).
57. Hodgkin, D. C., Pickworth, J., Robertson, J. H., Trueblood, K. N., Prosen, R. J., White, J. G., Bonnett, R., Cannon, J. R., Johnson, A. W., Sutherland, I., Todd, A. R., and Smith, E. L., The crystal structure of the hexacarboxylic acid derived from B_{12} and the molecular structure of the vitamin, *Nature (London)* **176:**325 (1955).
58. Hollowell, J. G., Coryell, M. É., Hall, W. K., Findley, J. K., and Thevaos, T. G., Homocystinuria as effected by pyridoxine, folic acid and vitamin B_{12}, *Proc. Soc. Exp. Biol. Med.* **129:**327 (1968).
59. Hom, B. L., Plasma turnover of ^{57}cobalt-vitamin B_{12} bound to transcobalamin I and II, *Scand. J. Haematol.* **4:**321 (1967).
60. Hommes, F. A., Comment, in: *Inborn Errors of Metabolism* (F.A. Hommes and C. J. VanDen Berg, eds.), pp. 127–130, Academic Press, London (1973).
61. Hommes, F. A., Kuipers, J. R. G., Elema, J. D., Jansen, J. F., and Jonxis, J. H. P., Propionicacidemia, a new inborn error of metabolism, *Pediat. Res.* **2:**519 (1968).
62. Hommes, F. A., Polman, H. A., and Reerink, J. D., Leigh's encephalomyelopathy: An enborn error of gluconeogenesis, *Arch. Dis. Child.* **43:**423 (1968).
63. Horrigan, D. L., and Harris, J. W., Pyridoxin-responsive anemia: Analysis of sixty-one cases, *Advan. Intern. Med.* **12:**103 (1964).
64. Horsting, M., and DeLuca, H. F., *In vitro* production of 25-hydroxycholecalciferol, *Biochem. Biophys. Res. Commun.* **36:**251 (1969).
65. Hsia, Y. E., Lilljeqvist, A. C., and Rosenberg, L. E., Vitamin B_{12}-dependent methylmalonicaciduria: Amino acid toxicity, long chain ketonuria, and protective effect of vitamin B_{12}, *Pediatrics* **46:**497 (1970).
66. Hsia, Y. E., Scully, K. J., And Rosenberg, L. E., Defective propionate carboxylation in ketotic hyperglycinaemia, *Lancet* **1:**757 (1969).
67. Hsia, Y. E., Scully, K. J., and Rosenberg, L. E., Inherited propionyl-CoA carboxylase deficiency in "ketotic hyperglycinemia," *J. Clin. Invest.* **50:**127 (1971).
68. Hunt, A. D., Jr., Stokes, J., Jr., McCrory, W. W., and Stroud, H. H., Pyridoxine dependency: Report of a case of intractable convulsions in an infant controlled by pyridoxine, *Pediatrics* **13:**140 (1954).
69. Itokawa, Y., and Cooper, J. R., The enzymatic synthesis of triphosphothiamin, *Biochim, Biophys. Acta* **158:**180 (1968).

70. Jaffe, I., Altman, K., and Merryman, P., Antipyridoxine effect of penicillamine in man, *J. Clin. Invest.* **43**:1869 (1964).

71. Jepson, J. B., Hartnup disease, in: *The Metabolic Basis of Inherited Disease* (J. B. Stanbury, J. B. Wyngaarden, and D. S. Fredrickson, eds.), 3rd ed., pp. 1486–1503, McGraw Hill, New York (1972).

72. Jusko, W. J., Khanna, N., Levy, G., Stern, L., and Yaffe, S. J., Riboflavin absorption and excretion in the neonate, *Pediatrics* **45**:945 (1970).

73. Kang, E. S., Snodgrass, P. J., and Gerald, P. S., Methylmalonyl coenzyme A racemase defect: Another cause of methylmalonic aciduria, *Pediat. Res.* **6**:875 (1972).

74. Katz, M., Lee, S. F., and Cooper, B. A., Vitamin B_{12} malabsorption due to a biologically inert intrinsic factor, *New Engl. J. Med.* **287**:425 (1972).

75. Katz, M., Mehlman, C. S., and Allen, R., Isolation and characterization of an abnormal human intrinsic factor, *J. Clin. Invest.* **53**:1274 (1974).

76. Kerwar, S. S., Spears, C., McAuslan, B., and Weissbach, H., Studies on vitamin B_{12} metabolism in HeLa cells, *Arch. Biochem. Biophys.* **142**:231 (1971).

77. Kim, Y. J., and Rosenberg, L. E., Studies of the mechanism of pyridoxine responsive homocystinuria. II. Properties of normal and mutant cystathionine synthase from cultured fibroblasts, *Proc. Natl. Acad. Sci. U. S. A.,* **71**:4821 (1974).

78. Knapp, A., Ueber eine neue Hereditare von vitamin B_6 abhangige Storung im tryptophan Stoffwechsel, *Clin. Chim. Acta* **5**:6 (1960).

79. Knappe, J., Mechanism of biotin action, *Ann. Rev. Biochem.* **39**:757 (1970).

80. Lanzkowsky, P., Congenital malabsorption of folate, *Am. J. Med.* **48**:580 (1970).

81. Lehniger, A., *Biochemistry,* Worth Publishers, New York (1970).

82. Lewy. J., Cabana, E. C., Repetto, H. A., Canterbury, J. M., and Reiss, E., Serum parathyroid hormone in hypophosphatemic vitamin D-resistant rickets, *J. Pediat.* **81**:294 (1972).

83. Lin. E. C. C., Civen, M., and Knox, W. E., Effect of vitamin B_6 deficiency on the basal and adapted levels of rat liver tyrosine and tryptophan transaminases, *J. Biol. Chem.* **233**:1183 (1958).

84. Lindblad, B., Lindstrand, K., Svanberg, B., and Zetterstrom, R., The effect of cobamide coenzyme in methylmalonic acidemia, *Acta Paediat. Scand.* **58**:178 (1969).

85. Litwack, G., and Rosenfield, S., Coenzyme dissociation, a possible determinant of short half-life of inducible enzymes in mammalian liver, *Biochem. Biophys. Res. Commun.* **52**:181 (1973).

86. Lonsdale, D., Faulkner, W. R., Price, J. M., and Smeby, R. R., Intermittent cerebellar ataxia associated with hyperpyruvic acidemia, hyperphenylalaninemia and hyperalaninuria, *Pediatrics* **43**:1025 (1969).

87. Luhby, A. L., Engle, F. J., Roth, E., and Cooperman, J. M., Relapsing megaloblastic anemia in an infant due to a specific defect in gastrointestinal absorption of folic acid, *Am. J. Dis. Child.* **102**:482 (1961).

88. Mahler, H. R., and Corder, E. H., Coenzymes, in: *Biological Chemistry,* 2nd ed., pp. 377–431, Harper and Row, New York (1971).

89. Mahoney, M. J., Hart, A. C., and Rosenberg, L. E., Methylmalonicacidemia: Biochemical heterogeneity in defects of 5'-deoxyadenosylcobalamin synthesis, *Proc. Natl. Acad. Sci. U. S. A.,* **72**:2799 (1975).

90. Mahoney, M. J., Hsia, Y. E., and Rosenberg, L. E., Non-ketotic hyperglycinemia and biotin responsiveness in propionicacidemia, (abst) *Ped. Res.* **5**:395 (1971).

91. Mahoney, M. J., and Rosenberg, L. E., Synthesis of cobalamin coenzymes by human cells in tissue culture, *J. Lab. Clin. Med.* **78**:302 (1971).

92. Mahoney, M. J., and Rosenberg, L. E., Inborn errors of cobalamin metabolism, in: *Cobalamin Biochemistry and Biochemical Pathology* (B. Babior, ed.), pp. 369–402 Wiley, New York (1975).

93. Mahoney, M. J., Rosenberg, L. E., Mudd, S. H., and Uhlendorf, B. W., Defective metabolism of vitamin B_{12} in fibroblasts from children with methylmalonicaciduria, *Biochem. Biophys. Res. Commun.* **44**:375 (1971).

94. May, C. D., Vitamin B_6 in human nutrition: A critique and an object lession, *Pediatrics* **14**:269 (1954).

95. Minot, G. R., and Murphy, L. P., Treatment of pernicious anemia by special diet, *J. Am. Med. Assoc.* **87**:470 (1926).

96. Mohamed, S. D., McKay, E., and Galloway, W. H., Juvenile familial megaloblastic anemia due to selective malabsorption of vitamin B_{12}, *Quart. J. Med.* **35**:433 (1966).

97. Morrow, G., III, Barness, L. E., Cardinale, G. J., Abeles, R. H., and Flaks, J. G., Congenital methylmalonic acidemia: Enzymatic evidence for two forms of the disease, *Proc. Natl. Acad. Sci. U. S. A.* **63**:191 (1969).

98. Mudd, S. H., Pyridoxine-responsive genetic disease, *Fed. Proc.* **30**:970 (1971).

99. Mudd, S. H., Edwards, W. A., Loeb, P. M., Brown, M. S., and Laster, L., Homocystinuria due to cystathionine synthase deficiency: The effect of pyridoxine, *J. Clin. Invest.* **49**:1762 (1970).

100. Mudd, S. H., Finkelstein, J. D., Irreverre, F., and Laster, L., Homocystinuria: An enzymatic defect, *Science* **143**:1443 (1964).

101. Mudd, S. H., Levy, H. L., and Abeles, R. H., A derangement in B_{12} metabolism leading to homocystinemia, cystathioninemia and methylmalonicaciduria, *Biochem. Biophys. Res. Commun.* **35**:121 (1969).

102. Mudd, S. H., Uhlendorf, B. W., Freeman, J. M., Finkelstein, J. D., and Shih, V. E., Homocystinuria associated with decreased methylenetetrahydrofolate reductase activity, *Biochem. Biophys. Res. Commun.* **46**:905 (1972).

103. Mudd, S. W., Uhlendorf, B. W., Hinds, K. R., and Levy, H. L., Deranged B_{12} metabolism: Studies of fibroblasts grown in tissue culture, *Biochem. Med.* **4**:215 (1970).

104. National Academy of Science's National Research Council, Food and Nutrition Board, *Recommended Dietary Allowances,* 7th ed., rev., National Academy of Science's Publication No. 1694, Washington, D. C., (1968).

105. Needham, J., Frederick Gowland Hopkins, *Perspect. Biol. Med.* **6**:2 (1962).

106. Newmark, P., Newman, G. E., and O'Brien, J. R. P., Vitamin B_{12} in the rat kidney: Evidence for an association with lysosomes, *Arch. Biochem. Biophys.* **141**:121 (1970).

107. Northrop, D. B., Transcarboxylase. IV. Kinetic analysis of the reaction mechanism, *J. Biol. Chem.* **244**:5808 (1969).

108. Nutrition Foundation, *Present Knowledge in Nutrition,* 3rd ed., Nutrition Foundation Inc., New York (1967).

109. Oberholzer, V. G., Levin, B., Burgess, E. A., and Young, W. F., Methylmalonic aciduria: An inborn error of metabolism leading to chronic metabolic acidosis, *Arch. Dis. Child.* **42**:492 (1967).

110. Pal, P. N., and Christensen, H. N., Uptake of pyridoxal phosphate by Ehrlich ascites tumor cells, *J. Biol. Chem.* **236**:894 (1961).

111. Pauling, L., Orthomolecular psychiatry, *Science* **160**:265 (1968).

112. Pawalkiewicz, J., Gorna, M., Fenrych, W., and Magas, S., Conversion of

cyanocobalamin *in vivo* and *in vitro* into its coenzyme form in humans and animals, *Ann. N.Y. Acad. Sci.* **112**:641 (1964).

113. Pincus, J. H., Itokawa, Y., and Cooper, J. R., Enzyme-inhibiting factor in subacute necrotizing encephalomyelopathy, *Neurology* **19**:841 (1969).

114. Pletsch, Q. A., and Coffey, J. W., Intracellular distribution of radioactive vitamin B₁₂ in rat liver, *J. Biol. Chem.* **246**:4619 (1971).

115. Pletsch, Q. A., and Coffey, J. W., Properties of the proteins that bind vitamin B₁₂ in subcellular fractions of rat liver, *Arch. Biochem. Biophys.* **151**:157 (1972).

116. Potts, J. T., Jr., and Deftos, C. J., Parathyroid hormone, calcitonin, vitamin D, bone and bone mineral metabolism, in: *Diseases of Metabolism* (P. K. Bondy, and L. E. Rosenberg, eds.), 7th ed., pp. 1225–1430, Saunders, Philadelphia (1974).

117. Prader, A., Illig, R., and Heierli, E., Eine besondere Form der pirmaren vitamin D-resisten Rachitis mit hypocalcemic und autosomal-dominant em Erbgang, *Helv. Paediat. Acta* **68**:227 (1966).

118. Requirements of ascorbic acid vitamin D, vitamin B₁₂, folate and iron, in: *Report of a Joint FAO/WHO Expert Group*, WHO Technical Report Series No. 452 (1970).

119. Requirements of vitamin A, thiamine, riboflavin and niacin, in: *Report of a Joint FAO/WHO Expert Group*, WHO Technical Report Series No. 362 (1967).

120. Rickes, E. L., Brink, N. G., Koniuszy, F. R., Wood, T. R., and Folkers, K., Crystalline vitamin B₁₂, 'Science **107**:396 (1948).

121. Rogers, L. E., Porter, F. S., and Sidbury, J. B., Thiamine-responsive megaloblastic anemia, *J. Pediat.* **74**:494 (1969).

122. Roof, B. S., Piel, C. F., and Gordon, G. S., Nature of defect responsible for familial vitamin D-resistant rickets (VDRR) based on parathormone (PTH) assay (abst.), *Clin. Res.* **20**:624 (1972).

123. Rosenberg, L. E., Inherited aminoacidopathies demonstrating vitamin dependency, *New Engl. J. Med.* **281**:145 (1969).

124. Rosenberg, L. E., Vitamin dependent genetic disease, in: *Medical Genetics* (V. A. McKusick and R. Claiborne, eds.), pp. 73–83, H P Publishers, New York (1973).

125. Rosenberg, L. E., Vitamin responsive inherited diseases affecting the nervous system, in: *Brain Dysfunction in Metabolic Disorders* (F. Plum, ed.), pp. 263–272, Raven Press, New York (1974).

126. Rosenberg, L. E., Lilljeqvist, A. C., and Allen, R. H., Transcobalamin II-facilitated uptake of vitamin B₁₂ by cultured fibroblasts: Studies in methylmalonica-ciduria (abst.), *J. Clin. Invest.* **52**:69 (1973).

127. Rosenberg, L. E., Lilljeqvist, A. C., and Hsia, Y. E., Methylmalonic aciduria: Inborn error leading to metabolic acidosis, long-chain ketonuria and intermittent hyperglycinemia, *New Engl. J. Med.* **278**:1319 (1968).

128. Rosenberg, L. E., Lilljeqvist, A. C., and Hsia, Y. E., Methylamlonic aciduria: Metabolic block localization and vitamin B₁₂ dependency, *Science* **162**:805 (1968).

129. Rosenberg, L. E., Lilljeqvist, A. C., Hsia, Y. E., and Rosenbloom, F. M., Vitamin B₁₂ dependent methylmalonicaciduria: Defective B₁₂ metabolism in cultured fibroblasts, *Biochem. Biophys. Res. Commun.* **4**:607 (1969).

130. Rosenberg, L. E., and Mahoney, M. J., Inherited disorders of methylmalonate and vitamin B₁₂ metabolism: A progress report, in: *Inborn Errors of Metabolism* (F. A. Hommes and C. J. Van Den Berg, eds.), pp. 303–320, Academic Press, London (1973).

131. Rosenberg, L. E., and Patel, L., Unpublished observations.

132. Schimke, R. N., McKusick, V. A., and Weilbaecher, R. G., Homocystinuria, in:

Amino Acid Metabolism and Genetic Variation (W. L. Nyhan, ed.), pp. 297–314, McGraw-Hill, New York (1967).

133. Scott, C. R., Hakami, N., Teng, C. C., and Sagerson, R. N., Hereditary transcobalamin II deficiency: The role of transcobalamin II in vitamin B_{12}-mediated reactions, *J. Pediat.* **81**:1106 (1972).

134. Scriver, C. R., Comment on vitamin B_6 deficiency and dependency syndromes, in: *Year Book of Pediatrics* (S. Gellis, ed.), 1963/1964 Series, Year Book Publishing, Chicago (1964).

135. Scriver, C. R., Vitamin B_6 deficiency and dependency in man, *Am. J. Dis. Child.* **113**:109 (1967).

136. Scriver, C. R., Vitamin-responsive inborn errors of metabolism, *Metabolism* **22**:1319 (1973).

137. Scriver, C. R., and Cullen, A. M., Urinary vitamin B_6 and 4-pyridoxic acid in health and in vitamin B_6 dependency, *Pediatrics* **36**:14 (1965).

138. Scriver, C. R., and Hutchison, J. H., The vitamin B_6 deficiency syndrome in human infancy, biochemical and clinical observation, *Pediatrics* **31**:240 (1963).

139. Scriver, C. R., Mackenzie, S., Clow, C. L., and Delvin, E., Thiamine-responsive maple syrup urine disease, *Lancet* **1**:310 (1971).

140. Scriver, C. R., and Rosenberg, L. E., Sulfur amino acids, in: *Amino Acid Metabolism and Its Disorders*, pp. 207–233, Saunders, Philadelphia (1973).

141. Scriver, C. R., and Rosenberg, L. E., The vitamin responsive aminoacidopathies, in: *Amino Acid Metabolism and Its Disorders*, pp. 453–478, Saunders, Philadelphia (1973).

142. Scriver, C. R., and Whelan, D. T., Glutamic acid decarboxylase (GAD) in mammalian tissue outside the central nervous system, and its possible relevance to hereditary vitamin B_6 dependency with seizures, *Ann. N. Y. Acad. Sci.* **166**:83 (1969).

143. Seashore, M. R., Durant, J. L., and Rosenberg, L. E., Studies of the mechanism of pyridoxine-responsive homocystinuria, *Pediat. Res.* **6**:187 (1972).

144. Shih, V. E., Salam, M. Z., Mudd, S. H., Uhlendorf, B. W., and Adams, R. D., A new form of homocystinuria due to $N^{5, 10}$-methylene tetrahydrofolate reductase deficiency (abst.), *Pediat. Res.* **6**:135 (1972).

145 Short, E. M., Binder, H. J., and Rosenberg, L. E., Familial hypophosphatemic rickets: Defective transport of inorganic phosphate by intestinal mucosa, *Science* **179**:700 (1973).

146. Siegal, L. Foot, J. L., and Coon, M. J., The enzymatic synthesis of propionyl coenzyme A holocarboxylase from *d*-biotinyl-5′-adenylate and the apocarboxylase, *J. Biol. Chem.* **240**:1025 (1965).

147. Smith, E. L., and Parker, L. F. J., Purification of anti-pernicious anemia factor, *Biochem. J.* **43**:VIII (1948).

148. Smith, H. W., Clearances involving tubular reabsorption and vitamin C, in: *The Kidney, Structure and Function in Health and Disease*, pp. 136–141, Oxford University Press, New York (1957).

149. Smith, L. H., Jr., and Williams, H. E., Treatment of primary hyperoxaluria, *Modern Treatment* **4**:522 (1967).

150. Snell, E. E., Chemical structure in relation to biological activity of vitamin B_6, *Vitam. Horm. (N.Y.)* **16**:77 (1958).

151. Snell, E. E., and Hashell, B. E., Metabolism of water-soluble vitamins: The metabolism of vitamin B_6, in: *Comprehensive Biochemistry*, Vol. 21 (M. Florkin and E. N. Stoitz, eds.), pp. 47–71, Elsevier, New York (1971).

152. Spurling, C. L., Sacks, M. S., and Jiji, R. M., Juvenile pernicious anemia, *New Engl. J. Med.* **271**:995 (1964).
153. Stickler, G. B., Jowsey, J., and Bianco, A. J., Possible detrimental effect of large doses of vitamin D in familial hypophosphatemic vitamin D resistant rickets, *J. Pediat.* **79**:68 (1971).
154. Stokke, O., Eldjarn, J., Norum, K. R., Steen-Johnson, J., and Halvorsen, S., Methylmalonic acidemia: A new inborn error of metabolism which may cause fatal acidosis in the neonatal period, *Scand. J. Clin. Lab. Invest.* **20**:313 (1967).
155. Stokke, O., Jellum, E., and Eldjarn, L., Beta-methylcrotonyl-CoA carboxylase deficiency, in: *Inborn Errors of Metabolism* (F. A. Hommes and C. J. Van Den Berg, eds.), pp. 321–337, Academic Press, London (1973).
156. Sydenstricher, V. P., Singal, S. A., Briggs, A. P., and DeVaughn, N. M., Preliminary observations on "egg white injury" in man and its cure with a biotin concentrate, *Science* **95**:176 (1942).
157. Tada, K., Sugita, K., Fujitani, K., Uesakai, T., Takada, G., and Omura, K., Hyperalaninemia with pyruvicemia in a patient suggestive of Leigh's encephalomyelopathy, *Tohoku J. Exp. Med.* **109**:13 (1973).
158. Tada, K., Yokoyama, Y., Nakagawa, H., and Arakawa, T., Vitamin B_6 dependent xanthurenic aciduria (the second report), *Tohoku J. Exp. Med.* **95**:107 (1968).
159 Tada, K., Yokoyama, Y., Nakagawa, H., Yoshida, T., and Arakawa, T., Vitamin B_6 dependent xanthurenic aciduria, *Tohoku J. Exp. Med.* **93**:115 (1967).
160. Tada, K., Yoshida, T., Konno, T., Wada, Y., Yokoyama, Y., and Arakawa, T., Hyperalaninemia with pyruvicemia, *Tohoku J. Exp. Med.* **97**:99 (1969).
161. Tan, C. H., and Hansen, H. J., Studies on the site of synthesis of transcobalamin II, *Proc. Soc. Exp. Biol. Med.* **127**:740 (1968).
162. Tang, T. T., Good, T. A., Dyken, P. R., Johnsen, S. D., McCreadie, S. R., Sy, S. T., Lardy, H. A., and Rudolf, F. B., Pathogenesis of Leigh's encephalomyelopathy, *J. Pediat.* **81**:189 (1972).
163. Uhlendorf, B. W., Conerly, E. B., and Mudd, S. H., Homocystinuria: Studies in tissue culture, *Pediat. Res.* **7**:645 (1973).
164. Vilter, R. W., Vitamin B_6–hydrazide relationship, *Vitam. Horm. (N.Y.)* **22**:797 (1964).
165. Vitols, E., Walker, G. A., and Huennekens, F. M., Enzymatic conversion of vitamin B_{12s} to a cobamide coenzyme, α-(5, 6-dimethylbenzimidazolyl) deoxyadenosylcobamide (adenosyl-B_{12}), *J. Biol. Chem.* **241**:1455 (1966).
166. Walker, G. A., Murphy, S., and Huennekens, F. M., Enzymatic conversion of vitamin B_{12} to adenosyl-B_{12}: Evidence for the existence of two separate reducing systems, *Arch. Biochem. Biophys.* **134**:95 (1969).
167. Walters, T. R., Congenital megaloblastic anemia responsive to N^5-formyltetrahydrofolic acid administration, *J. Pediat.* **70**:686 (1967).
168. Wang, F. K., Koch, J., and Stokstad, E. L., Folate coenzyme pattern, folate linked enzymes and methionine biosynthesis in rat liver mitochondria, *Biochem. Zeitsch.* **346**:458 (1967).
169. Williams, T. F., and Winters, R. W., Familial vitamin D resistant rickets with hypophosphatemia, in: *The Metabolic Basis of Inherited Disease* (J. B. Stanbury, J. B. Wyngaarden, and D. S. Fredrickson, eds.), 3rd ed., pp. 1465–1485, McGraw-Hill, New York (1972).
170. Wittenborn, J. R., Weber, E. S. P., and Brown, M., Niacin in the long term treatment of schizophrenia, *Arch. Gen. Psychiat.* **28**:308 (1973).

171. Wyngaarden, J. B., Genetic control of enzyme activity in higher organisms, *Biochem. Genet.* **4:**105 (1970).
172. Yaffe, S. J., and Filer, L. E., The use and abuse of vitamin A, *Pediatrics* **48:**655 (1971).
173. Yoshida, T., Tada, K., and Arakawa, T., Vitamin B_6-dependency of glutamic acid decarboxylase in the kidney from a patient with vitamin B_6 dependent convulsion, *Tohoku J. Exp. Med.* **104:**195 (1971).
174. Yoshida, T., Tada, K., Yokoyama, Y., and Arakawa, T., Homocystinuria and vitamin B_6 dependent type, *Tohoku J. Exp. Med.* **96:**235 (1968).

Chapter 2

Inherited Deficiency of Hypoxanthine-Guanine Phosphoribosyltransferase in X-Linked Uric Aciduria (the Lesch–Nyhan Syndrome and Its Variants)

J. Edwin Seegmiller

Department of Medicine, Division of Rheumatology
University of California, San Diego
La Jolla, California

INTRODUCTION

The amount of general interest in the inherited human X-linked neurological disease described by Lesch and Nyhan in 1964[192] in two brothers with choreoathetosis, spasticity, mental retardation, compulsive self-mutilation (Figs. 1 and 2), and a markedly excessive production of uric acid seems far greater than the clinical prevalence of the disease would warrant. However, the basis for this interest is not difficult to understand. Once the abnormal gene product was identified as a gross deficiency in activity of the enzyme hypoxanthine-guanine phosphoribosyltransferase (HPRT),[301] detailed study of this "experiment of nature" yielded insight into the operation of many genetic, biological, biochemical, physiological, and pathological processes that could be obtained in no other way. As with other such inborn errors of metabolism, the perturbation created by the abnormal gene product provided precise information on the role of the gene products not only at the primary level of enzyme activity but also at secondary and tertiary levels of cellular function. Description of the substantial amount of progress that has been made in elucidating the biochemical

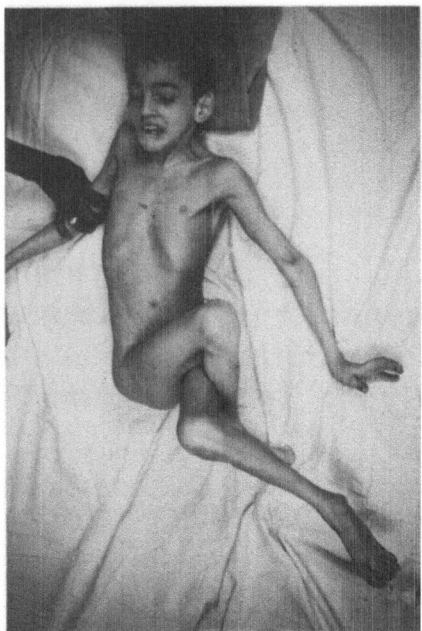

Fig. 1. Child with the Lesch–Nyhan syndrome.
From Seegmiller.[297]

mechanisms responsible for some of the disturbances of function comprises a portion of this review. More important are the possibilities that yet remain for identifying further steps in the discrete sequence of events leading from the abnormal gene product to disturbances in body biochemistry and function observed as clinical pathology.

The unusually large number and diversity of such secondary and tertiary effects, produced by the deficiency of the enzyme HPRT, and the wide degree of modulation in clinical expression, produced by different degrees of residual functional activity of HPRT resulting from the various mutations at the HPRT genetic locus in different families, readily account for the wide interest in this disorder by workers representing many disciplines. It has found wide use as a vehicle for the teaching not only of basic principles of genetics, somatic cell genetics, biochemistry, and regulation of metabolism but also of clinical pathology in a variety of subspecialties including metabolic rheumatology, urology, neurology, and hereditary diseases. However, its implications for the behavioral sciences have only recently begun to be

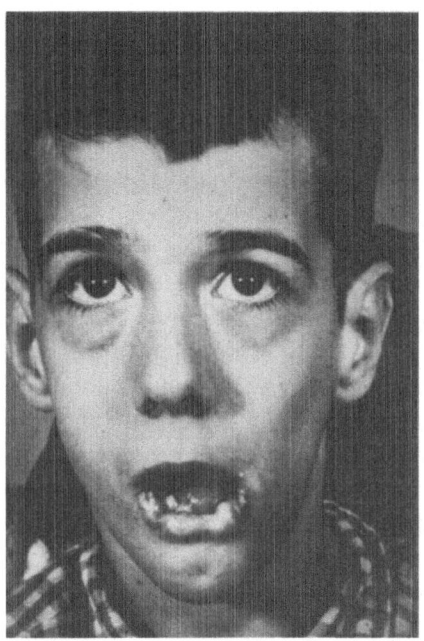

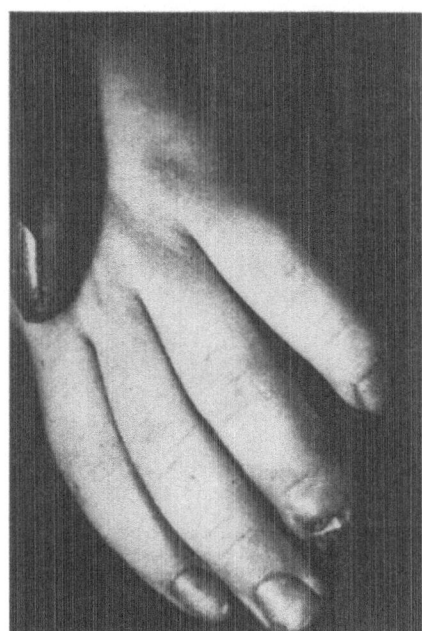

Fig. 2. Self-mutilation by biting in children with the Lesch–Nyhan syndrome. A: Loss of lip tissue. From Seegmiller.[290] B: Amputation of fingertip. From Nyhan.[240]

appreciated. A report of amelioration of the self-mutilation by adminis-tration of L-5-hydroxytryptophan to affected children gives promise of additional biochemical insights into this problem.[221]

Remarkable overproduction of uric acid is the most consistent feature of this group of mutations and provides the rational basis for inclusion of the complete spectrum of defects in the HPRT enzyme under the designation of "X-linked uric aciduria."[292] The excessive production first suggested that this disease might represent the mammalian counterpart[253] of a defect in a regulator genetic locus analogous to a mutation in the operator gene of bacterial systems first described by Jacob and Monod.[159] In keeping with this view was the simultaneous discovery of an increase in activity of a different, but related, enzyme, adenine phosphoribosyltransferase (APRT), in eryth-rocytes of affected children deficient in the enzyme HPRT.[301] The presence in the same cell of an increase in activity of one enzyme with a deficient activity of another enzyme provided an attractive model for a possible coordinate repression of one enzyme coupled with a derepression of another enzyme as a further analogy with the genetic regulation found in bacterial systems. However intellectually attractive the extrapolation of regulatory mechanisms from bacteria to mammal-ian cells may be, it seems premature. A wealth of evidence now favors the view that entirely different types of genetic regulatory mechanisms are present in eukaryotic cells. Evidence of the type of regulatory mechanisms found in bacterial cells remains to be conclusively demonstrated in the mammalian cell. Although regulator gene defects may exist, far simpler mechanisms have been found to account for the increased APRT activity of erythrocytes and the purine overproduction found in the Lesch–Nyhan syndrome and quite different mechanisms are apparently used for control of gene expression in mammalian cells.[336]

A large body of evidence has accumulated showing that the HPRT deficiency results from different types of mutations in the structural gene.[10,112,167,173,174,266,293,296] Although the possibility of a regulator gene defect causing HPRT deficiency now seems remote, the possibility in rare cases has been revived by evidence of such a defect in cells of other mammals.[13,183,303,343] The importance and extent of underlying genetic heterogeneity in the clinical expression of a disease are well shown by the Lesch–Nyhan syndrome and its variants.[177] Yet the occasional cases in which the enzyme assay may seem at variance with the clinical severity of the disease[36,39,40,93,97,191] have not all been fully explained.

The devastating neurological disease accompanying the severe deficiency of HPRT, seen in the Lesch–Nyhan syndrome,[192,240,242] provided the first indication of the importance of the HPRT enzyme to normal function of mammalian cells, particularly those in the central nervous system.[241,272,288,345] Likewise, the marked overproduction of uric acid by affected children was the first indication of the importance of the "salvage pathway" of purine metabolism, and particularly the HPRT enzyme, in the normal regulation of the rate of purine biosynthesis. Detailed study of the biochemical consequences of the enzyme defect has given new insight into the normal regulatory

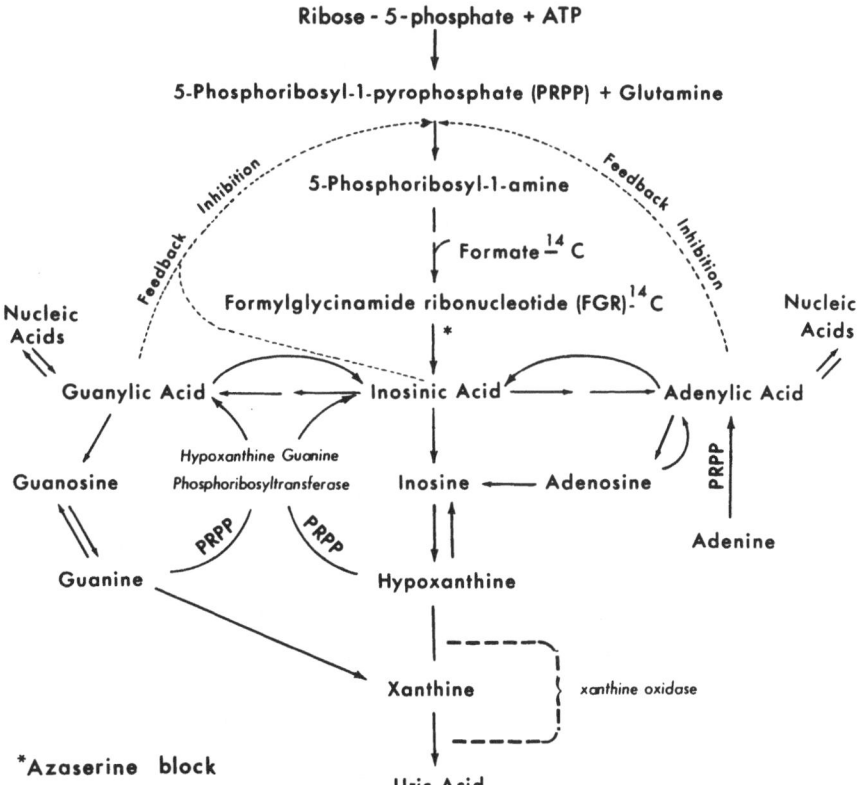

Fig. 3. Feedback control of purine biosynthesis. The location of the block produced by azaserine is indicated by the asterisk. From Seegmiller et al.[301]

mechanism (Fig. 3), in which the concentration of a rate-limiting substrate, phosphoribosylpyrophosphate (PP-ribose-P), provides the major modulation of the purine nucleotide synthetic rate[100,101,129,130,156,261,270] (Figs. 4 and 5). Evidence of additional regulatory mechanisms controlling the rate of PP-ribose-P generation has also been found,[122,287] but the precise mechanisms operating in human cells remain to be defined. Likewise, the mechanism responsible for the coordinate increase of three enzymes in addition to APRT in Lesch–Nyhan erythrocytes is but poorly understood.[256]

X-linked inheritance of the disorder has been firmly established by the demonstration of both normal and HPRT-deficient cells in fibroblasts[98,216,217,271,282] and in hair roots[104,114,305] cultured from heterozygous mothers of affected children as predicted by the Lyon hypothesis and has led more recently to detailed mapping of the HPRT locus on the X chromosome.[277] Yet erythrocytes[165] and leukocytes[74] from such mothers show only normal cells, presumably either from a selective process against the mutant precursor cells or from a nonrandom inactivation of

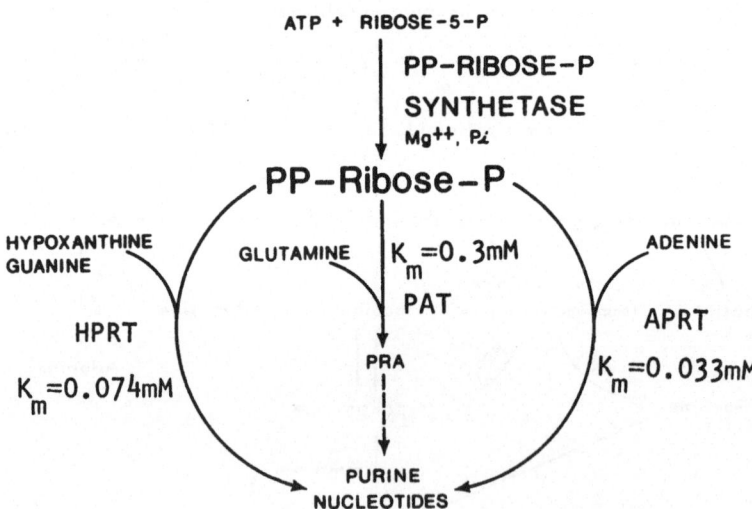

Fig. 4. Regulatory role of PP-ribose-P in control of purine nucleotide synthesis. Affinity constants for PP-ribose-P for each of the enzymes are indicated. Priority is given to the direct synthesis of nucleotides from free purine bases by the higher affinity of PP-ribose-P for adenine phosphoribosyltransferase (APRT) followed by hypoxanthine-guanine phosphoribosyltransferase (HPRT) in preference to enzymatic synthesis *de novo*. Modified from Becker *et al.*[28]

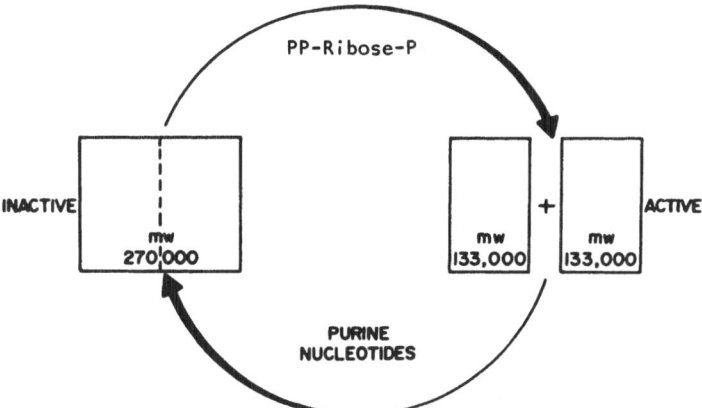

Fig. 5. Role of PP-ribose-P in the allosteric control of the activity of the enzyme PP-ribose-P glutamine amidotransferase. The ratio of the concentration of PP-ribose-P to purine nucleotide determines the overall activity of this enzyme. From Holmes *et al.*[156]

one of the X chromosomes.[204,244] Another curious finding, revealed by examination for heterozygosity in the mother, seems to be a smaller number of children affected as a result of new mutations than would be expected for genetic equilibrium.[105] Evidence has been obtained suggesting that "metabolic cooperation"[67,106,112,113,325,326] could be attenuating clinical expression in the heterozygote. An unresolved question is the extent to which more subtle aspects of the neurological disorder may be expressed in some heterozygotes.[292] Perhaps the most important practical outcome of identification of the abnormal gene in single cells has been the application of the same biochemical methods[271] to permit the prenatal diagnosis of fetal genotype and preventive control of this disease[56,290,299,341] as well as a number of other untreatable hereditary metabolic diseases[32,88,219,232,259] by prenatal diagnosis and gestational management.[32,108]

This chapter will summarize the work of a great many colleagues, many of them from my own laboratory, whose remarkable industry has provided key information in a remarkably short period of time since the primary metabolic defect was identified. I am especially indebted to contributions of Drs. William N. Kelley, Fred M. Rosenbloom, J. Frank Henderson, Martin L. Greene, Wilfred Y. Fujimoto, Theodore Friedmann, J. Anthony Boyle, C. H. Blank, K. O. Raivio, Alexander

Wood, Petrus Van Heeswijk, Ulrich Langenbeck, Michael A. Becker, George Nuki, Julia Lever, David Brenton, Kenneth Astrin, Michael Hershfield, Floyd Snyder, and Stephen Skaper. Each has made fundamental contributions to our understanding of this disease during the past 8 years while working in my laboratory and, in many cases, in later work as well. In addition, substantial contributions by other colleagues and collaborators are acknowledged in the bibliographical citations. Several reviews of the disease have been published.[48,69,108,124,164,167,173,181,229,242,243,292,293,295,296,321,343a,349]

CLINICAL PRESENTATION

Two brothers with athetoid cerebral palsy, mental retardation, reduced growth, and compulsive biting away of lips, tongue, and fingers, described by Lesch and Nyhan,[192] provided the first indication of the hereditary nature of this disease. In retrospect, it appears that sporadic cases of what may have been the same syndrome were described in the past.[44,63,267] The patient of Catel and Schmidt[63] was eventually shown to have a gross deficiency of the HPRT enzyme.[209,299] He differs from the usual patient, however, in being able to converse in three languages despite his dysarthric speech and shows very little evidence of mental retardation and no evidence of compulsive self-mutilation.[208,210,299] The patient of Riley[267] showed severe tophaceous gout at autopsy and evidence of self-mutilation.[55]

With the identification of a less severe defect of the same HPRT enzyme in three brothers with gouty arthritis from excessive production of uric acid and no detectable neurological problem,[177] another category of clinical presentation was defined. Subsequently identified were families with presentation of an attenuated neurological disease, kidney stones, and gout, correlated with enzyme defects slightly less severe than in patients showing the complete Lesch–Nyhan syndrome.[173,177] However, the correlation is not entirely consistent.[93]

Frequency

Although the precise frequency of the Lesch–Nyhan mutation is not known, it seems to be relatively common compared to many hereditary diseases. New cases are constantly being found but are usually no longer publishable unless they illustrate a new facet of the disorder.[243] Its occurrence is not limited to any race or country. On the basis of six known patients alive in the Canadian population of 21 million, Crawhall et al.[69] have estimated a frequency for Canada of one child born with the Lesch–Nyhan syndrome per 380,000 births.

In the past 10 years, over 90 cases have been reported in a total of 74 families,[2,39,40,43,49,50,56,72,80,93,97,115,132,149a,151,152,162,181,184,187,191,192,210,211, 212,220,226,228,233,240,262,266,269,283,285,317,329,337,339,340,341,342,343a] which is roughly half of the total cases known to Dr. Nyhan and to me. Yet deficiency of the HPRT enzyme accounts for only a small portion of gouty patients.[299] Five patients, three of them brothers, were found among 110 gouty patients admitted for metabolic studies at the National Institutes of Health.[299] Of 425 patients in an active gout clinic, HPRT deficiency was found in only seven.[352] In France, one case was found on screening 100 patients in a gout clinic.[2]

Complete Syndrome

Early Signs

Affected children appear entirely normal at birth, even though the primary enzyme defect and its metabolic accompaniment of overproduction of uric acid are present.[192,212,240,242,285] The subsequent development of clinical symptoms is essentially the same, in most cases, for the affected members of any given family. Yet from family to family the clinical symptoms observed and their sequence of development can vary greatly, depending, in general, on the severity of the impairment of functional activity of the mutant enzyme, with the most severe deficiency of the enzyme activity usually correlated with the most remarkable degree of overproduction of uric acid[173,181,292] and with clinical presentation of the most extreme form of the disease. Consequently, affected members of the same family usually show about the same extent of neurological involvement, with a marked attenuation of the neurological dysfunction in those families showing more residual activity of the mutant enzyme. Those patients who show complete attenuation of the neurological dysfunction still show evidence of overproduction of uric acid. As a consequence, they tend to develop renal calculi composed of uric acid and gouty arthritis with onset in early adult life as their major problem.[173,177]

Exceptions have been noted, however, in which a discordancy exists between the clinical presentation and the degree of enzyme defect measured in erythrocyte lysates *in vitro*.[39,97,115,191,203] In two cases,[39] studied in more detail, a K_m mutation accounted for the normal enzyme activity measured *in vitro*.[36,39,40,203]

The marked overproduction of uric acid—four to eight times the normal amount—is present from birth (Fig. 6). The first clinical sign of the disease can therefore arise from this metabolic abnormality. The presence of a reddish-orange to brown "sand" of precipitated uric acid in the diaper of the affected child[240,243,299] has been the earliest abnormality noted by a number of mothers, but only in retrospect, as it had not been considered of sufficient concern for them to seek medical advice. In some cases, affected children are inconsolably colicky babies, and uncontrollable repeated vomiting has been the most prominent feature of some of these infants. Affected children are therefore especially vulnerable to dehydration, which often leads to the development of obstructive symptoms of the urinary tract. This may

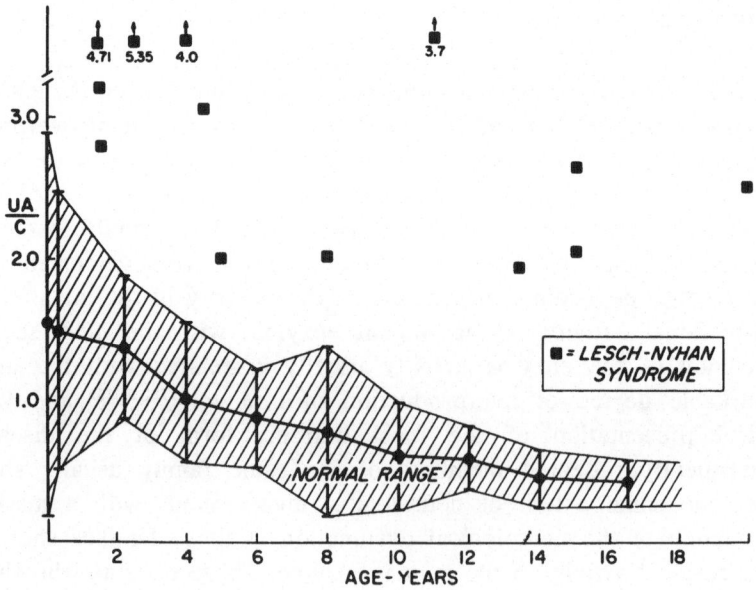

Fig. 6. Uric acid/creatinine ratio found in urine from a group of normal children at various ages and from patients with the Lesch–Nyhan syndrome. From Kaufman *et al.*[163]

take the form of hematuria, frank renal colic with passage of calculi, or development of anuria from obstruction in the renal tubules. The obstructive symptoms of the urinary tract have been documented in older children in whom the diagnosis has already been made, but might well account for some of the episodes of unexplained fever, nausea, and vomiting observed in earlier stages of the disease. Growth retardation below the third percentile is often found, yet patients show normal pituitary and thyroid function.[311] Presumably the HPRT deficiency in cartilage produces the defect in growth and osseous maturation. Associated congenital abnormalities of Hirschprung's disease,[254] bilateral cryptorchidism,[288,309] and imperforate anus[283] have also occasionally been noted.

Neurological Symptoms

The first neurological symptoms are usually noted around 6–8 months of age with a failure to achieve the normal milestones and are initially in the form of muscle weakness and flaccidity.[240,242,243] In a few patients known to have the disease, the first detectable signs of motor weakness were observed by 3 months of age.[43,192,212,283,285] In some instances, a child who has been able to sit up without support has subsequently lost this ability. The first symptom is often an inability to hold the head upright. The period of muscle flaccidity and weakness is followed by development of muscle spasticity, choreoathetosis, and hemiballismic movements. During the first year, hypertonicity appears in all patients. Athetoid and choreic movements develop late in the first year, and by 1 year of age most patients show extrapyramidal signs as well as an increase in deep tendon reflexes, sustained ankle clonus, extensor plantar response, and scissoring of the lower extremities. Contractures, club feet, and dislocated hips are frequent results of the hypertonicity. Some degree of mental retardation is present in virtually all patients when measured with conventional psychological tests. Nevertheless, these patients appear to be very bright and alert, fully aware of their surroundings, and interact in an engaging manner with those around them. In fact, most individuals who have worked with affected children share the clinical impression that they are far less retarded than their scores on conventional psychological tests would indicate. They characteristically become the favorite patients of attendants and are very perceptive and responsive individuals. The severe neurological dysfunction produces markedly dysarthric speech, and they are unable to walk or care for themselves. They therefore lead a bed-and-wheelchair existence and require full-time nursing care.

Behavioral Characteristics

The most unusual feature of this syndrome is in the behavioral abnormalities, consisting of compulsive self-mutilation and aggression toward others (Figs. 1 and 2). Self-mutilation takes the form of biting away the lips, tongue, and ends of the fingers in a compulsive manner which is obviously quite beyond the ability of the patients to control. They are fully sensitive to pain and are quite aware of the painful consequences of the self-mutilation, which they try to avoid by eliciting the help of those around them to protect their hands by placing them in restraints or placing bandages or gloves over them. When this has been done, the patients appear to be quite content but respond with great anxiety or even terror at the prospect of having the restraints removed and their hands freed. Actual amputation of the distal phalanges by biting has been noted[192] (Fig. 2B). In some of the patients, the self-mutilation may take other forms such as flinging themselves from the bed, if unrestrained, or injuring their arms or legs in wheelchairs unless sharp protuberances are padded. One patient, in whom the injury from biting was eliminated by extraction of all teeth, subsequently injured himself by poking his fingers into his eyes whenever a hand became free.[299] However, in other cases extraction of teeth has had an overall beneficial effect.[299] Many of the children also show a curious aggressive behavior to those around them, both in action and, as they learn some limited degree of communication, in verbal abuse. Despite their choreoathetosis, some of the children have shown a remarkable ability in removing and flinging, with one motion, an examining physician's or attendant's eyeglasses across the room, all accomplished with a fiendish delight. They seem to regard even a painful accident of an individual close to them as an occasion for great glee.

The behavioral abnormality is the least constant symptom of the disease. The age at onset varies greatly from one patient to another. Erosion of the underside of the tongue has been noted upon eruption of the lower incisors at about 8 months of age,[285] while in other patients the self-mutilation did not occur until 14 years of age and in other cases not at all. In still other patients, self-mutilation is present intermittently. Although this urge to self-mutilation seems to violate the fundamental biological principles of self-preservation, detailed study of one 14-year-old patient with almost daily observations over a period of 2 years gave quite a different interpretation of this behavior. During this time, we learned to understand his dysarthric speech and found that everything he said was entirely appropriate. Furthermore, we found that he was fully aware of all aspects of his environment and he could give us his own subjective understanding of the causes of the self-mutilating behavior. He stated that the impulse to bite his fingers came upon him only when he was emotionally upset and worried. This brought to mind the common habit among many people of biting their lips or biting their fingernails under periods of emotional stress and suggested the possibility that the bizarre behavior of these children was merely an exaggeration of this relatively common compulsive reaction.

The hospital course of that patient seemed to bear out his observations. During a period of very tranquil existence in which all of his needs were met and he was surrounded by a loving, concerned nursing and professional staff, he announced that he would not need his restraints and indeed he went for as long as 6 months at a time without needing them. However, when he was exposed to stress from his concern over an intercurrent illness of his mother he immediately requested the resumption of restraints for his hands. This observation suggests that the abnormal behavior may provide a specific example of the influence of genetic predisposition on the reaction to environmental stress.

Many patients, as they grow older, show, in addition, a curious reaction to emotional states of anger or excitement that may be voluntary, at least in part. The response consists of spasms lasting a minute or so and producing opisthotonus with arching of the back, laryngeal stridor, and, in some cases, temporary cyanosis. The sudden onset can produce injury from the head striking hard objects in the vicinity.[240,242,243]

Hematological Abnormality

A megaloblastic macrocytic anemia unresponsive to vitamin B_{12} or to folic acid is another relatively unusual but troublesome accompaniment of the syndrome, reported so far in eight patients.[63,152,208,211,339,340] Although a detailed study of this complication has so far been reported for only one child,[198,339,340] it also developed in one of the two brothers originally studied by Nyhan after the children were placed in a mental institution.[299] Many more patients with either the complete syndrome and or one of its variants show a tendency to macrocytosis and somewhat lowered blood levels of folic acid.[115,173]

Clinical Variants of the Syndrome

General Correlations

In addition to the complete syndrome described above, variants of the syndrome have been described[173,177,181,292] that differ primarily in the degree of neurological involvement and the degree of overproduction of uric acid. The severity of the clinical symptoms can, in most cases, be correlated with the severity of the functional impairment of the mutant enzyme. Correlated with the increasing quantities of residual enzyme found in the various families is an attenuation of the neurological dysfunction to a much more marked extent than the overproduction of purines. Consequently, individuals with around 1% or more of residual activity of the enzyme in their erythrocytes have been found who show no detectable neurological dysfunction and merely the symptoms produced by the overproduction of uric acid.[173] These include renal calculi—in some cases with onset in childhood—a marked tendency to infections of the urinary tract, and progressive renal damage, which in some cases has led to uremia and death in the third or fourth decade of life. As might be expected, patients with less severe deficiencies tend to develop gouty arthritis much earlier in life than the general gouty population. Onset in the second decade of life is not unusual. Around 50 patients with variants of the Lesch–Nyhan syndrome have been detected to date.[2,93–95,124,173,177,184,299,352] They all show the X-linked pattern of inheritance.

The enzyme defect has served a useful function of identifying, in addition, a wide range of neurological dysfunctions with clinical expression including such seemingly divergent disorders as the spino-cerebellar syndrome with mental retardation in one sibling and a mild spastic quadriplegia in his older brother.[173,177] Other patients have

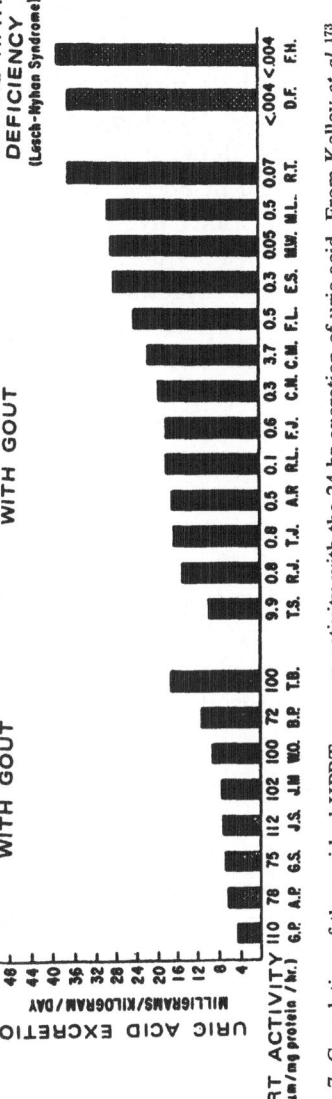

Fig. 7. Correlation of the residual HPRT enzyme activity with the 24-hr excretion of uric acid. From Kelley *et al.*[173]

shown dysarthric speech, seizure disorders, mild spasticity, and a high incidence of mental retardation. Without the biochemical difference to link them, the task of relating such diverse clinical neurological presentations to the same common underlying genetic disorder would have been extremely difficult, if not impossible. Patients with less severe degrees of enzyme deficiency still show an excessive rate of purine biosynthesis, although its degree appears to be attenuated substantially by mutations showing increasing amounts of residual enzyme activity, as indicated in Fig. 7. The precise percent of normal HPRT enzyme activity at which overproduction of uric acid is no longer observed has not been fully defined. Yu et al.[352] have described a gouty patient who had 30% of normal HPRT enzyme activity in his erythrocytes yet excreted a normal quantity of uric acid in the single 24-hr urine collected. Becker and Sweetman[34] have found a gouty patient with around 60% of normal HPRT activity who still showed an increased amount of uric acid in his 24-hr urine. This finding is in keeping with the fact that all of the HPRT-deficient cell lines selected in vitro from a single parental lymphoblast line showed some degree of excessive activity in the first few enzymatic steps of purine biosynthesis.[194,237] The group of six clones retaining around 57–63% of parental HPRT activity showed, for the most part, modest increases in purine synthesis, with three clones showing a rate 20–30% above controls and three additional clones showing higher rates: 1.9, 2.1, and 2.8 times control values, respectively.[194,237]

Possible Attenuated Behavioral Abnormalities

The possibility of behavioral abnormalities in patients with the less severe neurological symptoms deserves more detailed investigation. Although occasional patients have been reported who had served a prison term or demonstrated other antisocial behavior,[173] this type of history is not prominently mentioned. Geerdink et al.[115] report a curious, less blatant, variation of the self-destructive compulsion which was recounted by a 32-year-old man with a 17-year history of gouty arthritis, excessive uric acid production, and reportedly no detectable HPRT enzyme. Neurological deficit was limited to an unsteady gait, dysarthria, dysdiadokokinesis, and involvment of both the tongue and mandible with clumsy motor performance. He had serious learning problems in primary school but was able to support himself as an unskilled controller. He admitted having the urge to put his hands in the cogwheels of machines and had done that on one occasion, losing the tip of the middle finger. He also had an uncontrollable impulse to jump from a motorcycle at full speed, sustaining injuries to the mouth. He also admitted having an urge to carry out "crazy maneuvers" and jump from a car at high speeds, resulting in one serious motoring accident. He also is tempted to jump from a tree when he sees one and has an urge to push nails into an electric-plug socket or pull the cord of an emergency brake on a train. He admitted to a difficult time controlling other impulses such as the desire to fondle women who are strangers. Yet his psychological test profile did not show an aggressive personality structure. Some of the tests were indicative of an organic brain disorder. His older brother had the same syndrome but developed intermittent attacks of gout beginning at age 10.

Pathology

Routine autopsy examination conducted on at least ten patients has revealed very little additional information regarding the disease process. The consistent gross and histological findings have been those expected. In addition to retarded growth and self-mutilation, the kidneys have been shrunken and usually contained urate crystals. The abnormality in brain tissue failed to be shown by conventional histological stains.[72,152,254,273,342] Likewise, electron microscopy failed to reveal any characteristic morphological changes in the brain of an affected fetus delivered by hysterotomy[188] which nevertheless also showed the gross enzyme defect.[341]

Demyelination, vascular lesions, degranulation of the Purkinje fibers, and numerous small infarcts found in both cerebral and cerebellar white matter, as well as deposits staining with the de Galantha stain, were all nonspecific accompaniments of terminal uremia.[283] More severe clinical presentation in another patient was correlated at autopsy with marked thinning of the cerebral cortex with necrosis of nerve cells, internal hydrocephalus producing a cystic dilation of the ventricle, diffuse demyelination, generalized glial proliferation, and atrophy of the medulla, but no significant changes in the basal ganglia.[342]

Autopsy of one of Dr. Nyhan's original patients[192] revealed a brown pigment on the cortical surface of the brain which failed to be detected in histological sections.[272,273] Although he had experienced only one acute attack of gout, and that in the knee, his kidneys nevertheless showed histological changes characteristic of far-advanced gouty nephropathy.[312] A severe gouty nephropathy has been a prominent finding in other patients. Frequently encountered contributing causes of death are uremia and pneumonia.

BIOCHEMICAL CHARACTERISTICS

Children afflicted with the complete Lesch–Nyhan syndrome show the highest rate of purine synthesis yet found in man. In their 24-hr urine, they excrete four to eight times the normal amount of uric acid based on body weight.[48,167,192,240,242,243,301] They also excrete a twenty-fold increase in the purine precursor 4-amino-5-imidazole carboxamide[24,234] and its riboside,[24] substances usually found in the urine in conditions of folic acid or vitamin B_{12} deficiency.[147] Hypoxanthine and xanthine, the oxypurine precursors of uric acid, are also excreted in sixfold excess, with a ratio of hypoxanthine to xanthine of 2.0–2.5 compared to a ratio of 0.3 in unaffected children.[20,24,89,328,329] The possible diagnostic value of the latter difference has not been exploited because of the lack of a method commonly available for oxypurine determination.[182] Although marked hyperuricemia is a consequence, in most patients, of the excessive production of uric acid, occasional patients will show a serum urate concentration in the normal range, particularly those patients with a compensating polyuria.

Primary Enzyme Defect

A gross deficiency of the enzyme hypoxanthine-guanine phosphoribosyltransferase (HPRT) is found in all patients with the complete Lesch–Nyhan syndrome.[301] The enzyme deficiency is most conveniently demonstrated in hemolysates of washed erythrocytes using either hypoxanthine or guanine as substrate. Although initially some patients appeared to have no measurable enzyme, more detailed studies have shown its presence. With use of larger amounts of hemolysate in the assay, residual activity, ranging from less than 0.01% to 0.79% of normal with hypoxanthine as a substrate or from less than 0.001% to 0.61% of normal with guanine as a substrate, was found.[10,173,266,301,330] Using a gel electrophoretic system, Bakay and Nyhan[14] have been able to demonstrate small, but definitely detectable, amounts of enzyme activity in hemolysates of all affected children tested.[15] Likewise, Mizuno et al.[220] and Sorenson[315] have reported low but measurable levels (see below).

Complete Syndrome

Virtually all patients with the complete clinical expression of the Lesch–Nyhan syndrome show markedly deficient enzyme activity in erythrocyte lysates using the usual assay procedure (see below) on the order of less than 0.1% of normal activity. However, considerable heterogeneity is found in detailed studies of the characteristics of the residual enzyme activity (Table I), suggesting that a great many types of structural abnormalities of enzyme may be present in the various families and underlie the variation in activity (see below). As shown in Table II, the HPRT enzyme is normally present in all tissues of the body and is most abundant in brain, particularly the basal ganglia, and is also relatively high in placenta, gonads, erythrocytes, fibroblasts,[112] leukocytes,[21,145] spleen,[255] and platelets.[160] Virtually all of the activity resides in the cytosol.[167] A small amount of activity has been reported in cell membranes and has been assigned a possible transport function.[150] HPRT activity is grossly deficient in all tissues of affected children at autopsy.[56,272]

Clinical Variants

In general, patients showing more than 1% of normal activity of HPRT enzyme in their erythrocyte lysates have little or no neurological dysfunction and tend to have clinical problems related to their excessive uric acid production. Again, considerable evidence of genetic heterogeneity has been found on careful examination of the properties of the residual enzyme (see below).

TABLE I. Specific Activity of Phosphoribosyltransferase in Erythrocyte Hemolysates in Hyperuricemic Subjects[a]

Subject	Number studied	Phosphoribosyltransferase activity (nmoles/mg protein/hr)		
		Hypoxanthine (mean ± s.D.)	Guanine (mean ± s.D.)	Adenine (mean ± s.D.)
Normal	32	103 ± 18	103 ± 21	31.1 ± 6.0
Hyperuricemia				
Normal uric acid production	6	99 ± 13	106 ± 10	31.2 ± 6.9
Excessive uric acid production				
Normal HPRT activity	10	103 ± 18	104 ± 22	30.4 ± 5.3
X-linked uric aciduria				
Virtually complete deficiency HPRT (Lesch–Nyhan syndrome)	15	<0.01	<0.004	62 (normal 22)
Incomplete deficiency HPRT				
J. family				
F. J.		1.3	0.6	46
R. J.		1.5	0.8	43
T. J.		1.8	0.8	56
L. family				
F. L.		11.8	0.5	74
M. L.		8.7	0.5	64
S. family				
T. S.		9.9	9.5	39
D. family				
A. D.		12.2	17.3	33
G. family				
J. G.		9.4	8.8	32
R. G.		9.2	7.5	38
S_2. family				
G. S.		0.03	0.009	58

[a] From Kelley et al.[173,177]

TABLE II. Specific Activity of Hypoxanthine-Guanine and Adenine Phosphoribosyltransferases in Human Necropsy Tissue

Tissue	Phosphoribosyltransferase activity (nmoles/mg protein/hr)						
	Adult tissues[a]			Control fetus[b]		Lesch–Nyhan fetus[b]	
	Hypo-xanthine	Guanine	Adenine	Hypo-xanthine	Adenine	Hypo-xanthine	Adenine
Brain							
Frontal lobe	497	736	12	48.9	26.4	0.9	64
Basal ganglia	843	1137	43	—	—		
Midbrain						1.5	129
Spinal cord	42	57	4	—	—	5.0	161
Cerebellum	463	660	68	42.8	17.3	1.1	>115
Liver	41	66	155	50.7	116	1.1	>99
Spleen	36	60	50	—	—		
Kidney	28	48	11	—	—	<0.3	>103
Muscle	1	5	15	33.9	50.7	1.5	130
Ovary	143	194	46				
Pancreas	42	51	5				
Jejunum	18	27	9				
Adrenal	35	58	31				
Erythrocytes	103	103	31	39.9	20.7	0.9	>36
Leukocytes	128	183	211				
Lesch–Nyhan syndrome—basal ganglia	<4	<4	71				

[a] From Kelley et al.[173] and Rosenbloom et al.[272]
[b] From Van Heeswijk et al.[341]

Disparities between Clinical Manifestations and Enzyme Activity

Several families have recently been described in which only minimal neurological symptoms, if any, were present despite an absence of detectable enzyme in erythrocytes.[39,40,97,115,203,205] In each of these cases, the lower limits of activity detectable by the method used have not been stated. In general, special procedures are required to detect small quantities of enzyme activity. While carrying out these special precautions, Emmerson[93] has found two nongouty brothers, aged 25 and 28, with HPRT activity in erythrocyte lysates of 0.018% and 0.007% of normal activity despite a complete absence of illness including neurological symptoms in the 28-year-old sibling. However, their older brother produced excessive amounts of uric acid with evidence of impaired renal function and died at age 25 from complications of severe tophaceous gout of 7 years' duration. Furthermore, both brothers had a serum urate of 8.8 mg/100 ml and the younger brother excreted 1300 mg of uric acid in his 24-hr urine while on a purine-free diet, had a normal creatinine clearance despite having passed renal calculi, and had a history of temporal lobe epilepsy. Nevertheless, the enzyme activity was still only ten times greater than that found by Emmerson in a child with classical Lesch-Nyhan syndrome. Both brothers are obvious candidates for development of gouty arthritis and would be particularly vulnerable to dehydration or to any attrition of renal function in the future. Impairment of renal function can greatly accelerate the development of gouty symptoms, which in turn can lead to additional renal impairment. The ability to detect such disease susceptibility before development of any clinical symptoms illustrates the great potential for a more definitive form of preventive medicine provided by the identification of the abnormal gene product.[295]

The lack of a consistent finely graded correlation between the amount of residual enzyme in erythrocyte lysates and the severity of neurological symptoms is not surprising when one considers the many unknown sequential factors involved in the production of the neurological disease from the HPRT deficiency. Variations in even the first step of the sequence, the activity of the HPRT enzyme, might well account for the disparity in some cases. For example, the activity of the enzyme as measured in erythrocytes may not reflect precisely the activity existing in the brain cells. Fibroblast lysates from all Lesch–Nyhan patients tested have shown substantially more enzyme than is detectable in erythrocytes, with values in the range of 2–3% of normal activity.[112] Furthermore, the rate of denaturation of the enzyme could be substantially less in the brain than in erythrocytes. A possible model of the latter proposal has already been demonstrated.[112] Changes observed in the HPRT activity of children with the Lesch–Nyhan syndrome produced by the dietary content of purines[5,6] further complicate attempts to make fine clinical correlations with residual enzyme activity.

The converse type of disparity in which the full clinical syndrome is present in a patient with seemingly normal activity of the HPRT of peripheral erythrocytes has been described by Benke and Herrick[39] and Etienne et al.[97] The patient of Benke proved to have a substantial enzyme deficiency with an increase in K_m for substrates,[36,40] analogous to that described by McDonald and Kelley.[203,205] Only at low substrate concentration was the defect demonstrable. Comparable studies are yet to be done on the mutation described by Etienne et al.[61] An alternative possibility is the presence of a kinetic variant of enzyme producing a small activity in intact cells of the central nervous system that is not detectable under the conditions selected for assay of hemolysate in vitro. Still another possibility is the action of a modifier gene that has no effect on the enzyme activity per se but does produce other metabolic alterations that effectively attenuate the sequence of biochemical reactions leading to a disturbance in neuronal function.

Effects of Diet on HPRT Activity

The detailed evaluation of the significance of low levels of enzyme activity was further complicated by the discovery of a rather wide range of variability in HPRT activity in the same patient at different times.[5,6,9] However, activities remained substantially less than 1% of normal. Eventually the cause of the variability was found to be the purine content of the diet. A diet free of purines caused a progressive three- to ninefold increase in enzyme activity over 1- to 3-week periods, while addition oi adenine to the diet produced a decrease from 0.008% to less than 0.001% of normal in some cases. The mechanism of the alteration remains obscure.

Secondary Enzyme Disturbances

Erythrocytes of all patients with the Lesch–Nyhan syndrome show a curious increase in activity of several other enzymes.

Adenine Phosphoribosyltransferase

A two- to threefold increase in activity of a related enzyme, adenine phosphoribosyltransferase (APRT), was discovered quite inadvertently when it was selected quite arbitrarily for use as a control enzyme in assays.[167,173,301] A variety of confirmatory studies[22,23,275,320,353] support the conclusion that the increased APRT activity results from a stabilization against the normal attrition with aging of erythrocytes produced by a high intracellular concentration of PP-ribose-P.[125] The fact that crude hemolysates of normal subjects and Lesch–Nyhan patients,[22] as well as purified APRT, show the same stabilization by PP-ribose-P against thermal inactivation[125] which is lost by treatment of lysates with adenine suggests that bound PP-ribose-P is directly responsible for the stabilization.[22] Compared to normal adults, newborn infants show nearly twofold increases in APRT activity in erythrocytes, also associated with a 2.4-fold increase in concentration of PP-ribose-P.[51] A 4000-fold purified preparation of APRT from human erythrocytes showed multiple peaks on Sephadex column chromatography or polyacrylamide gel electrophoresis but only one peak if treated first with PP-ribose-P.[324,334,335,350,351] Antibody to the purified enzyme was used to demonstrate the same amount of cross-reacting APRT protein in erythrocytes of normal and HPRT-deficient cells, suggesting the presence of an enzyme of higher specific activity.[350] In keeping with this view, the same authors have shown loss of both immunologically reactive protein and APRT activity at the same rate from aging erythrocytes of both normal subjects and Lesch–Nyhan patients. Obviously the two views of the cause of the increased APRT activity are not mutually exclusive.

Inosinic Acid Dehydrogenase

Another curious correlation is an increase in activity of the enzyme inosinic acid dehydrogenase also found in Lesch–Nyhan erythrocytes by Pehlke *et al.*[256] The increase was attributed to an unidentified dialyzable inhibitor normally present in erythrocytes but absent from erythrocytes of patients with the Lesch–Nyhan syndrome.[154] Lommen *et al.*[197] have presented evidence that the increased inosinic acid dehydrogenase activity of HPRT-deficient erythrocytes results from its complete insensitivity to the inhibition normally produced by 2,3-diphosphoglycerate in erythrocytes. The molecular basis for the lack of responsiveness remains to be determined.

Orotate Phosphoribosyltransferase and Orotate Decarboxylase

Activity of two enzymes of pyrimidine metabolism, orotate phosphoribosyltransferase and orotate decarboxylase, is elevated two- to tenfold in erythrocytes of affected children and shows another twofold increase, as in a group of gouty patients, in response to allopurinol therapy.[25] No evidence of stabilization by PP-ribose-P or other dialyzable factors was found to account for the increased activity. These increases of pyrimidine enzyme activity are limited to erythrocytes and are not found in leukocytes or cultured fibroblasts.[26]

PP-Ribose-P Glutamine Amidotransferase

A possible increase in activity of the enzyme PP-ribose-P glutamine amidotransferase of cultured fibroblasts of Lesch–Nyhan patients was inferred in studies of Rosenbloom *et al.*[270] More direct evidence of such an increase in activity of this enzyme has been reported by Reem[263] using a cell-free preparation of lymphoblast lines cultured from a normal subject and from a child with Lesch–Nyhan syndrome. She reports a 50% increase in activity with glutamine as a substrate by measuring the incorporation of ^{14}C-formate into the reaction product formylglycinamide ribonucleotide (FGAR) accumulating in the presence of azaserine. Substitution of ammonia for glutamine resulted in a four- to fivefold increase in FGAR formation in the normal lymphocyte and a ninefold increase in the mutant cells. These increases, presumably of amidotransferase activity in mutant cells, contradict earlier work showing, by a different assay system, the same amount of amidotransferase activity for normal and HPRT-deficient lymphoblast lysates.[346] The significance of the increased activity observed with ammonia as a substrate[264] under physiological conditions of growth in intact cells is doubtful since ammonia is substantially less effective than glutamine in supporting growth of both normal and HPRT-deficient fibroblasts[260,261] or lymphoblasts.[308]

There is no doubt that the functional activity of glutamine PP-ribose-P amidotransferase enzyme is increased in HPRT-deficient cells, but it appears to be the consequence of an aberrant regulatory mechanism from increased intracellular PP-ribose-P (see below) rather than from an intrinsic increase in amount of the enzyme. No alteration in activity of PP-ribose-P synthetase has been found in fibroblasts cultured from Lesch–Nyhan patients.[31,100]

Properties of the Normal Enzyme

The enzyme HPRT normally catalyzes the reaction

$$\text{PP-ribose-P} + \text{Hypoxanthine} \xrightarrow{\text{Mg}^{2+}} \text{Hypoxanthine-ribose-5-P} + \text{PP}_i$$

Guanine also serves as a substrate while xanthine is used at a rate only 0.3% of that with hypoxanthine.[176] The enzyme is conventionally regarded as a scavenging system for the thrifty "salvage" of purine bases into nucleotides at a substantial saving in energy cost to the cell over the energy used to synthesize a purine nucleotide *de novo*.[140,142,229] A possible role of the enzyme in membrane transport of purine bases in bacteria has been proposed.[150]

Specificity

The purine analogues 6-mercaptopurine, 6-azahypoxanthine, allopurinol, 8-azaguanine, and 6-thioguanine are also substrates. The HPRT enzyme fails to react with adenine, uracil, azathioprine, oxipurinol, or uric acid.[68,138,140,186,225] The structural requirements for a purine compound to bind to the enzyme are an oxo or thio group in position 6 but not an amino group. However, binding is enhanced by an amino group at position 2 and diminished by a hydroxyl group. Certain purines methylated at the 1 position are bound but not those methylated at other nitrogens of the purine ring. Only PP-ribose-P can serve as a phosphoribosyl donor, and it is competitively inhibited by purine nucleotide products of the reaction. Fructose-1,6-diphosphate also inhibits the enzyme, as does magnesium at concentrations greater than 20 mM, unless very high concentrations of PP-ribose-P are present. The nucleotide reaction products of the enzyme also are very effective inhibitors.[141]

Reaction Mechanism and Kinetics

Kinetics of the reaction are complex and highly dependent on the concentration of magnesium.[141,167,186] The usual hyperbolic curve obtained with a normal enzyme on plotting activity vs. substrate is changed to a sigmoidal curve at low ratios of magnesium to PP-ribose-P. The sequence of the reaction is also dependent on the magnesium concentration. PP-ribose-P binds to the enzyme first and purine nucleotide is released last,[141] but the magnesium concentration determines the order of the intervening events.[186] Relatively low magnesium, only slightly in excess of the PP-ribose-P concentration, results in the formation of a ternary complex of enzyme PP-ribose-P-purine base, while at high magnesium concentrations an enzyme–ribosylphosphate intermediate is formed with release of pyrophosphate (a "ping-pong" mechanism).[141] The purine base then adds to the enzyme–ribosylphosphate intermediate with release of the purine nucleotide product.

Purification and Structure

The purification of the enzyme has been beset with problems, primarily due to its marked instability with increasing purity. Stabilization of activity required the addition of dithiothreitol, dimethylsulfoxide, sucrose, albumin, and the magnesium salt of PP-ribose-P at different stages in enzyme purification.[4]

The HPRT enzyme purified 8000-fold to homogeneity from normal washed human erythrocytes by Arnold et al.[4,8] showed by chromatography on Sephadex G100 the same molecular weight of 68,000 found in the native impure preparation with a Stokes radius of 36 Å. It was composed of two presumably identical subunits of 34,000 molecular weight. A variety of electrophoretic or chromatographic variants have been found by various investigators.[4,17,76,224] Rubin et al.[276] found two peaks of HPRT activity on DEAE-cellulose chromatography of partially purified enzyme preparations using isoelectric focusing. Arnold and Kelley[4,167] consistently found three peaks at isoelectric points 5.65 ± 0.06, 5.8 ± 0.06, and 6.1 ± 0.09, each with the same molecular weight, specific activity, and product inhibition.[8] A modest difference in the amino acid composition of two of the peaks obtained from isoelectric focusing was found.[8] The purified variants showed some degree of interconvertibility from one to the other form *in vitro*, suggesting a labile equilibrium.

Several lines of evidence suggest that the electrophoretic heterogeneity originates in nongenetic posttranscriptional alterations of enzyme protein.[167,173,224] The loss of enzyme in all tissues of man as a result of a single genetic event argues against multiple genes coding for the enzyme.[272] Furthermore, since the gene is located on the X chromosome and the electrophoretic variants found by isoelectric focusing[4,167] were all isolated from erythrocytes of male donors, multiple alleles cannot account for the observed heterogeneity.

HPRT enzyme purified 650-fold from rat brain by Gutensohn[133,134] was around 50% pure and showed a similar molecular weight but a subunit of 26,000 molecular weight. A 540-fold purification of HPRT from Chinese hamster brain by Olsen and Milman[250] showed a molecular weight of 78,000–85,000 composed of three subunits with a molecular weight of 25,000. Using a similar procedure, Olsen and Milman[251] have isolated from human blood HPRT enzyme with a subunit molecular weight of 26,000 which they find as a minor component of the enzyme preparation of Arnold and Kelley.

Properties of the Mutant Enzyme

Activity of HPRT

Initial studies of the activity of mutant forms of HPRT in erythrocytes suggested two classifications: (1) complete absence of activity in patients with the Lesch–Nyhan syndrome and (2) partial activity in patients presenting clinically with gout and kidney stones. With the discovery of patients with, in addition, a mild neurological disease and very low but detectable enzyme activity, a third category was added.[173,177] The subsequent discovery of detectable but low levels of HPRT activity, first in the fibroblasts[112] and then, with use of improved methods, in erythrocytes of even severely affected children,[15] presented problems for the original classification. These observations, coupled with the increase in number and diversity of patients identified, have led to a blurring of the boundaries between the groups of the original classification. We now realize that HPRT activity of patients with different clinical presentations can overlap to some extent. Despite the overlap, the general view of the diseases originally conceived may still be true. The patients with the higher enzyme activities tend, in general, to have less neurological involvement and a greater likelihood of developing only the gouty diathesis. The spectrum of impairment in enzyme activity found in erythrocytes of the various mutations ranges from barely detectable to 60% of normal.[34,93,173,224]

Kinetics and Stability

In addition to the variations in enzyme activity, the various mutations present a wide range of differences in other properties as well. In one child with the complete syndrome described by McDonald and Kelley,[203,205] the mutant HPRT showed a reduced affinity for all substrates with apparent K_m or $S_{0.5}$ values for hypoxanthine, guanine, or PP-ribose-P around ten times greater than normal, as shown in Table III. In addition, the enzyme showed a sigmoid curve when activity was plotted against PP-ribose-P concentration. As a consequence of the high K_m, the mutant enzyme showed essentially normal activity when exposed to the saturating concentrations of hypoxanthine and PP-ribose-P that are usually used in the routine determination (Table IX). Yet the child's clinical presentation showed the usual evidence of a grossly deficient enzyme function which obtains at the physiological concentrations of substrates present within the patient's cells *in vivo*.[167,203]

A similar type of K_m mutation reported by Benke *et al.*[36,40] registered as normal activity of HPRT enzyme when measured in the routine determination using saturating concentrations of substrates. This type of mutation was responsible for the erroneous conclusion that the patient had a new form of metabolic overproduction of uric acid.[39] Whether or not other similar reports of normal HPRT enzyme activity in patients with clinical symptoms of the Lesch–Nyhan syndrome[97] will fall into the same category remains to be demon-

TABLE III. Comparison of the Kinetic Constants of Normal and Mutant Hypoxanthine-Guanine Phosphoribosyltransferase for PP-Ribose-P[a]

Enzyme source		Apparent K_m (mg PP-ribose-P) (M)	Apparent K_m (guanine) (M)	Apparent K_m (hypoxanthine) (M)	V_{max} of phosphoribosyltransferase activity (nmoles/mg/hr)	
Cell	Type				Guanine	Hypoxanthine
Erythrocyte	Normal	2.5×10^{-4}	5.0×10^{-6}	1.7×10^{-5}	98 ± 14^c	97 ± 19^b
	Mutant	$3.2^b \times 10^{-3}$	4.8×10^{-5}	1.8×10^{-4}	12.1	94.4
Fibroblast	Normal	1.0×10^{-4}			141 ± 17^d	
	Mutant	$>2.0^b \times 10^{-3}$			10.4	

[a] From McDonald and Kelley.[203]
[b] Values depict $S_{0.5}$ rather than K_m.
[c] Mean ± s.d. in 119 subjects.
[d] Mean ± s.d. in 13 normal cell strains.

strated. An increase in both growth response and HPRT enzyme activity of six fibroblast lines from Lesch–Nyhan patients was observed on increasing the magnesium content of the media.[38] Erythrocyte lysate from a Lesch–Nyhan patient showed no significant alteration in affinity for magnesium ion; however, no kinetic data were obtained on the enzyme in the actual fibroblast strains used in the study.[3,35,38] Faster electrophoretic migration of mutant HPRT was found in hemolysates of all six patients examined[15] despite Der Kaloustian's failure to find electrophoretic variants in 382 normal blood samples tested on starch gel.[84] Patients with a less severe deficiency have also shown differences in electrophoretic mobility.[17,173]

Additional indices of the mutational events have been evaluated. In some patients, HPRT enzyme shows substantial differences in activity toward hypoxanthine as compared to guanine as a substrate.[93,173,177] Unexpected differences between degree of HPRT deficiency and ability of the cells to grow in the presence of the purine analogue 8-azaguanine[237,284,303] could well reflect in part an analogous discordance in the ability of the mutant HPRT to react with azaguanine as compared to hypoxanthine. The realization that mutations exist with such a differential effect on various substrates makes complete reliance on such phenomena as azaguanine resistance (see below) to connote HPRT deficiency potentially misleading.

Considerable variation in stability of the different mutant enzymes has been found. Cells from some families showed an increase in thermal stability and others a decreased stability as compared to normal erythrocyte lysates.[173,177] A quite similar instability of mutant HPRT has been shown upon heating extracts of fibroblasts.[112] Seven of eight mutant fibroblast strains studied by Kelley and Meade[174] showed an increased heat lability. Stability of mutant enzyme under the physiological conditions existing *in vivo* has also been assessed by determining the amount of residual enzyme activity in erythrocytes that have been separated on the basis of age by passage through a density gradient. In contrast to the loss of APRT activity that occurs with aging of the erythrocyte, normal HPRT shows no such decline. On the other hand, the mutant HPRT of three of five Lesch–Nyhan patients showed a substantial decline with aging of the erythrocytes *in vivo*. An entirely different method for evaluating the stability of HPRT has been used by Balis *et al.*[21] In two families, they have shown undetectable activities of HPRT in erythrocytes (less than 0.1% of normal) while leukocytes from the same patients showed 10–20% of normal activity. Upon incubation *in vitro*, the same patients' leukocytes showed a marked loss of HPRT enzyme over a 96-hr period while control leukocytes showed a substantial increase in activity. Evidently the greater life span of the erythrocyte as compared to the leukocyte, and its inability to synthesize additional enzyme, permits a greater time for natural instability of mutant enzyme to become apparent. This observation suggests the possibility that simultaneous determination of enzyme activity in leukocytes and erythrocytes would allow detection of an unstable mutant enzyme.[21] It also holds forth the exciting possibility that agents able to stabilize or reactivate the mutant enzyme may be found and used for therapy.

Immunological Assessment

Antibody prepared against the HPRT enzyme, purified from normal human erythrocytes, has been used to determine whether or not the mutant cells contain a normal amount of HPRT protein that is enzymatically inactive but nevertheless capable of reacting with the antibody. All HPRT-deficient human cells so far tested have shown a normal amount of cross-reacting material,[7,10,21,226,227,276] thus eliminating from consideration the possibility of any of them being caused by a deletion mutation. The decrease in enzyme activity produced by incubating with antibody-containing serum and centrifugation is strong evidence that the antibody was indeed directed against active enzyme protein. Only in certain HPRT-deficient animal cell lines, including the mouse line A9 and the RAG line, is cross-reactive material absent.[303] By immunodiffusion, Arnold and Kelley[7] and Müller and Stemberger[227] demonstrated the same cross-reactive material in hemolysates of normal and Lesch–Nyhan cells.

Further comparisons of the normal and mutant protein in erythrocytes fractionated by age revealed no loss of immunoreactive HPRT protein from either the normal or mutant cells with aging *in vivo* despite the instability of the activity of mutant enzyme in comparison to the normal.[7] By contrast, the decrease in HPRT activity seen after heat treatment at 82°C is accompanied by a corresponding decrease in the amount of cross-reactive material (see below), presumably from denaturation of the enzyme proteins, suggesting that the loss of activity with aging observed in erythrocytes *in vivo* and that observed with heating are not entirely comparable processes.[7]

Activation

The simple mixing of normal and mutant HPRT enzyme failed to restore activity.[301] However, Bakay and Nyhan[18] have noted that exposure of the crude or partially purified mixture of normal and mutant enzyme to interaction with macromolecules by passage through a molecular sieve (Sephadex G25) or by electrophoresis on polyacrylamide gel resulted in a substantial increase in total activity. With use of ^{125}I for labeling of normal HPRT, he was able to show the transfer of label to the mutant HPRT, suggesting the possibility that activation may have occurred through recombination of normal and mutant subunits of the enzyme.[15,18]

Structural Gene Mutation

An impressive array of evidence has accumulated favoring the view that a structural gene mutation is responsible for the decrease in HPRT enzyme activity observed in this group of patients. The fact that small quantities of enzyme have been detected in all affected patients when a sufficiently sensitive method has been used[15,19] in erythrocyte hemolysates as well as in fibroblasts[112,174] provides a strong argument against the disorder resulting from genetic deletion. More direct evidence of structural gene mutations is provided by the wide range of enzyme activities observed in the different families,[93,173,177] the large differences in stability of the enzyme, both in erythrocytes *in vivo* and in response to heating *in vitro*,[112,173] and the differences in kinetic behavior with absence of product inhibition in some patients. The response of various mutant lines to these modalities provides a reasonable approach to classifying the various mutations in this enzyme, as shown in Table IV.[167] The consistent finding of cross-reactive material to antibody produced in response to purified human HPRT enzyme in all patients studied to date is additional evidence against this being a deletion or a regulator gene mutation.[303]

The possibility of a regulator gene in human cells has been raised by the appearance of a rodent HPRT enzyme from HPRT-deficient

TABLE IV. Proposed Classification of Human HPRT Mutations[a]

	Product inhibition[b]	Thermal stability[b]	Prototype (cell strain)[c]
Normal	+	+	
Mutant			
Type 1	+	+	193
Type 2	+	−	182, 197, 198, 199
Type 3	−	−	121

[a] From Kelley and Arnold.[167]
[b] +, Normal; −, abnormal.
[c] Cell strains described by Kelley and Mead.[174]

rodent cell lines following a variety of interspecies fusions including fusion with human cells (see below).[13,16,71,343] If such deletions or regulator gene mutations do indeed occur in the human species, they have not yet been detected. The possibility that complete absence of HPRT enzyme would be incompatible with full development during intrauterine life should be considered. Conceivably, cells other than the hematopoietic precursors (see section on heterozygote detection) might be subject to some further selective disadvantage by HPRT deficiency at crucial stages of intrauterine development. If this were so, the deletion defect would be expressed as an increased frequency of spontaneous abortion of 50% of male fetuses, with a resulting statistical predominance of female offspring in families carrying the gene. Such severe deletions, however, should be readily demonstrable by skin biopsy or hair root analysis in suspected heterozygotes who might also have gout (see below).

Mechanism of Excessive Rate of Purine Synthesis

The excessive rate of uric acid production of affected children reflects an excessive rate of purine synthesis presumably in virtually all body cells, rather than being linked to a single organ. An exception is the mature erythrocytes, all of which have lost the enzyme complement required for carrying out the *de novo* synthesis of purine nucleotides, although they have a full complement of enzymes including HPRT involved in the "salvage" pathway of purine nucleotide synthesis as well as most of the enzymes required for purine nucleotide interconversion with the exception of that required for the conversion of inosinic acid to adenylic acid.[79]

Cultured Fibroblasts

The demonstration that fibroblasts cultured from affected patients show an increased activity of the early enzymatic reactions of purine

TABLE V. Incorporation of ^{14}C-Formate into Formylglycinamide Ribonucleotide (FGAR) in Fibroblasts Cultured from Normal Subjects, from Patients with X-Linked Uric Aciduria, and from Patients with Gout[a]

Cells	Source		FGAR (cpm)
	Sex	Age (yr)	
Normal			
R. S.	Male	23	1710
G. C.	Male	21	1980
W. M.	Male	17	1870
G. R.	Female	15	1380
	Mean		1740
X-linked uric aciduria			
Lesch–Nyhan syndrome with virtually complete HPRT deficiency			
D. F.	Male	15	7320
F. H.	Male	15	8060
M. W.	Male	8	7100
J. S.	Male	3	7310
	Mean		7450
Gout with uric acid overproduction and normal HPRT			
B. P.	Male	27	6470
T. B.	Male	49	6320
	Mean		6400
Gout with normal uric acid production and normal HPRT. (R. McJ.)	Male	58	1620

[a] From Rosenbloom et al.[270] and Henderson et al.[146]

biosynthesis has greatly simplified the detailed study of the mechanism of this aberration.[270,301] A very useful index of the rate of these reactions is provided by the incorporation of ^{14}C-formate into the formylglycinamide ribonucleotide (FGAR) which accumulates as a result of the block to further metabolism produced by addition of the glutamine antagonist azaserine, as shown in Fig. 3.[42,193] The rate of ^{14}C-formate incorporation into FGAR found in HPRT-deficient fibroblasts was increased four- to sixfold over normal, an amount quite comparable to the degree of overproduction of uric acid found in the affected children (Table V). A ^{14}C-formate incorporation into nucleic acids, nucleotides, nucleosides, and free bases can also be used to evaluate synthesis *de novo*.[310] HPRT-deficient cells excrete hypoxanthine into the growth medium; consequently, hypoxanthine will show the highest specific activity.[65 a,310]

Feedback Control Mechanism

A feedback control mechanism has been proposed for regulation of the rate of purine biosynthesis from studies in both bacterial[121,140] and mammalian systems.[138,140,202,270,349] In this mechanism (Figs. 3 and 5), purine nucleotides act as allosteric inhibitors of the first and presumed rate-limiting reaction of purine biosynthesis catalyzed by the enzyme PP-ribose-P glutamine amidotransferase. The enzyme from human sources shows inhibition of activity by purine nucleotides both in crude cell extracts of lymphoblasts[348] and in a preparation purified some thirtyfold from human placenta.[153,155,156] Synthesis of purines *de novo* is also inhibited in patients *in vivo* by exogenous purines.[41,300]

As shown in Fig. 3, the HPRT enzyme is part of a cyclic mechanism for reutilization of free purine bases before their irreversible degradation to uric acid. Failure of the recharging part of the cycle through a decreased activity of HPRT enzyme could well result in a bleeding away of free purine bases and conceivably produce a lowering of the intracellular concentration of purine nucleotides and thereby release *de novo* synthesis from feedback inhibition. Such a mechanism has been proposed by Greene and Ishii[123] and by Sorenson.[315] Despite the attractiveness of the concept, no actual differences in the total intracellular concentration of adenine and guanine nucleotides were found in normal or mutant cultured fibroblasts.[270] Recent studies in which guanylic acid and guanosine diphosphate were also measured separately have also failed to reveal any significant differences in purine nucleotide concentrations.[58]

Allosteric Activation of Rate-Limiting Enzyme by Increased Concentrations of PP-Ribose-P

Another possible mechanism is suggested by the fact that the HPRT enzyme and the presumed rate-limiting enzyme PP-ribose-P glutamine amidotransferase share a common substrate, PP-ribose-P. Failure to utilize it in the HPRT reaction could reasonably result in its accumulation. Increased intracellular concentrations of PP-ribose-P have indeed been found in HPRT-deficient fibroblasts,[270] lymphoblasts,[237,346] neuroblastoma,[345] and erythrocytes,[129,285] and at the present time the increased PP-ribose-P concentration appears to be the principal mechanism responsible for the excessive rate of FGAR synthesis found in the three cultured cell lines. Studies on partially purified human PP-ribose-P glutamine amidotransferase demonstrated the effectiveness of PP-ribose-P in enhancing the rate of this presumably limiting enzyme.[142,153,155,156] Evidently, treatment of the enzyme with purine mononucleotides results in formation of an aggregated dimer of the enzyme showing lesser activity while treatment of the aggregate with PP-ribose-P results in a disaggregation with restoration to the more active monomeric form as shown in Fig. 5. Since children with the Lesch–Nyhan syndrome show a tenfold increase in the PP-ribose-P content of their erythrocytes, as well as more moderate increases in their leukocytes and cultured cells,[100,129,270,285,346] these data provide a very plausible molecular basis for the increased rate of purine synthesis observed in this disease, with the ratio of PP-ribose-P to purine nucleotide being the crucial determinant of the degree of activity of this presumed rate-limiting enzyme.

Corroborative Genetic Evidence of Primary Role of PP-Ribose-P

Further evidence has been found from another genetic disease in support of a primary role for PP-ribose-P concentration in regulation of purine biosynthesis. A small portion of patients with excessive purine

TABLE VI. Intracellular Concentration of Phosphoribosylpyrophosphate (PP-Ribose-P) in Fibroblasts of Patients with Excessive Purine
Synthesis[a]

Cell line	PP-ribose-P (nmoles/g)
Normal	0.853
Virtually complete deficiency of HPRT (Lesch–Nyhan syndrome)	3.59
Gout with normal HPRT	
B. P.	1.52
T. B.	1.34

[a] From Rosenbloom et al.[270] and Henderson et al.[146]

biosynthesis and normal HPRT enzyme activity have shown an increased intracellular concentration of PP-ribose-P in cultured fibroblasts[146,148,149,171] (Table VI). Since fibroblasts cultured from two such patients failed to show the normal degree of inhibition by feedback inhibitors, a primary defect in the responsiveness of the amidotransferase to feedback inhibition was proposed.[146] Subsequent studies, however, have shown that one of the two patients has a 2½- to threefold increase in activity of the enzyme PP-ribose-P synthetase in both erythrocytes and fibroblasts.[27–31]

The presence of an enhanced rate of purine synthesis was shown in both the patient and his gouty brother as well as in fibroblasts cultured from one of the brothers. Both erythrocytes and fibroblasts showed an enhanced rate of generation of PP-ribose-P and an increase in its intracellular concentration. The presence of the same increase in activity of the enzyme in erythrocytes of a clinically unaffected daughter who nevertheless excreted increased quantities of uric acid in the 24-hr urine suggests that it was dominantly inherited. This enzyme defect represents an unusual type of metabolic and genetic abnormality also in being associated with an increase in specific activity rather than a decrease in activity of an enzyme. The increased activity shown at all concentrations of inorganic phosphate and a normal responsiveness to purine nucleotide feedback inhibitors distinguishes it from an analogous but different mutational defect in the same enzyme observed earlier in another family.[85,319,322,323] The increased rate of purine synthesis found in patients with glycogen storage disease type I from a primary deficiency of glucose-6-phosphatase has also been postulated to result from an increased concentration of PP-ribose-P within the liver, but such an increase remains to be demonstrated.[33,171,292,294]

Corroborative Pharmacological Evidence of Primary Role of PP-Ribose-P

Further evidence of the importance of PP-ribose-P in control of the rate of purine biosynthesis has been found from the effect of various pharmacological agents that are able to diminish the intracellular concentration of PP-ribose-P. Orotic acid also consumes PP-ribose-P and produces a lowering of the intracellular concentration of PP-ribose-P correlated with a diminished rate of purine biosynthesis both in fibroblasts cultured *in vitro*[170] and in patients *in vivo*.[172] Nicotinic acid produces a concurrent lowering of the intracellular concentration of PP-ribose-P correlated with a diminished rate of purine synthesis *de novo* in cultured human fibroblasts.[57] Administration of allopurinol *in vivo*[103] and *in vitro*[169,180] diminishes both the intracellular concentration of PP-ribose-P and the rate of purine synthesis *de novo*. Conversely, a variety of substances that increase the intracellular concentration of PP-ribose-P also increase the rate of purine synthesis. These include glucose in high concentrations, methylene blue, inorganic phosphate, and certain trophic hormones.[181,287,292]

One of the additional consequences of an increased intracellular concentration of PP-ribose-P may be an increased rate of pyrimidine biosynthesis *de novo*. The rate of the first reaction of pyrimidine biosynthesis catalyzed by the enzyme carbamyl phosphate synthetase is substantially increased by PP-ribose-P.[333] An increased intracellular concentration of pyrimidine nucleotides, some four to six times normal, has been found in HPRT-deficient lymphoblasts cultured *in vitro*[238] and may very well be one of the secondary disturbances in metabolism created by the primary enzyme defect.

Role of PP-Ribose-P in Establishing Priorities in Purine Metabolism

The HPRT enzyme had been regarded by biochemists as merely providing a thrifty mechanism for the efficient reutilization of preformed purines.[140,229] At least six ATP molecules are expended in the synthesis of an intact purine nucleotide *de novo*, compared to just one via the salvage pathway. Therefore, a system to assure the preferential reutilization of purine nucleotides would obviously be of advantage to the energy economy of the cell. The importance of this enzyme, however, to normal function of the neurological system and to normal activity of the control mechanisms of purine biosynthesis was not appreciated until the clinical consequences of their deficit were observed in children affected with the Lesch–Nyhan syndrome. Considerable evidence has accumulated that certain organs of the body, including erythrocytes and bone marrow, must acquire supplemental nutrition with purine compounds formed within the liver and transported by the bloodstream to organs requiring them.[142,144,189,199,229] A mechanism built into the various PP-ribose-P-utilizing enzymes establishes very effectively the priority system. The enzyme APRT, as measured in cultured lymphoblasts,[348] has the highest affinity for PP-ribose-P with a K_m of 33 μM. The HPRT enzyme has the next lowest affinity with a K_m of 74 μM, and PP-ribose-P glutamine amidotransferase shows the lowest affinity with a concentration at half-maximal velocity $S_{0.5}$ of 300 μM, while the normal intracellular concentration of PP-ribose-P in lymphoblasts and other nucleated cells is on the order of $10 - 100$ μM[12,100,310] so that in the intracellular economy of limited availability of PP-ribose-P the purine reutilization pathway takes precedence over the *de novo* synthetic pathway. This relative priority of reactions is reflected in the fact that adenine is more effective than hypoxanthine or guanine in inhibiting purine synthesis *de novo* or in depleting PP-ribose-P.[138,140,270] The competition for PP-ribose-P and its determining role in giving priority to the reutilization pathway are indicated in Fig. 4.

Mechanism of Neurological Dysfunction

When compared with the state of knowledge of the mechanism by which the abnormal gene product leads to an excessive rate of purine biosynthesis, the state of our knowledge of the mechanism by which the enzyme defect produces the neurological dysfunction is very rudimentary. It is a particularly significant problem since this appears to be the only primary enzyme defect known in which a stereotyped form of behavior is produced.[240–243] An extension of our knowledge to include the detailed mechanisms producing such behavior could greatly increase our understanding of the genetic basis of behavior. The lack of detectable specific organic pathology in the brain of affected children at autopsy examination (see above) suggests a basic abnormality of function rather than structure. A reasonable hypothesis is that a reversible biochemical imbalance may be responsible for the disordered brain function.

Uric Acid and Oxypurines

The possibility that the high uric acid content of body fluids might in some way be responsible for the neurological dysfunction seems to be a particularly attractive hypothesis since uric acid is largely excluded from the cerebrospinal fluid to values less than 10% of those found in serum under normal conditions. However, the cerebrospinal fluid of affected children showed concentrations of uric acid that were not significantly different from those found in control subjects, as shown in Table VII.[272] Since uric acid is not normally formed within the central nervous system because of the absence in the brain tissue of xanthine oxidase, the possibility remained that the oxypurine precursors of uric acid, hypoxanthine, and xanthine might be present in increased amounts. This proved to be the case, with the concentration of oxypurines in the cerebrospinal fluid of affected children substantially higher than that of control subjects.[272] Furthermore, the cerebrospinal fluid of affected children showed a content of oxypurine significantly higher than that found in their plasma while the reverse situation obtained in control subjects. This was the first indication that the overproduction of purines observed in cultured cells and in the patients 24-hr urine might also be present in the nervous system. Subsequent studies have revealed excessive synthesis of purine nucleotides in a cultured line of HPRT-deficient mouse neuroblastoma cells.[345] Further evidence against uric acid or oxypurines playing a significant role in the genesis of the neurological dysfunction has been obtained from studies of patients receiving allopurinol. This drug inhibits the enzyme xanthine oxidase and thereby decreases the content of uric acid in both serum and urine and greatly increases the oxypurine content of both the plasma and the cerebrospinal fluid, yet its administration to children with the Lesch–Nyhan syndrome makes

TABLE VII. Oxypurine and Uric Acid Concentration in Plasma and Cerebrospinal Fluid of Patients with X-Linked Uric Aciduria[a]

Subjects	Number studied	Uric acid (mg/100 ml)			Oxypurines (mg/100 ml)		
		CSF	Plasma	Ratio CSF/plasma	CSF	Plasma	Ratio CSF/plasma
Control	7	0.29	4.28	0.07	0.13	0.18	0.72
Virtually complete HPRT deficiency	5	0.32	8.15	0.04	0.55	0.20	2.75
Incomplete HPRT deficiency	4						
F. L.		1.25	14.05	0.09	0.32	0.12	2.67
M. L.		0.39	9.77	0.04	0.45	0.15	3.00
T. J.		0.72	7.47	0.10	0.44	0.19	2.32
C. M.		1.25	10.9	0.11	0.23	—	—

[a] From Kelley et al.[173] and Rosenbloom et al.[272]

no detectable change in the severity of the neurological symptoms.[233,242,243,289] Even when started shortly after birth, allopurinol failed to prevent onset of neurological symptoms at the expected time.[212] The possibility that purine compounds may act in a manner similar to L-dopa has also been suggested.[258]

Pharmacologically Induced Self-Mutilation

A self-mutilating behavior in experimental animals that resembles in many ways the behavior of affected children can be produced by administering a variety of drugs. The methylated xanthines are effective. Caffeine in very high doses given to rats that are maintained on a semistarvation diet[52,240,257,288] or administration of theophylline to rabbits[239] produces a compulsive self-mutilation in which the animals bite away the tissues of their paws and feet.[52,240] The same symptoms in an exaggerated form leading to complete self-amputation of paws can be produced by administering amphetamines to rats pretreated with reserpine.[299] The mechanism by which these drugs produce this curious behavior is not known. The fact that either methylated xanthines or oxypurines can produce an increase in cyclic AMP in certain tissues suggests the possibility that this mechanism might be involved; however, no evidence has yet been presented that such a mechanism is indeed operating.

HPRT Enzyme Activity in Brain

Although the precise mechanism by which the HPRT mutation results in aberrant function of the central nervous system is not known, the available evidence suggests that it is from an intrinsic defect within the cells rather than being a secondary result of a circulating humoral agent. Determination of the distribution of HPRT enzymes within various organs of the body as shown in Table II has demonstrated the very high activity in the brain, particularly in the basal ganglia, of patients coming to autopsy or aborted fetuses.[56,272] However, in an autopsy of a patient with the Lesch–Nyhan syndrome and of an aborted fetus, the HPRT enzyme was undetectable in all tissues of the body that were measured, including the brain and the basal ganglia, despite substantial activity of the control enzymes APRT and guanase.[56,272] With more sensitive methods, however, small amounts of residual enzyme activity (Table II) were detectable in the brain and various tissues of an aborted fetus affected with the Lesch–Nyhan syndrome.[341]

It is worth noting in this connection that the clinical symptoms observed in these patients are generally referable to dysfunction of the basal ganglia, suggesting that this particular tissue is particularly susceptible to impaired function in the presence of deficient enzyme activity. The precise mechanism by which the HPRT activity leads to deficient neuronal function is quite unknown at the present time. Recent studies in which HPRT activity was found in synaptosomes have suggested a possible neurotransmitter function for the HPRT enzyme.[133,134]

Adrenergic Dysfunction

The overresponse of children with Lesch–Nyhan syndrome to emotions of excitement or anger has suggested an excessive adrenergic response to some observers.[292] In like manner, the self-mutilation, agitation, and "sham rage" produced by the methylated purines caffeine and theophylline as well as amphetamines furthered this type of speculation.[52,228,240] More definitive evidence of an adrenergic overactivity has been provided by Rockson et al.,[267a] who demonstrated a significantly increased activity of the enzyme dopamine-β-hydroxylase in the plasma of all six patients tested who showed choreoathetosis and self-mutilation, while four less severely affected patients who showed neither of these symptoms despite deficient HPRT enzyme showed dopamine β-hydroxylase activities of plasma within the normal range. Since this enzyme is released into the synaptic cleft along with the neurotransmitter norepinephrine, the increased activity of the enzyme in plasma is thought to reflect an increased activity of the sympathetic nervous system. An additional aberration in response of affected children showing self-mutilation was their failure to develop an increase in arterial pressure in response to the cold pressor test.[267a] These observations provide the first reproducible correlation of an experimental variable with the self-mutilating behavior. The amelioration of the self-mutilating behavior by administration of L-hydroxytryptophan suggests that a relative deficit of serotonin may well be involved.[221] The ability to develop cell lines originating from the nervous system and carrying the HPRT deficiency suggests a possible approach to be made for the elucidation of this problem.[345]

GENETIC SIGNIFICANCE

Genetic Heterogeneity

The many variations found not only in the clinical presentation of X-linked uric aciduria but also in the properties and activity of the mutant gene product, the HPRT enzyme, undoubtedly reflect to a large extent the wide range of mutational events that have occurred in this single gene. Together they emphasize the importance of genetic heterogeneity to both clinical medicine and basic genetics.[173] The diversity of clinical expression of these different mutations impinges on a wide range of clinical specialties. Consequently, the initial clinical presentation of patients with HPRT deficiency may draw the attention of not only the pediatrician but also the psychiatrist, neurologist, dentist, urologist, or rheumatologist, depending to a considerable extent on the locus within the gene of the mutational event and the consequent clinical expression.

The unifying influence of genetics in bringing together in one basic explanation the pathology of concern to such widely diverse practitioners of medicine holds an unusual germ of hope. Conceivably, further progress in identifying other disorders at the genetic level may lead to a unification and simplification in concept for disease states of significance to divergent areas of medicine that today seem entirely unrelated in pathogenesis.

X-Linked Inheritance

Pedigree

Although the pedigrees of affected males in families carrying the Lesch–Nyhan syndrome as shown in Fig. 8 are compatible with an X-

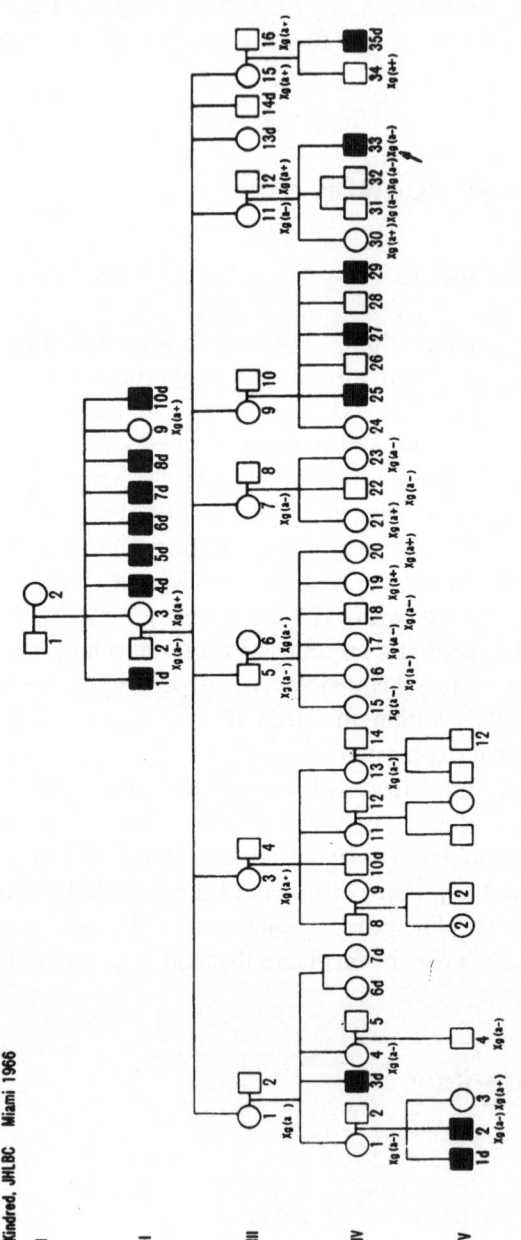

Fig. 8. Pedigree of family with the Lesch–Nyhan syndrome. From Greene et al.[128]

linked recessive pattern of inheritance,[192,240,242,246] they are equally compatible with a dominant inheritance with expression only in males. Failure of affected males to reproduce rules out the crucial test for distinguishing these two types of inheritance, that of absence of male-to-male transmission in X-linked diseases. Therefore, other evidence of X linkage was sought at a cellular level.

Demonstration of Single Active X Chromosome

The concept of the single active X chromosome in female somatic cells, first proposed by Dr. Mary Lyon in 1961[200] and independently by Dr. Ernest Beutler,[47] required the random inactivation of one of the two X chromosomes in female somatic cells at an early stage of embryonic development to form the Barr body (Fig. 9). A consequence would be the presence in somatic cells of heterozygous females of both normal and mutant cell phenotypes presenting as a mosaic. Such mosaicism had previously been demonstrated in the coat colors of female cats and mice,[200] and in the human X-linked disorders glucose-6-phosphate dehydrogenase deficiency[75] and granulomatous disease of childhood.[344] Fibroblasts cultured from the mothers of children with the Lesch–Nyhan syndrome and incubated with ³H-hypoxanthine also

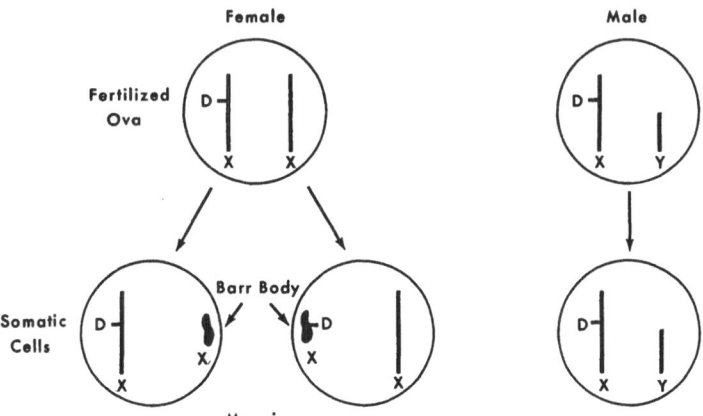

Fig. 9. The Lyon hypothesis. Compensation for the two X chromosomes in female cells is achieved by random inactivation at an early stage of fetal development to form the "Barr body" characteristic of female cells. Females heterozygous for an X-linked disorder "D" will therefore show mosaicism in their somatic cells. From Seegmiller.[292]

show both normal and mutant cells by direct autoradiography[271] (Fig. 10A), upon cloning,[216,282] or by selection using azaguanine.[98,217] The normal and mutant phenotypes have also been demonstrated in hair follicles of carrier females.[104,105,114,119,305] The inactivation of the X

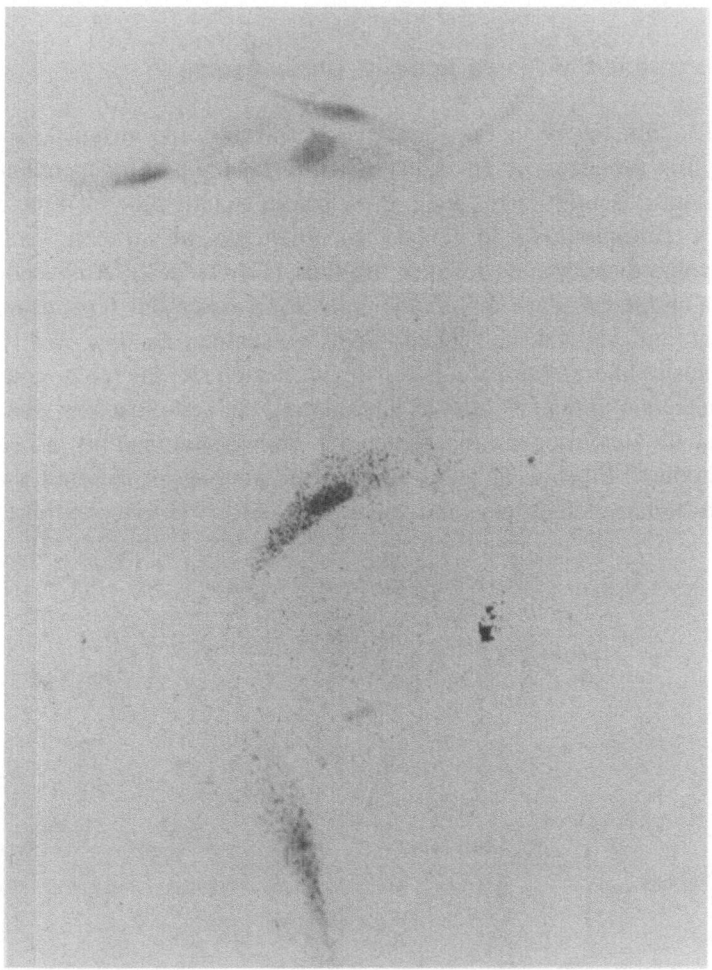

Fig. 10a

Fig. 10. Autoradiographs showing mosaicism in (A) fibroblasts cultured from a heterozygous mother and (B) amniotic cells cultured from a heterozygous fetus, 17 weeks' gestation. HPRT enzyme is required for

chromosomes occurs at a very early stage of development, well before the 17 weeks of gestation at which a heterozygous fetus was detected by culture of amniotic cells (Fig. 10B)[111] and is very stable with no detectable reactivation over many generations in culture.

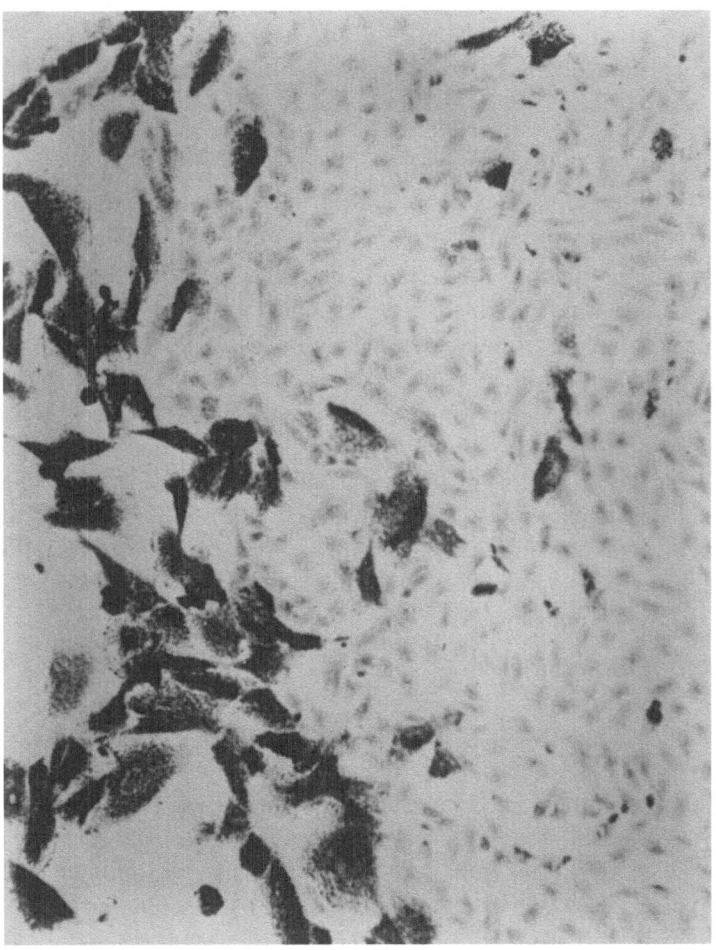

Fig. 10b

incorporation of tritiated hypoxanthine into cellular nucleic acid. Normal cells show incorporation by the presence of dense silver granules overlying the cells. Mutant cells show no such granules. From Fujimoto *et al.*[111]

Mapping of the X Chromosome

HPRT enzyme has also been used in genetic mapping of the X chromosome. The HPRT locus and the Xg locus were sufficiently distant that no linkage could be detected in eight informative matings in a total of 30 families[128] or in a single pedigree from the Netherlands.[80] Neither was it within linkage distance of Deutan color blindness in an Australian kindred.[95] Nabholz et al.,[230] using the progressive loss of human chromosomes from mouse–human hybrid cells, found the expected evidence of X linkage, which was confirmed by similar studies of Ruddle et al.[274,277–280] and others.[304] Studies using a 14/X translocation have provided evidence that the HPRT locus is on the long arm of the X chromosome between the locus for phosphoglycerate kinase (PGK) on the more proximal portion of the arm relative to the centromere and glucose-6-phosphate dehydrogenase on the more distal portion of the arm.[279] Evidence of a similar relationship of these genes has been obtained from studies of cells in a 19/X translocation by Gerald.[278] Relationship to banding patterns has also been determined. These results are somewhat at variance with those obtained by Grzeschik et al.,[131] who concluded that the HPRT and G6PD loci are located on the short arm of the X chromosome, based on studies of an infrequent segregation of HPRT and G6PD from the PGK locus in hybrids using human cells with the 14/X translocation, although assignment of these loci to the long arm was not entirely ruled out.

Chemical Selection

The varied uses found for the HPRT deficiency, by somatic cell geneticists, in the study of basic biological phenomena and genetic mechanisms have made this mutation a standard working tool in a wide variety of applications.[46,196,304] Fundamental to such use has been the ability to separate the normal from the mutant cell or to identify the phenotype by simple observations of growth in selective media.

Selective Survival of HPRT-Deficient Cells

Specific chemicals added to the growth medium permit the selective growth of either normal or the HPRT-deficient cells from a mixture of the two. The selective survival of HPRT-deficient cells in the presence of the purine analogues 6-thioguanine, 6-mercaptopurine, 8-azahypoxanthine, or 8-azaguanine actually permitted the isolation of this mutation in cultured lines of mammalian cells a number of years before the human mutation was identified clinically.[59,195,196,331,332] In order for the purine analogue to exert its lethal effects, it must be converted to the toxic purine nucleotide form by the HPRT enzyme.[142] Therefore, cells deficient in HPRT are able to survive doses of the analogue that are lethal to normal cells. This selective system has thus permitted the isolation of HPRT-deficient cells in a wide variety of types of mammalian cells,[46,59,86,118,252,284,345] including some human cells.[1,81,82,194,284] With use of azaguanine selection, most of the mutations show an incomplete deficiency of the enzyme, while use of 6-thioguanine as selective agent purportedly results in a higher proportion of more severe enzyme deficiencies. 6-Mercaptopurine has proven to be a less reliable selective agent.[299]

Selection against HPRT-Deficient Cells

Reverse selection systems directed against the HPRT-deficient cell have also been developed. Two chemical systems are both based on the fact that the mutant cells are dependent on purine synthesis via the *de novo* pathway for their continued survival in culture. Therefore, agents added to the culture medium that will inhibit purine synthesis *de novo* will permit growth only of normal cells containing the HPRT enzyme, provided that hypoxanthine or guanine is present in the culture medium. Cells so treated are, in a manner, analogous to auxotrophic mutants in bacteria and require preformed purines and appropriate enzymes for utilization of the purines in order to survive. Inhibition of *de novo* synthesis can be accomplished with the drug aminopterin, a folic acid antagonist which therefore confers an additional requirement for exogenous thymidine to be added to the growth medium along with increased quantities of glycine.[59,195,196,331,332] This mixture comprises the so-called HAT medium.

An alternative method for inhibiting purine synthesis *de novo* is by addition of the glutamine analogue azaserine.[42,113,193,302,306,307] The enzyme carrying out the amidation of formylglycinamide ribonucleotide is around ten times more sensitive to inhibition by azaserine than are the other glutamine-requiring reactions of purine synthesis *de novo*.[193] Either of these agents has been proven effective in permitting selective survival of normal cells in the presence of HPRT-deficient cells. The use of HPRT-deficient cells in studies involving cell fusion provides a convenient method for eliminating one parental cell type.[302,304,306] DeMars has proposed an ingenious scheme for obtaining a mouse strain deficient in HPRT by selecting for HPRT-deficient sperm *in vivo* through treating male mice with 8-azaguanine.[81] In initial unsuccessful trials, the dose required to inhibit spermatogenesis was very close to the lethal dose.[299] Using the above selective system, DeMars and Held[82] found a natural mutation rate of 5×10^{-6} per cell division in human fibroblasts.

Significance of Metabolic Cooperation

When used for selection of fibroblasts, the discrimination of either of these chemical systems of selection is blunted by the phenomenon of "metabolic cooperation"[106,113,325,326] in which the mutant cells growing in contact with the normal cells gain the ability to incorporate labeled nucleotides into their nucleic acids. In dense cultures of fibroblasts, the resulting cellular contact and metabolic cooperation thus permit survival of some mutant cells in the presence of azaserine or HAT medium by the "kiss of life," and in azaguanine- or thioguanine-selective systems the same cellular contact results in the "kiss of death" for any mutant cells in contact with normal cells.[113] Consequently, the fibroblast cultures must be appropriately disperse for fully effective selection to be accomplished by use of these selective agents.

Evidence of metabolic cooperation between cell types other than fibroblasts has also been presented.[248] Normal peripheral lymphocytes preincubated with ^{3}H-hypoxanthine washed and mixed with HPRT-deficient lymphocytes resulted in a substantial labeling of all cells shown by autoradiography, some being more heavily labeled than others. By use of normal female lymphocytes, specific identification of the HPRT-deficient male cells with substantial labeling was made possible by staining with quinacrine mustard to identify the fluorescent F body, i.e., the Y chromosome. A similar labeling occurred in HPRT-deficient lymphocytes or fibroblasts after mixing and intimate contact with normal erythrocytes prelabeled with ^{3}H-hypoxanthine. Surprisingly, contact of HPRT-deficient fibroblasts with cell membranes from both HPRT-deficient and normal erythrocytes or fibroblasts also purportedly resulted in a significant uptake of ^{3}H-inosinic acid from the medium into the deficient cell.[248] The explanation for the latter observation remains an enigma.

A variety of mechanisms have been proposed to account for metabolic cooperation. A cell-to-cell transfer of enzyme has been proposed based on a model system in which HPRT-deficient cells were grown in the presence of HPRT enzyme.[11] Evidence of a direct transfer of purine nucleotides has also been obtained.[67] Metabolic cooperation has been demonstrated between the HPRT-deficient and normal fibroblasts cultured from females heterozygous for the Lesch–Nyhan syndrome (see below) and could well provide a physical basis, at least in part, for the attenuation of the clinical symptoms of the disease in carrier females.[112]

Somatic Cell Genetics

Cell Fusion

The fusion of dissimilar cells in culture which occurs at low frequency spontaneously is greatly facilitated by inactivated Sendai virus. This procedure has proved to be a powerful technique for elucidating a variety of different types of biological problems, many of which are beyond the scope of this review. The facile combinations of human genes within the various cell types that are now possible give promise of greatly enhancing the degree of sophistication with which the human genome can be examined.[306] The selective loss of human chromosomes in man–mouse hybrids has allowed substantial progress to be made in assigning specific genes to the various chromosomes.[277,278,279]

The question of whether or not a tetraploid cell would tolerate two active X chromosomes was answered by fusion of glucose-6-phosphate dehydrogenase (G6PD) deficient fibroblasts with a ninefold greater number of HPRT-deficient cells using inactivated Sendai virus and a selective system consisting of azaserine and hypoxanthine to permit only normal cells to survive.[302,307] The fibroblasts severely deficient in glucose-6-phosphate dehydrogenase were cultured from a patient showing the Mediterranean variant with an accompanying hemolytic anemia. The G6PD deficiency was demonstrated histochemically by the failure to form granules using tetrazolium blue dye, and the HPRT deficiency was demonstrated autoradiographically by the failure to incorporate ^{3}H-hypoxanthine. Clones of cells that grew up from the fusion showed evidence of both enzymes, indicating that both X chromosomes remained active. In a similar manner, HPRT-deficient male fibroblasts having G6PD type A transformed with SV40 virus and fused to WI38 female fibroblasts having G6PD type B showed G6PD types A and B and the AB heteropolymeric form of G6PD in the tetraploid cells, indicative of two active X chromosomes.[70]

Genetic Control of HPRT Expression

Cell fusion of different species has also produced a correction of HPRT deficiency and has, in addition, introduced a new method for studying regulation of HPRT gene expression.[53] After fusion of mouse A9 cells deficient in HPRT with nucleated chick erythrocytes and selection with HAT medium, Schwartz et al.[286] recovered cells with HPRT enzyme that showed electrophoretic characteristics similar to those of chick HPRT. Furthermore, the resulting cells showed only mouse chromosomes and expressed no chick cell surface antigens and had a high rate of reversion to HPRT-deficient cells. Similar results were obtained when A9 cells were fused with frog erythrocytes or when HPRT-deficient Chinese hamster cells were fused with chick erythrocytes.[53] Presumably only a small cytologically unidentifiable segment of the chicken or frog genome has been incorporated by the recipient cells.[53,286] Klinger and Shin[183] subsequently showed that the rapid reversion to HPRT-deficient cells resulted from modulation of enzyme expression by presence or absence of aminopterin in the growth medium rather than by selection of cell revertants. Evidently, the avian gene for HPRT that is normally expressed constitutively becomes inducible by aminopterin when integrated into a mammalian cell. Whether a similar modulation of gene expression can account for the lack of correlation between the cell ploidy and the frequency of formation of surviving colonies after 8-azaguanine and other types of chemical selection noted by Harris[137] and by Metzger-Freed[214] remains to be determined. Selective transfer of heterologous genetic material into a mammalian cell has also been achieved with isolated chromosomes.[201] Shin[303] found no evidence of HPRT protein in two stable HPRT-deficient mouse cell lines A9 and RAG that would cross-react with antibody to normal mouse HPRT despite a small but detectable amount of residual enzyme activity in A9 that was clearly different from the normal in heat lability and substrate affinity. Since both cell lines show a low frequency of reversion to the normal phenotype, he proposes that A9 results from a missence mutation in the HPRT gene, while RAG carries a recessive regulatory mutation. A significant degree of restoration of mouse HPRT enzyme activity has also been obtained by fusion of HPRT-deficient mouse 1R cells with chick embryo fibroblasts[13] or with human HPRT-deficient fibroblasts.[71] A possible regulator gene activity in the human cells is one of several possible explanations of these results. A marked increase in HPRT activity in response to phytohemagglutinin stimulation of the lymphocytes from the peripheral blood of a patient with Lesch–Nyhan syndrome[78,79] was demonstrated by De Bruyn and Oei. Such an effect might well be expected if the newly synthesized enzyme is active but very unstable at 38°C. Whatever the cause, HPRT enzyme reappeared on attempted hybridization with a human cell line.[343]

A number of attempts have been made to use cell fusion of HPRT-deficient fibroblast lines from different families to detect genetic complementation. Fujimoto et al.[110] were unsuccessful in finding any restoration of HPRT activity by fusing all combinations of fibroblasts from eight unrelated families. Hösli et al.[157] attempted a similar complementation analysis in families.

Preventive Control through Prenatal Diagnosis

Detailed studies of the biochemical and genetic basis of the disease have provided the means for implementing a preventive program for its control. Successful demonstration of X-linked inheritance at a cellular level by proof of the presence of both the normal and mutant cell phenotypes in heterozygous females as predicted by the Lyon hypothesis[271] provided a diagnostic test that could be used with cultures of amniotic cells obtained by amniocentesis around the midpoint of gestation[111] (Fig. 10), thus opening the possibility of preventive control of this disease through prenatal diagnosis and gestational management.[73,83,108,219] In fact, the feasibility of this preventive approach has now been demonstrated. We have monitored 17 pregnancies at risk for the Lesch–Nyhan syndrome and have detected six affected male fetuses, in each case sufficiently early that the parents' desire to terminate the pregnancy could be met.[56,299,341] Affected twins have also been identified *in utero* but at too late a stage in the pregnancy to permit its termination.[83] The urate content of amniotic fluid has not been consistently helpful in diagnosis.[56,87,213,222,299] The application, in a similar manner, of other biochemical tests of abnormal gene products in cultured amniotic cells has now opened the possibility of prenatal diagnosis and similar preventive control of over 50 previously untreatable serious metabolic diseases[32,88,219,231,259] in the short space of 6 years since the initial demonstration of the feasibility of applying biochemistry to determination of fetal genotype *in utero*.

Characteristics of the Heterozygous State

The mosaicism of normal and mutant cells characteristic of the heterozygous state for HPRT deficiency as a consequence of the random inactivation of one X chromosome is found in fibroblasts, epithelial cells, and hair follicles (see above) but shows a curious sparing of the hematopoietic system. As a consequence, mothers of children with the Lesch–Nyhan syndrome show normal activity of HPRT in their erythrocytes[143,165,173] and in their leukocytes,[74] making the standard HPRT enzyme assay of blood samples of no value for identification of heterozygous family members. Erythrocytes from a carrier female whose cultured fibroblasts showed heterozygosity for an electrophoretic variant of another X-linked marker, glucose-6-phosphate dehydrogenase, nevertheless showed only one type of glucose-6-phosphate dehydrogenase in her red blood cells.[244] In a similar manner, McDonald and Kelley[204] found no evidence of the mutant enzyme in erythrocytes from the mother of a child with Lesch–Nyhan syndrome who himself showed a readily detectable enzyme with low affinity for substrates. These results could result either from a specific inactivation of the defective X chromosome or from a selective elimination of hematopoietic precursor cells of mutant phenotype at an early stage of fetal development. The latter theory appears to be the more reasonable of the two. However, the survival of the same cells in affected children poses an unexplained problem. McKeran *et al.*[207] report fewer and smaller colonies of myeloid progenitor cells growing *in vitro* from bone marrow of affected patients. Only in females carrying a mutation for substantially less severe deficiencies of the enzyme associated with marked attenuation of the clinical symptoms do we find evidence of intermediate levels of the enzyme in peripheral erythrocytes or leukocytes, although they still show evidence of an excessive rate of purine biosynthesis.[92,94,96]

Another curious observation is an increased thermal stability of APRT enzyme in heterozygotes.[94,139,143,173,330] The observation by Gordon *et al.*[120] of an increase in concentration of PP-ribose-P of erythrocytes of some but not all heterozygotes probably does not fully explain the stabilization since it was correlated fairly well with a diminished activity of HPRT in erythrocytes of the heterozygotes. By contrast, the erythrocytes of the heterozygotes with heat-stable APRT first described showed normal HPRT activity.[139,143]

The frequency of mothers of affected children showing heterozygosity for HPRT deficiency is substantially greater than would be expected from theoretical considerations.[105] Since children with the full syndrome fail to reproduce, equilibrium of the gene pool of the population would require one-third of the cases of HPRT deficiency to be new mutations to compensate for the genes thereby lost.

The random nature of the inactivation of the X chromosome (see above) makes it possible that heterozygous females could vary widely in not only the number of mutant cells in their body but also the relative proportion of normal and mutant cells in various organs. Sufficient involvement of the central nervous system to give rise to impairment in neurological function is therefore theoretically possible. However, to date only one mentally retarded heterozygous female has been observed and another such female showed a tremor on writing.[299] But these considerations suggest that mothers of affected children should have a careful examination of neurological functions for detection of subtle abnormalities. The fact that heterozygous females show excessive incorporation of glycine-1-^{14}C into urinary uric acid despite, in many cases, a normal concentration of urate in the serum provides additional evidence that a substantial portion of the heterozygote's body cells are mutant.[92,94,96,173]

Pharmacological Consequences of HPRT Deficiency

The role of the HPRT enzyme in converting a variety of purine analogues to their metabolically active ribonucleotide form provides the basis for a variety of aberrant responses to these substances. In fact, an unexplained failure of the drug azathioprine to produce a decrease in purine synthesis in children with the Lesch–Nyhan syndrome[179,313,314,316] provided the first clinical indication that led eventually to the identification of the primary enzyme defect.[179,247,272,301] Gouty patients who overproduce uric acid show a marked diminution in total purine synthesis when treated with azathioprine in moderate doses,[313] as do those with normal production, when tested by glycine-1-^{14}C incorporation into urinary uric acid;[179] whereas children with the Lesch–Nyhan syndrome fail to show this inhibition of purine synthesis.[301,316] Likewise, fibroblasts cultured *in vitro* from affected children fail to show the normal inhibition of *de novo* purine synthesis in response to 6-mercaptopurine, an intermediate to which azathioprine is degraded, at least in part, during its metabolism in the human subject.[270,301] In the search for the cause of this difference in response, the gross deficiency of the enzyme HPRT was hypothesized and eventually proven.[301]

The deficiency of HPRT also produces a number of other aberrant responses. As might be expected, in normal lymphocytes 6-mercaptopurine prevents the stimulation of incorporation of tritiated hypoxanthine into nucleic acids in response to exposure to phytohemagglutinin. By contrast, lymphocytes from children with the Lesch–Nyhan syndrome fail to be inhibited by 6-mercaptopurine.[60] Evidently, the HPRT enzyme is required for conversion of 6-mercaptopurine to the inhibitory nucleotide form required presumably for turning off purine synthesis and thereby preventing new DNA formation and cell division.

Detailed studies of the aberrant response of patients with X-linked uric aciduria to allopurinol have provided insight into one of its unexpected beneficial secondary effects.[178] The primary effect of allopurinol in blocking xanthine oxidase activity[91,182,281,318] is not altered by deficiency of HPRT activity. However, it does alter a secondary response. In most patients who overproduce uric acid, treatment with allopurinol not only blocks uric acid formation but, as a secondary beneficial therapeutic effect, also substantially diminishes the excessive rate of purine synthesis.[65,91,182,281] As a consequence, all patients with HPRT deficiency show in their 24-hr urine essentially a stoichiometric substitution of the oxypurine precursors of uric acid, hypoxanthine, and xanthine for the deficit in uric acid excretion produced by allopurinol, as shown in Fig. 11.

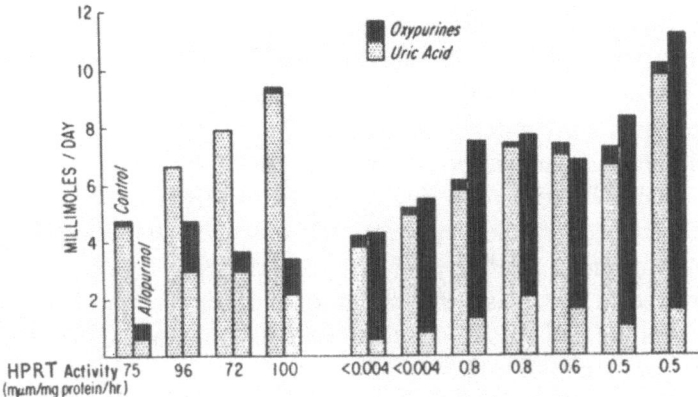

HPRT Activity 75   96   72   100   <0.004 <0.004 0.8   0.8   0.6   0.5   0.5
(mμm/mg protein/hr)

Fig. 11. Effect of allopurinol on total purine excretion in patients who produce excessive quantities of uric acid and its relationship to erythrocyte hypoxanthine-guanine phosphoribosyltransferase (HPRT) activity in each patient. The total height of each bar represents total purine excretion, oxypurines plus uric acid, in millimoles per day. From Kelley et al.[173]

The mechanism of the inhibition of total purine synthesis by allopurinol is not precisely known, but it must require a functionally active HPRT enzyme. Three possible mechanisms have been considered, each one requiring HPRT enzyme. Allopurinol administration produces a substantial decrease in intracellular concentration of PP-ribose-P in erythrocytes both *in vivo*[103] and *in vitro* and in cultured fibroblasts[168,169,180] that is dependent on the presence of HPRT enzyme.[100–102] The resulting ribonucleotide of allopurinol formed by the HPRT enzyme is then dephosphorylated and excreted as the ribonucleosides.[185] A decreased rate of purine nucleotide synthesis could thereby result from PP-ribose-P depletion as with other substances that deplete intracellular PP-ribose-P.[100,129,180,285]

The observation that allopurinol ribonucleotide is itself a potent inhibitor of the presumed rate-limiting reaction of purine biosynthesis catalyzed by the enzyme glutamine PP-ribose-P amidotransferase provides a second possible mechanism for the inhibitory action.[153,202] Inhibition of the same enzyme by the natural nucleotides of hypoxanthine, xanthine, adenine, or guanine is the basis for the postulated feedback control mechanism for controlling the rate of purine biosynthesis.[140] The higher extracellular concentrations of hypoxanthine and xanthine produced by allopurinol administration could well serve to activate this natural feedback mechanism by increasing the formation of the natural nucleotide inhibitors and further depleting the intracellular PP-ribose-P as a third possible mechanism. In each case, HPRT enzyme would be required.

Another curious response of the HPRT-deficient state is still unexplained. The rate of purine synthesis of HPRT-deficient children is increased even further by very high doses of allopurinol.[327] In an analogous manner, relatively small doses of hypoxanthine or guanine administered to fibroblasts *in vitro* produce a stimulation of the rate of purine synthesis in HPRT-deficient cells but an inhibition of purine synthesis in normal fibroblasts.[180,270]

DIAGNOSIS OF X-LINKED URIC ACIDURIA

Clinical Signs

The earliest clinical sign of the complete Lesch–Nyhan syndrome is one that is generally regarded as inconsequential. Neither parents nor physicians commonly regard the appearance of brownish-orange "sand" in the diapers as an ominous sign, yet such a history is obtained by specific questioning of the mothers in a remarkably high proportion of the cases. Obviously, more professional and public education is needed to alert both physicians and parents to the possible significance of this most unusual sign. The simple screening test described below should be applied to the urine of any child who shows such sand.

Complete Lesch–Nyhan Syndrome

The complete clinical syndrome of diminished growth, mental retardations, spasticity, choreoathetosis, and compulsive self-mutilation of the hands, fingers, lips, and tongue is sufficently unusual that, in most cases, a presumptive diagnosis can be made on clinical appearance alone. If the patient has a history of renal lithiasis, passage of sludge in the urine composed of uric acid, recurrent unexplained fever, episodes of anuria, hematuria, uncontrollable vomiting, and a family history of similarly afflicted males among maternal relatives, the likelihood of a correct diagnosis is enhanced. A possible history of attacks of acute monarticular arthritis in either the patient or maternal relatives should also be explored, although gouty arthritis is a rather infrequent accompaniment of the disorder in childhood. However, in occasional patients it can be the most prominent feature of the disease.[63,267] In view of the remarkably large production of uric acid and sustained hyperuricemia, a more frequent clinical presentation of this facet of the disease might be expected. Presumably the explanation lies in the failure of most children to survive into adult life when susceptibility to development of gout becomes greater.[292,349] In the less severely affected families, the clinical presentation may be limited to uric acid renal lithiasis.

Variant Expression

The major difficulty in diagnosis is found in the highly variable degree of clinical expression of some features of the syndrome from one family to another. The compulsive self-mutilation, although the most dramatic and compelling feature of the disease, is also the least consistently expressed. The fact that attenuation of the neurological symptoms of mental retardation, choreoathetosis, and spasticity is also found in certain families makes reliance on clustering of clinical presentation a very unreliable method for detection of variant forms of the disease and increases the need for more frequent use of laboratory tests beginning with relatively simple ones.

Laboratory Tests

Urine Examination

The most consistent feature of the disorder present in all affected patients remains the excessive production of uric acid, which accounts for its eponym of "X-linked uric aciduria" to cover the full range of clinical presentation. Therefore, laboratory tests that evaluate or reflect the excessive uric acid production must be used in a routine screening manner if all cases of HPRT deficiency are to be detected. Routine laboratory results supporting the diagnosis are the presence of uric acid crystalluria and hyperuricemia. The most reliable routine test generally available is the determination of the uric acid and creatinine contained in the 24-hr urine. Children with the Lesch–Nyhan syndrome show a 24-hr excretion of uric acid ranging from 20 to 70 mg per kilogram of body weight.

Screening Test

Since 24-hr urine collections are difficult to obtain, particularly from small children and infants, a screening test applied to morning or random urine samples has been evaluated.[163] The ratio of uric acid to creatinine is substantially elevated, with a range in the newborn period substantially greater than 2.7.[163] As shown in Fig. 6, normal infants show a rapid decline during the first year of life, a less precipitous further decline during the next decade, and a relatively constant ratio after age 15 into adult life with a mean value of 0.35 and with 0.60 as the upper range of normal, as shown in Table VIII.

TABLE VIII. Urinary Uric Acid/Creatinine Ratio as an Index of Purine Overproduction[a]

Classification	Number of patients	Mean ± s.d.	Range
Normal control subjects	41	0.34 ± 0.10	0.21–0.59
Gout	89	0.36 ± 0.14	0.15–0.73
Excrete < 600 mg urinary uric acid per 24 hr	64	0.32 ± 0.11	0.15–0.73
Excrete > 600 mg urinary uric acid per 24 hr	25	0.45 ± 0.14	0.28–0.73
Hyperuricemia[b]	41	0.53 ± 0.30	0.25–1.77
Blood dyscrasias	10	0.75 ± 0.45	0.33–1.77
Glycogen storage disease	6	0.74 ± 0.28	0.37–1.17
Other	25	0.39 ± 0.10	0.25–0.64
Nongouty arthritis	10	0.38 ± 0.11	0.27–0.58
Other conditions[c]	15	0.40 ± 0.15	0.26–0.80
Patients with gout and partial HPRT deficiency	8	1.06 ± 0.43	0.62–2.00
Complete HPRT deficiency	13	3.19 ± 1.00	1.98–5.35

[a] From Kaufman et al.[163]

[b] Patients with hyperuricemia but no clinical gout and those with hyperuricemia associated with another disorder, e.g., leukemia or glycogen storage disease.

[c] Including obesity, Fanconi's syndrome, Werner's syndrome, histidinemia, Wilson's disease, hyperlipoproteinemia, diabetes mellitus, Down's syndrome, and erythroderma ichthyosiforme congenitum in one 7-year-old girl.

The values obtained for uric acid/creatinine ratio are substantially higher than normal for all children with the Lesch–Nyhan syndrome.[163] Cerebral palsy clinics, mental retardation clinics, and neurology clinics might very appropriately include the ratio of uric acid to creatinine in a casual urine sample as part of the routine workup of patients. In addition to the screening test performed on liquid urine samples, a modification has been described in which urine is blotted onto Schuell No. 903 filter paper either after passage or, for infants or young children not toilet trained, by placing the filter paper in an appropriate position inside the diaper.[206] The paper is then dried for shipping and storage, and the uric acid and creatinine are determined after elution in a small volume of phosphate buffer.[206] A pilot procedure for examining urine from patients in mental hospitals and mental retardation and cerebral palsy clinics is currently under way.[90] Additional screening tests that have been described include a determination of the concentration of uric acid in urine, with any sample showing a concentration greater than 0.9 mg/ml being subject to creatinine analysis as well.[45] A microbiological test system, based on the high hypoxanthine content of urine of affected children, has also been proposed but has not yet been fully tested.[232]

Blood Examination

Hyperuricemia is present in well over 90% of patients.[136] An occasional patient may have normal serum urate concentration at times. Therefore, a serum urate in the normal range does not completely rule out the Lesch–Nyhan syndrome.

Once a high ratio of uric acid to creatinine has been detected in the urine screening test, the diagnosis should be unequivocally confirmed by demonstration of a gross deficiency of HPRT enzyme activity in washed erythrocyte lysate. A qualitative screening test using blood samples obtained by fingerstick blotted onto filter paper and dried before shipping has also been described for possible institutional use.[109] The normal enzyme activity of erythrocytes in heparinized blood samples is stable at room temperature for several days, thus allowing the bloods to be shipped via air mail or air express to a central laboratory equipped and staffed to perform the quantitative assay. Samples are stable for a longer period of time if stored in the refrigerated state. If the determination is to be postponed, the washed erythrocytes are best stored frozen along with a control sample from a normal subject. The increased activity of APRT is confirmatory evidence as well as an internal control.

Methods for HPRT Enzyme Determination

A large number of methods have been described for measuring the HPRT enzyme. Most procedures involve reacting the enzyme with ^{14}C-labeled hypoxanthine or guanine and PP-ribose-P in the presence of magnesium ion, followed, after deproteinization, by the physical separation of the ^{14}C-nucleotide formed and counting in a liquid scintillation counter. A variety of separation procedures have been devised. Although we initially[301] used high-voltage electrophoresis on paper in a 0.05 M borate buffer, pH 9.0, we have since found that chromatography on thin-layer cellulose sheets developed with carrier nucleotides in 1.6 M LiCl for 10 min is more convenient and requires less laboratory space.[56] Nucleotides are visualized by inspection under ultraviolet light, cut out, and counted. A micromethod has been described by Hösli et al.[157] and used for analysis of enzyme content of single cells. A spectrophotometric method has also been described based on the assessment of comsumption during the reaction of hypoxanthine or guanine determined spectrophotometrically with xanthine oxidase.[235,299] Qualitative screening tests for use with blood samples spotted onto filter paper and dried have been devised both with[109] and without[54] radioactive substrate. A rapid system for detection of mutant cells uses the ratio of incorporation of hypoxanthine or guanine as compared to adenine.[73,265] A very sensitive automated procedure using gel electrophoresis has been developed by Bakay et al.[14,19] in which the insoluble lanthanum salt of nucleotides is formed. It determines both APRT and HPRT and detects electrophoretic variants. The wide variety of concentrations of reactants, as well as pH of buffer, that have been used for the assay by various investigators are listed in Table IX. Inspection of Table IX, Table III, and Fig. 4 shows the desirability, if K_m mutations are to be detected, of doing determinations of mutant enzyme activity at low substrate concentrations as well as at the usual saturating concentrations.

The determinations of HPRT activity in disrupted fibroblasts and

TABLE IX. Concentration of Reagents Used by Various Investigators in HPRT Assay Compared to Affinity Constants

Buffer used	Hypoxanthine used (mM)	Guanine used (mM)	PP-ribose-P used (mM)	Magnesium used (mM)	Source
55 mM Tris-HCl, pH 7.4	0.6	0.14	1.0	5.0	Kelley et al.[177]
—	0.1	0.1	1.0–10	1.0	McDonald and Kelley[203]
40 mM Tris buffer	0.56	—	0.9	4.0	Boyle et al.[56]
55 mM Tris-HCl buffer, pH 8.5	0.4	0.2	2.0	5.0	Emmerson et al.[94]
—	0.18	0.18	—	—	Kogut et al.[184]
225 Tris HCl pH 7.7	0.1	—	5.0	0.6–5.0	Benke et al.[38]
50 mM Tris, pH 7.4	0.6	0.14	1.0	5.0	Benke et al.[40]
100 mM Tris-HCl, pH 7.4	10	—	0.25	10.0	Francke et al.[104]
10 mM Tris-HCl, pH 7.4	0.005–0.010	—	0.25	10	Bakay and Nyhan[15]
55 mM Tris buffer, pH 7.4	0.6	0.14	1.0	5.0	Seegmiller et al.[301]

in other cell lines are complicated by the presence of the 5'-nucleotidase, which degrades the inosinic acid formed to inosine.[112,174] Nucleotidase activity can be inhibited to some extent by thymidine triphosphate.[112] An alternative solution is to measure the incorporation of ^{14}C-hypoxanthine or guanine into both nucleotides and nucleosides, using as a control for the activity of phosphorylase a reaction mixture containing ethylenediaminetetraacetic acid to inhibit the HPRT reaction.[57]

Excessive production of uric acid has been found in a variety of other disorders, including autistic behavior in a child,[245] encephalopathy,[158] seizures,[66] benign symmetrical lipomatosis,[127] and peripheral neuropathy.[268]

Heterozygote Detection

The most essential component of a preventive program for control of the disease through prenatal diagnosis is identification and genetic counseling of all female relatives of child-bearing age to alert them to the need for amniocentesis if they are to avoid producing an affected child. All female relatives of child-bearing age should be tested for heterozygosity. A 3-mm full-thickness skin biopsy specimen, taken with local anesthesia after skin preparation with PHisohex and alcohol, should immediately be placed in a tube of sterile culture medium and shipped to a specially designated laboratory prepared to culture fibroblasts and perform autoradiography to detect the presence of both normal and mutant cells characteristic of the heterozygote as shown in Fig. 10. Whenever possible, mutant cells from the propositus should be used along with normal cells and cells being tested each plated in individual compartments on the same slide for comparison in the autoradiographic procedure.[56] If, for some reason, culture medium is not immediately available, AB-positive human serum is a perfectly adequate substitute for maintaining viability during shipment.[299] Azaguanine selection has also been used to demonstrate the presence of mutant cells in cultured skin fibroblasts[98,217] but is best accompanied by enzyme determination as well. Biopsy samples remain viable at room temperature in medium for at least 7 days and probably longer if refrigerated.

Examination of hair follicles is also a practical approach for heterozygote detection.[104,105,114,305] Its utility has been expanded with the demonstration that it can also be performed on desiccated samples after shipment since the enzyme remains active in the dried state.[104] Hair samples are plucked from the head and inspected to make certain that the bulb-shaped root is attached to the shaft. About 30 root bulbs with 2 or 3 cm of the hair shaft are then placed in a sterile bottle and shipped by mail or air express to a central laboratory for HPRT enzyme assay of each one. Enzyme activity of hair root bulbs remains stable for up to 14 days when they are stored dry at room temperature and for at least 2 months when frozen.

Both of the above procedures are tedious, however, and involve a great deal of laboratory effort, and a more simple method for heterozygote detection is needed. Nevertheless, they are at least 90% effective in our hands in identifying heterozygotes. From theoretical considerations of the random nature and the very early stage in fetal development of the X inactivation, certain areas of the body could very well fail to show mosaicism, thus, in theory, reducing the reliability of the test for heterozygosity. Since the risk of amniocentesis to either fetus or mother is extremely small, we recommend that each pregnancy of all female relatives should be monitored until the full reliability of the heterozygote detection systems can be more thoroughly evaluated.

TREATMENT

General Measures

Nutrition

Many children with the Lesch–Nyhan syndrome show evidence of nutritional deprivation, particularly if they have been residing in an understaffed institution. A complete inability to feed themselves, coupled with their tendency to regurgitate, undoubtedly contributes to this state. With excellent nursing care, adequate nutrition, and a secure, loving environment, the tendency to both self-mutilation and spasticity is diminished.

Physical Measures

Contractures appear to respond to physical therapy to some extent. A variety of approaches have been used to prevent the children from biting their fingers, including use of large bandages or mittens over the hands or restraining the hands by tying them to the bed or wheelchair. The most satisfactory approach to this problem, in our experience, has been to construct loosely fitting, wraparound splints for the elbows. Plastic or wooden ribs are placed in fabric pockets with Velcro or snap fasteners to allow adjustment to the desired tightness. Such splints permit the children to use their hands and arms but prevent them from bringing their hands to their mouths.

Dental

A dentist can often be of substantial help in eliminating sites of chronic irritation in the mouth by removing the sharp edges from offending teeth or extracting them.

Medications

Although no drugs have yet been found to treat effectively all of the symptoms of the disease, some aspects can be controlled quite effectively with medications. The drug allopurinol, a xanthine oxidase inhibitor, is very effective in controlling the clinical problems resulting from excessive uric acid production and hyperuricemia.[281,289,318] For most patients, a dose of 10 mg per kilogram of body weight produces a dramatic decrease in the serum urate concentration.[289] The ultimate dose should be precisely adjusted to bring the serum urate eventually to the normal range. The uric acid precursors hypoxanthine and xanthine replace a substantial portion of the uric acid excreted in the daily urine (see above), thus reducing the tendency to form renal calculi composed of uric acid.[178,182,210,223,281] Such treatment is also capable of diminishing significantly the size of renal calculi composed of uric acid.[210,242,299] The fact that xanthine is less soluble than is uric acid in urine results in some tendency to form urinary concretions composed of xanthine. In three patients this has appeared as gravel in the urine[126,242,298,314] and in four additional patients as frank calculi.[210,220,299] This tendency can be diminished by assuring a high fluid intake of at least 50 ml/kg/day. Some additional benefit may also result from alkalinizing the urine. As noted above, allopurinol fails to diminish the rate of total purine synthesis in patients with the Lesch–Nyhan syndrome as it does in patients with excessive uric acid production from other causes.[178] Its metabolic product oxypurinol inhibits *de novo* purine synthesis in HPRT-deficient fibroblasts[180] but remains to be fully evaluated for this effect *in vivo*, where it conceivably could reduce the tendency to form xanthine concretions.

Unfortunately, the most disabling feature of the disease, the neurological dysfunction, remains beyond rational therapy. The drug diazepam (Valium) appears to help reduce the spasticity and athetosis as with other forms of cerebral palsy.[289] Allopurinol begun as early as 4 days of age failed to alter the development of the neurological dysfunction in two patients,[212,242] and improvement first attributed to allopurinol[233] has not been observed with other patients and most likely resulted from general improvement in nutrition and nursing care.[242,292] The use of a variety of additional agents has been attempted. A drug that is a very potent inhibitor of excessive purine synthesis of the cultured mutant fibroblasts, 6-methylmercaptopurine ribonucleoside,[270] produced toxic symptoms at a dose that was ineffective in diminishing excessive purine synthesis in an affected child.[299] 2,6-Diaminopurine has also been attempted as treatment without benefit.[299] Although improvement has been reported after administration of monosodium glutamate,[116,117] the results obtained are difficult to distinguish from the generally beneficial effects produced by a secure environment and improved nutrition. It is worth noting that monosodium glutamate may not be without potential danger in treatment of developing infants, since it produces brain lesions and obesity in developing mice.[249]

The report of requirements for increased folic acid and adenine for optimal growth of HPRT-deficient fibroblasts[83] led to a clinical evaluation of treatment with these two agents.[37,41] Identical twins with the Lesch–Nyhan syndrome identified prenatally were both treated from the first day of life with 15 mg of folic acid per day, with one of them receiving, in addition, adenine at 10 mg/kg/day. The central nervous system dysfunction developed in both children.[41] In another child, adenine treatment from 20 days of age, at maximally tolerated doses of 60 mg/kg/day, along with allopurinol for the first year of life failed to prevent development of neurological dysfunction.[285] Older children showed no significant clinical improvement in the disease,[236,242,285] and an older child developed acute renal failure during treatment with adenine.[64,236]

Detailed evaluation failed to demonstrate any beneficial effects on motor performance from exchange blood transfusion or administration of adenine and allopurinol, tetrabenazine, thiopropazate, or chlorpromazine.[343a] Increased magnesium intake also produced no improvement.[38]

Despite its failure in preventing the neurological problems, adenine has nevertheless been effective in correcting the megaloblastic macrocytic anemia in one child with HPRT deficiency.[338,339,340] Treatment also corrected to normal the low concentration of adenine nucleotides found in the peripheral erythrocytes.[198,338]

A new approach to treatment of the abnormal behavior has been tried with promising results by Mizuno and Yugari.[221] L-5-Hydroxytryptophan at a dose of 1–7 mg/day was effective in alleviating the self-mutilating behavior for periods of 12–15 hr in all four patients with the Lesch–Nyhan syndrome to whom it was administered.[221] Mizuno and Yugari postulate that HPRT deficiency may be associated with a decrease or imbalance in serotonin levels in areas of the brain which causes the self-mutilating behavior that is correctable by L-5-hydroxytryptophan administration. Alterations in brain serotonin content of mice can be produced by dietary treatment, since the decarboxylase for converting L-5-hydroxytryptophan to serotonin is not rate limiting.[99] This interesting observation needs corroboration, but it could very well lead to a more rational approach for treatment of this disease.

In the absence of a completely effective treatment for the neurological aspects of the Lesch–Nyhan syndrome, the preventive program through prenatal diagnosis and the selective abortion of affected male fetuses (see above) does permit mothers carrying the defective gene to produce the nonaffected children that they desire. Extensive study of family pedigrees to trace all relatives carrying the abnormal gene therefore becomes an important aspect of the activities of any physician who is involved in caring for these children.

BIBLIOGRAPHY

1. Albertini, R. J., and DeMars, R., Diploid azaguanine-resistant mutants of cultured human fibroblasts, *Science* **169**:482–485 (1970).
2. Amor, B., Delbarre, F., Auscher, C., and de Gery, A., Hypoxanthine-guanine phosphoribosyl transferase deficiency, our experience, *Advan. Exp. Med. Biol.* **41A**:271–279 (1974).
3. Arnold, W. J., Magnesium in the Lesch–Nyhan syndrome, *New Engl. J. Med.* **290**:631 (1974).
4. Arnold, W. J., and Kelley, W. N., Human hypoxanthine-guanine phosphoribosyl-transferase, *J. Biol. Chem.* **246**:7398–7404 (1971).
5. Arnold, W. J., and Kelley, W. N., Dietary-induced variation of hypoxanthine-guanine phosphoribosyltransferase activity in patients with Lesch–Nyhan syndrome, *J. Clin. Invest.* **52**:970–973 (1973).
6. Arnold, W. J., and Kelley, W. N., Hypoxanthine-guanine phosphoribosyltransfer-ase (HGPRT) deficiency: Effect of dietary purines on enzyme activity, *Advan. Exp. Med. Biol.* **41A**:203–209 (1974).
7. Arnold, W. J., and Kelley, W. N., Hypoxanthine-guanine phosphoribosyltransfer-ase (HGPRT) deficiency: Immunologic studies on the mutant enzyme, *Advan. Exp. Med. Biol.* **41A**:177–185 (1974).
8. Arnold, W. J., Lamb, R. V., III, and Kelley, W. N., Human hypoxanthine-guanine phosphoribosyltransferase (HGPRT): Purification and properties, *Advan. Exp. Med. Biol.* **41A**:5–14 (1974).
9. Arnold, W. J., Meade, J. C., and Kelley, W. N., Dietary-induced variation of hypoxanthine-guanine phosphoribosyltransferase (HGPRT) activity in patients with the Lesch–Nyhan syndrome, *Am. J. Hum. Genet.* **24**:32a (1972).
10. Arnold, W. J., Meade, J. C., and Kelley, W. N., Hypoxanthine-guanine phosphori-bosyltransferase: Characteristics of the mutant enzyme in erythrocytes from patients with the Lesch–Nyhan syndrome, *J. Clin. Invest.* **51**:1805–1812 (1972).
11. Ashkenazi, Y. E., and Gartler, S., A study of metabolic cooperation utilizing human mutant fibroblasts, *Exp. Cell Res.* **64**:9–16 (1971).
12. Astrin, K. H., 1974, Purine metabolism in cultured human lymphoid cells, doctoral thesis, University of California, San Diego.
13. Bakay, B., Croce, C., Koprowski, H., and Nyhan, W. L., Restoration of hypoxanthine phosphoribosyltransferase activity in mouse 1R cells after fusion with chick-embryo fibroblasts, *Proc. Natl. Acad. Sci. U.S.A.* **70**:1998–2002 (1973).
14. Bakay, B., and Nyhan, W. L., The separation of adenine and hypoxanthine-guanine phosphoribosyltransferase isoenzymes by disc gel electrophoresis, *Biochem. Genet.* **5**:81–90 (1971).
15. Bakay, B., and Nyhan, W. L., Electrophoretic properties of hypoxanthine-guanine phosphoribosyl transferase in erythrocytes of subjects with Lesch–Nyhan syn-drome, *Biochem. Genet.* **6**:139–146 (1972).
16. Bakay, B., Nyhan, W. L., Croce, C. M., and Kaprowski, H., 1975, Reversion in expression of hypoxanthine-guanine phosphoribosyltransferase following cell hybrid-ization, *J. Cell Sci.* **17**:567–578 (1975).
17. Bakay, B., Nyhan, W. L., Fawcett, N., and Kogut, M. D., Isoenzymes of hypoxanthine-guanine phosphoribosyltransferase in a family with partial deficiency of the enzyme, *Biochem. Genet.* **7**:73–85 (1972).

18. Bakay, B., and Nyhan, W. L., Activation of variants of hypoxanthine-guanine phosphoribosyltransferase by the normal enzyme, *Proc. Natl. Acad. Sci. U.S.A.* **69**:2523–2527 (1972).
19. Bakay, B., Telfer, M. A., and Nyhan, W. L., Assay of hypoxanthine-guanine and adenine phosphoribosyl transferases: A simple screening test for the Lesch–Nyhan syndrome and related disorders of purine metabolism, *Biochem. Med.* **3**:230–243 (1969).
20. Balis, M. E., Krakoff, I. H., Berman, P. H., and Dancis, J., Urinary metabolities in congenital hyperuricosuria, *Science* **156**:1122–1123 (1967).
21. Balis, M. E., Yip, L. C., Yu, T.-F., Gutman, A. B., Cox, R., and Dancis, J., Unstable HPRTase in subjects with abnormal urinary oxypurine excretion, *Advan. Exp. Med. Biol.* **41A**:195–202 (1974).
22. Bashkin, P., Sperling, O., Schmidt, R., and Szeinberg, A., Resistance of erythrocyte adenine phosphoribosyltransferase in the Lesch–Nyhan syndrome to destabilization to heat by hypoxanthine, *Advan. Exp. Med. Biol.* **41A**:215–220 (1974).
23. Bashkin, P., Sperling, O., Scnmidt, R., and Szeinberg, A., Erythrocyte adenine phosphoribosyltransferase in the Lesch–Nyhan syndrome, *Israel J. Med. Sci.* **9**:1553–1558 (1974).
24. Beardmore, T. D., and Kelley, W. N., Ultraviolet-absorbing compounds in urine from patients with hereditary disorders of purine and pyrimidine metabolism, *Clin. Chem.* **17**:795–801 (1971).
25. Beardmore, T. D., Meade, J. C., and Kelley, W. N., Increased activity of two enzymes of pyrimidine biosynthesis *de novo* in erythrocytes from patients with the Lesch–Nyhan syndrome, *J. Lab. Clin. Med.* **81**:43–52 (1973).
26. Becker, M. A., Argubright, K. F., Fox, R. M., and Seegmiller, J. E., Oxipurinol-associated inhibition of pyrimidine synthesis in human lymphoblasts, *Mol. Pharmacol.* **10**:657–668 (1974).
27. Becker, M. A., Kostel, P. J., Meyer, L. J., and Seegmiller, J. E., Human phosphoribosylpyrophosphate synthetase: Increased enzyme specific activity in a family with gout and excessive purine synthesis, *Proc. Natl. Acad. Sci. U.S.A.* **70**:2749–2752 (1973).
28. Becker, M. A., Meyer, L. J., Kostel, P. J., and Seegmiller, J. E., Increased PP-ribose-P synthetase activity: A genetic abnormality leading to excessive purine production and gout, *Advan. Exp. Med. Biol.* **41A**:307–315 (1974).
29. Becker, M. A., Meyer, L. J., Wood, A. W., and Seegmiller, J. E., Gout associated with increased PRPP synthetase activity (abst.), *Arthritis Rheum.* **15**:430 (1972).
30. Becker, M. A., Meyer, L. J., Wood, A. W., and Seegmiller, J. E., Gout with purine overproduction due to increased phosphoribosylpyrophosphate synthetase activity, *Am. J. Med.* **55**:232–242 (1973).
31. Becker, M. A., Meyer, L. J., Wood, A. W., and Seegmiller, J. E., Purine overproduction in man associated with increased phosphoribosylpyrophosphate synthetase activity, *Science* **179**:1123–1126 (1973).
32. Becker, M. A., and Seegmiller, J. E., Prenatal diagnosis of inborn errors of metabolism, in: *Molecular Pathology*, Bell Museum of Pathology, ed. R. A. Good, S. B. Day and J. J. Yunis. Springfield: Charles C. Thomas, pp. 511–546 (1975).
33. Becker, M. A., and Seegmiller, J. E., Genetic aspects of gout, *Ann. Rev. Med.* **25**:15–28 (1974).
34. Becker, M. A., and Sweetman, L., Gout with mild hypoxanthine guanine

phosphoribosyltransferase deficiency due to diminished affinity for purine substrate (abst.), *Clin. Res.*, **23**:26A (1975).

35. Benke, P. J., Letter to editor, *New Engl. J. Med.* **290**:631 (1974).
36. Benke, P. J., Personal communication.
37. Benke, P. J., and Anderson, J., Use of folic acid, adenine, and bicarbonate in new born twins with Lesch–Nyhan syndrome, *Proc. Soc. Pediat. Res.* 3:356 (1969).
38. Benke, P. J., Herbert, A., and Herrick, N., *In vitro* effects of magnesium ions on mutant cells from patients with the Lesch–Nyhan syndrome, *New Engl. J. Med.* **289**:446–450 (1973).
39. Benke, P. J., and Herrick, N., Azaguanine-resistance as a manifestation of a new form of metabolic overproduction of uric acid, *Am. J. Med.* **52**:547–555 (1972).
40. Benke, P. J., Herrick, N., and Hebert, A., 1975, Hypoxanthine guanine phosphoribosyltransferase variant with altered kinetic properties, *J. Clin. Invest.*, **52**:2234–2240 (1973).
41. Benke, P. J., Herrick, N., Smitten, L., Aradine, C., Laessig, R., and Wolcott, G. J., Adenine and folic acid in the Lesch–Nyhan syndrome, *Pediat. Res.* 7:729–738 (1973).
42. Bennett, L. L., Jr., Schabel, F. M., Jr., and Skipper, H. E., Studies on the mode of action of azaserine, *Arch. Biochem. Biophys.* **64**:423–436 (1956).
43. Berman, P. H., Balis, M. E., and Dancis, J., Congenital hyperuricemia: An inborn error of purine metabolism associated with psychomotor retardation, athetosis and self-mutilation, *Arch. Neurol.* **20**:44–53 (1969).
44. Bernstein, S., Gout in early life, *J. Mt. Sinai Hosp. N.Y.* **14**:747–763 (1947).
45. Berry, H. K., and Granger, M., Uric acid excretion in infants and children, *Clin. Chim. Acta* **32**:377–383 (1971).
46. Beudet, A. L., Roufa, D. J., and Caskey, C. T., Mutations affecting the structure of hypoxanthine guanine phosphoribosyltransferase in cultured Chinese hamster cells; *Proc. Natl. Acad. Sci. U.S.A.* **70**:320–324 (1973).
47. Beutler, E., Biochemical abnormalities associated with hemolytic states, in; *Mechanisms of Anemia* (I. M. Weinstein and E. Beutler, eds.), pp. 195–236, McGraw-Hill, New York (1962).
48. Bland, J. H., ed., Proceedings of the seminars on Lesch–Nyhan syndrome, *Fed. Proc.* **27**:1021–1112 (1968).
49. Bluestone, R., Lesch–Nyhan syndrome and juvenile gout (2 cases). *Proc. Roy. Soc. Med.* **61**:1119–1120 (1968).
50. Bonavita, V., Cotrufo, R., Rizzuto, R., Terzian, H., and Vio, M., La sindrome di Lesch–Nyhan: Studio clinico-metabolico di un caso (1), *Acta Neurol. (Napoli)* **28**:350–364 (1973).
51. Borden, M., Nyhan, W. L., and Bakay, B., Increased activity of adenine phosphoribosyltransferase in erythrocytes of normal newborn infants, *Pediat. Res.* **8**:31–36 (1974).
52. Boyd, E. M., Dolman, M., Knight, L. M., and Sheppard, E. P., The chronic oral toxicity of caffeine, *Can. J. Physiol. Pharmacol.* **43**:995–1007 (1965).
53. Boyd, Y. L., and Harris, H., Correction of genetic defects in mammalian cells by the input of small amounts of foreign genetic material, *J. Cell Sci.* **13**:841–861 (1973).
54. Boyle, J. A., and Seegmiller, J. E., Unpublished procedure.
55. Boyle, J. A., in: *Clinical Rheumatology* (J. A. Boyle and W. W. Buchanan, eds.), pp. 225–226, Blackwell, Oxford (1971).

56. Boyle, J. A., Raivio, K. O., Astrin, K. H., Schulman, J. D., Graf, M. L., Seegmiller, J. E., and Jacobsen, C. B., Lesch–Nyhan syndrome: Preventive control by prenatal diagnosis, *Science* 169:688–689 (1970).

57. Boyle, J. A., Raivio, K. O., Becker, M. A., and Seegmiller, J. E., Effects of nicotinic acid on human fibroblast purine biosynthesis, *Biochim. Biophys. Acta* 269:179–183 (1972).

58. Brenton, D., Nuki, G., Astrin, K., and Seegmiller, J. E., Unpublished observation.

59. Brockman, R. W., Kelley, G. G., Stutts, P., and Copeland, V., Biochemical aspects of resistance to 6-mercaptopurine in human epidermoid carcinoma cells in culture, *Nature (London)* 191:469–471 (1961).

60. Brown, R. S., Kelley, W. N., Seegmiller, J. E., and Carbone, P. P., The action of thiopurines in lymphocytes lacking hypoxanthine-guanine phosphoribosyltransferase, *J. Clin. Invest.* 47:12a (1968).

61. Cartier, P. Personal communication.

62. Caskey, C. T., Ashton, D. M., and Wyngaarden, J. B., The enzymology of feedback inhibition of glutamine phosphoribosylpyrophosphate amidotransferase by purine ribonucleotides, *J. Biol. Chem.* 239:2570–2579 (1964).

63. Catel, V. W., and Schmidt, J., Uber familiare gichtische Diathese in Verdendung mit zerebralen und renalen Symptomen bei einem Kleinkind, *Deutsch. Med. Wochenschr.* 84:2145–2147 (1959).

64. Ceccarelli, M., Ciompi, M. L., and Pasero, G., Acute renal failure during adenine therapy in Lesch–Nyhan syndrome, *Advan. Exp. Med. Biol.* 41B:671–675 (1974).

65. Chalmers, R. A., Krömer, H., Scott, J. T., and Watts, R. W. E., A comparative study of the xanthine oxidase inhibitors allopurinol and oxipurinol in man, *Clin. Sci.* 35:353–362 (1968).

65a. Chan, T. S., Ishii, K., Long, C., and Green, H., Purine excretion by mammalian cells deficient in adenosine kinase, *J. Cell Physiol.* 81:315–322 (1973).

66. Coleman, M., Reversal of organic brain syndrome with seizures and hyperuricosuria subsequent to allopurinol therapy, *Trans. Am. Neurol. Assoc.* 96:113–117 (1971).

67. Cox, R. P., Krauss, M. R., Balis, M. E., and Dancis, J., Evidence for transfer of enzyme product as the basis of metabolic cooperation between tissue culture fibroblasts of Lesch–Nyhan disease and normal cells, *Proc. Natl. Acad. Sci. U.S.A.* 67:1573–1579 (1970).

68. Craft, J. A., Dean, B. M., Watts, R. W. E., and Westwick, W. J., Studies on human erythrocyte IMP: Pyrophosphate phosphoribosyltransferase, *Eur. J. Biochem.* 15:367–373 (1970).

69. Crawhall, J. C., Henderson, J. F., and Kelley, W. N., Diagnosis and treatment of the Lesch–Nyhan syndrome, *Pediat. Res.* 6:504–513 (1972).

70. Croce, C. M., and Bakay, B., Presence of two active X-chromosomes in hybrids between normal human and SV40-transformed fibroblasts from patients with the Lesch-Nyhan syndrome. *Exptl. Cell Res.* 87:422–425, 1974.

71. Croce, C. M., Bakay, B., Nyhan, W. L., and Koprowski, H., Reexpression of the rat hypoxanthine phosphoribosyltransferase gene in rat–human hybrids, *Proc. Natl. Acad. Sci. U.S.A.* 70:2590 (1973).

72. Crussi, F. G., Robertson, D. M., and Hiscox, J. L., The pathological condition of the Lesch–Nyhan syndrome, *Am. J. Dis. Child.* 118:501 (1969).

73. Dancis, J., The prenatal detection of hereditary defects, *Obstet. Gynecol. Surv.* 24:1351–1353 (1969).

74. Dancis, J., Berman, P. H., Jansen, V., and Balis, M. E., Absence of mosaicism in the lymphocyte in X-linked congenital hyperuricosuria, *Life Sci. Pt. II* **7**:587 (1968).
75. Davidson, R. G., Nitowsky, H. M., and Childs, B., Demonstration of two populations of cells in the human females heterozygous for glucose-6-phosphate dehydrogenase variants, *Proc. Natl. Acad. Sci. U.S.A.* **50**:481–485 (1963).
76. Davies, M. R., and Dean, B. M., The heterogeneity of erythrocyte IMP: Pyrophosphate phosphoribosyl transferase and purine nucleoside phosphorylase by isoelectric focusing, *FEBS Letters* **18**:283–286 (1971).
77. De Bruyn, C. H. M. M., and Oei, T. L., Lesch–Nyhan syndrome: Incorporation of hypoxanthine in stimulated lymphocytes, *Exp. Cell Res.* **79**:450–452 (1973).
78. De Bruyn, C. H. M. M., and Oei, T. L., Incorporation of ³H-hypoxanthine in PHA^x stimulated HG-PRT deficient lymphocytes, *Advan. Exp. Med. Biol.* **41A**:229–235 (1974).
79. De Bruyn, C. H. M. M., and Oei, T. L., Purine metabolism in intact erythrocytes from controls and HGPRT deficient individuals, *Advan. Exp. Med. Biol.* **41A**:223–228 (1974).
80. De Bruyn, C. H. M. M., Oei, T. L., Geerdink, R. A., and Lommen, E. J. P., An atypical case of hypoxanthine-guanine phosphoribosyltransferase deficiency (Lesch–Nyhan syndrome). II. Genetic studies, *Clin. Genet.* **4**:353–359 (1973).
81. DeMars, R., Genetic studies of HG-PRT deficiency and the Lesch–Nyhan syndrome with cultured human cells, *Fed. Proc.* **30**:944–955 (1971).
82. DeMars, R., and Held, K. R., The spontaneous azaguanine-resistant mutants of diploid human fibroblasts, *Humangenetik* **16**:87–110 (1972).
83. DeMars, R., Sarto, G., Felix, J. S., and Benke, P., Lesch–Nyhan mutation: Prenatal detection with amniotic fluid cells, *Science* **164**:1303–1305 (1969).
84. Der Kaloustian, V. M., Byrne, R., Young, W. J., and Childs, B., An electrophoretic method for detecting hypoxanthine-guanine phosphoribosyltransferase variants, *Biochem. Genet.* **3**:299–302 (1969).
85. de Vries, A., and Sperling, O., Accelerated erythrocyte 5-phosphoribosyl-1-pyrophosphate synthesis: A familial abnormality associated with excessive uric acid production and gout. *Pahlavi Med. J.* **3**:512, 1972.
86. Deys, B. F., Demonstration of X-linkage of G6PD, HGPRT, and PGK in the horse by means of mule–mouse somatic cell hybrids, doctoral thesis, University of Leyden (1972).
87. Doran, T. A., Bjerre, S., and Porter, C. J., Creatinine, uric acid, and electrolytes in amniotic fluid, *Am. J. Obstet. Gynecol.* **106**:325–332 (1970).
88. Dorfman, A., ed., *Antenatal Diagnosis*, University of Chicago Press, Chicago (1972).
89. Dörner, K., and Manzke, H., Einfache Bestimmung von Purinen durch präparative Dünnschichtchromatographie, *Z. Klin. Chem. Klin. Biochem.* **1**:57–58 (1971).
90. Dyer, C., and Seegmiller, J. E., Unpublished observation.
91. Emmerson, B. T., Discussion session. I. Biochemistry and metabolism: Symposium on allopurinol, *Ann. Rheum. Dis.* **25**:621–622 (1966).
92. Emmerson, B. T., Urate metabolism in heterozygotes for HGPRTase deficiency, *Advan. Exp. Med. Biol.* **41A**:287–290 (1974).
93. Emmerson, B. T., and Thompson, L., The spectrum of hypoxanthine-guanine phosphoribosyltransferase deficiency, *Quart. J. Med.* **42**:423–440 (1973).
94. Emmerson, B. T., Thompson, C. J., and Wallace, D. C., Deficiency of hypoxan-

thine-guanine phosphoribosyltransferase: Intermediate enzyme deficiency in heterozygote red cells, *Ann. Intern. Med.* **76**:285–287 (1972).

95. Emmerson, B. T., Thompson, L., Wallace, D. C., and Spence, A., Hypoxanthineguanine phosphoribosyltransferase and deutan colour blindness: The relative positions of these loci on the X-chromosome, *Advan. Exp. Med. Biol.* **41A**:281–283 (1974).

96. Emmerson, B. T., and Wyngaarden, J. B., Purine metabolism in heterozygous carriers of hypoxanthine-guanine phosphoribosyltransferase deficiency, *Science* **166**:1533–1535 (1969).

97. Etienne, J.-C., Champanie, J.-P., Pascalis, G., and Gougeon, J., Encéphalopathie hypèruricosurique avec auto-mutilations, *Rev. Rheum.* **40**:265–270 (1973).

98. Felix, J. S., and DeMars, R., Detection of females heterozygous for the Lesch–Nyhan syndrome by 8-azaguanine resistant growth of cultured human fibroblasts, *J. Lab. Clin. Med.* **77**:596–604 (1971).

99. Fernstrom, J. D., Modification of brain serotonin by the diet, *Ann. Rev. Med.* **25**:1–8 (1974).

100. Fox, I. H., and Kelley, W. N., Phosphoribosylpyrophosphate in man: Biochemical and clinical significance, *Ann. Intern. Med.* **74**:424–433 (1971).

101. Fox, I. H., and Kelley, W. N., Human phosphoribosylpyrophosphate (PP-ribose-P) synthetase: Properties and regulation, *Advan. Exp. Med. Biol.* **41A**:79–86 (1974).

102. Fox, I. H., and Kelley, W. N., Pharmacological alterations of intracellular phosphoribosylpyrophosphate (PP-ribose-P) in human tissues, *Advan. Exp. Med. Biol.* **41A**:93–99 (1974).

103. Fox, I. H., Wyngaarden, J. B., and Kelley, W. N., Depletion of erythrocyte phosphoribosylpyrophosphate in man: A newly observed effect of allopurinol, *New Engl. J. Med.* **283**:1177–1182 (1970).

104. Francke, U., Bakay, B., and Nyhan, W. L., Detection of heterozygotes for the Lesch–Nyhan syndrome by electrophoresis of hair root lysates, *J. Pediat.* **82**:472–478 (1973).

105. Francke, U., Gartler, S., Migeon, B., Davies, J., Seegmiller, J. E., Bakay, B., and Nyhan, W. L., The occurrence of new mutants in the X-linked recessive Lesch–Nyhan disease. Submitted *Am. J. Hum. Genet.* 1975.

106. Friedmann, T., Seegmiller, J. E., and Subak-Sharpe, J. H., Metabolic cooperation between genetically marked human fibroblasts in tissue culture, *Nature (London)* **220**:272–274 (1968).

107. Frost, P., Weinstein, G. D., and Nyhan, W. L., Diagnosis of Lesch–Nyhan syndrome by direct study of skin specimens, *J. Am. Med. Assoc.* **212**:316–318 (1970).

108. Fujimoto, W. Y., An approach to the control of PRT deficiency through antenatal diagnosis, *Arch. Intern. Med.* **130**:207–211 (1972).

109. Fujimoto, W. Y., Greene, M. L., and Seegmiller, J. E., X-linked uric aciduria with neurological disease and self-mutilation: Diagnostic test for the enzyme defect, *J. Pediat.* **73**:920–922 (1968).

110. Fujimoto, W. J., Thompson, B., and Seegmiller, J. E., Unpublished observation.

111. Fujimoto, W. Y., Seegmiller, J. E., Uhlendorf, B. W., and Jacobson, C. B., Biochemical diagnosis of an X-linked disease *in utero*, *Lancet* **2**:511–512 (1968).

112. Fujimoto, W. Y., and Seegmiller, J. E., Hypoxanthine-guanine phosphoribosyltransferase deficiency: Activity in normal, mutant, and heterozygote cultured human skin fibroblasts, *Proc. Natl. Acad. Sci. U.S.A.* **65**:577–584 (1970).

113. Fujimoto, W. Y., Subak-Sharpe, J. H., and Seegmiller, J. E., Hypoxanthine-

guanine phosphoribosyltransferase deficiency: Chemical agents selective for mutant or normal cultured fibroblasts in mixed and heterozygote cultures, *Proc. Natl. Acad. Sci. U.S.A.* **68**:1516–1519 (1971).

114. Gartler, S. M., Scott, R. C., Goldstein, J. L., Campbell, B., and Sparkes, R., Lesch–Nyhan syndrome: Rapid detection of heterozygotes by use of hair follicles, *Science* **172**:572 (1971).

115. Geerdink, R. A., DeVries, W. H. M., Willemse, J., Oei, T. L., and DeBruyn, C. H. M. M., An atypical case of hypoxanthine-guanine phosphoribosyltransferase deficiency (Lesch–Nyhan syndrome). I. Clinical studies, *Clin. Genet.* **4**:348 (1973).

116. Ghadimi, H., Role of the deficiency state in clinical manifestations of Lesch–Nyhan syndrome (L-NS), *Pediat. Res.* **3**:355 (1969).

117. Ghadimi, H., Bhalla, C. K., and Kirchenbaum, D. M., The significance of the deficiency state in Lesch–Nyhan disease. *Acta Paediat. Scand.* **59**:233 (1970).

118. Gillen, F., Roufa, D. J., Beaudet, A. L., and Caskey, C. T., 8-Azaguanine resistance in mammalian cells. I. Hypoxanthine-guanine phosphoribosyl transferase, *Genetics* **72**:239 (1972).

119. Goldstein, L. L., Marks, J. F., and Gartler, S. M., Expression of two X-linked genes in human hair follicles of double heterozygotes, *Proc. Natl. Acad. Sci. U.S.A.* **68**:1425 (1971).

120. Gordon, R. B., Thompson, L., and Emmerson, B. T., Erythrocyte PRPP concentrations in heterozygotes for HGPRTase deficiency, *Advan. Exp. Med. Biol.* **41A**:291 (1974).

121. Gots, J. S., and Benson, C. E., Genetic control of bacterial purine phosphoribosyl-transferases and an approach to gene enrichment, *Advan. Exp. Med. Biol.* **41A**:33 (1974).

122. Green, C. D., and Martin, D. W., Jr., A direct effect of cyclic GMP on purified phosphoribosyl pyrophosphate synthetase and its antagonism by cyclic AMP, *Cell* **2**:241 (1974).

123. Greene, H., and Ishii, K., On the existence of a guanine nucleotide trap, the role of adenosine kinase and a possible cause of excessive purine production in mammalian cells, *J. Cell Sci.* **11**:1073 (1972).

124. Greene, M. L., Clinical features of patients with the "partial" deficiency of the X-linked uric aciduria enzyme, *Arch. Intern. Med.* **130**:193 (1972).

125. Greene, M. L., Boyle, J. A., and Seegmiller, J. E., Substrate stabilization: Genetically controlled reciprocal relationship of two human enzymes, *Science* **167**:887 (1970).

126. Greene, M. L., Fujimoto, W. Y., and Seegmiller, J. E., Urinary xanthine stones— A rare complication of allopurinol therapy, *New Engl. J. Med.* **280**:426 (1969).

127. Greene, M. L., Glueck, C. J., Fujimoto, W. Y., and Seegmiller, J. E., Benign symmetric lipomatosis (Launois–Bensaude adenolipomatosis) with gout and hyperli-poproteinemia, *Am. J. Med.* **48**:239 (1970).

128. Greene, M. L., Nyhan, W. L., and Seegmiller, J. E., Hypoxanthine-guanine phosphoribosyltransferase deficiency and Xg blood group, *Am. J. Hum. Genet.* **22**:50 (1970).

129. Greene, M. L., and Seegmiller, J. E., Erythrocyte 5-phosphoribosyl-1-pyrophos-phate (PRPP) in gout: Importance of PRPP in the regulation of human purine synthesis, *Arthritis Rheum.* **12**:666 (1969).

130. Greene, M. L., and Seegmiller, J. E., Elevated erythrocyte phosphoribosylpyro-phosphate in X-linked uric aciduria: Importance of PRPP concentration in the regulation of human purine biosynthesis, *J. Clin. Invest.* **48**:32a (1969).

131. Grzeschik, K. H., Allderdice, P. W., Grzeschik, A., Opitz, J. M., Miller, O. J., and Siniscalco, M., Cytological mapping of human X-linked genes by use of somatic cell hybrids involving an X-autosome translocation, *Proc. Natl. Acad. Sci. U.S.A.* **69**:69 (1972).

132. Gusmano, R., Perfumo, F., Gilli, G., and Basile, G. C., La malattia di Lesch–Nyhan, *Minerva Pediat.* **26**:241 (1974).

133. Gutensohn, W., Purification and characterization of a neural hypoxanthine-guanine phosphoribosyltransferase (HGPRT), *Advan. Exp. Med. Biol.* **41A**:19 (1974).

134. Gutensohn, W., and Guroff, G., Hypoxanthine-guanine phosphoribosyltransferase from rat brain (purification, kinetic properties, development and distribution), *J. Neurochem.* **19**:2139–2150 (1972).

135. Gutensohn, W., and Guroff, G., Rapid assay for phosphoribosyltransferase, *Anal. Biochem.* **47**:132 (1972).

136. Harkness, R. A., and Nicol, A. D., Plasma uric acid levels in children, *Arch. Dis. Childh.* **44**:773–778 (1969).

137. Harris, M., Mutation rates in cells at different ploidy levels, *J. Cell Physiol.* **78**:177–184 (1971).

138. Henderson, J. F., Feedback inhibition of purine biosynthesis in ascites tumor cells, *J. Biol. Chem.* **237**:2631–2635 (1962).

139. Henderson, J. F., Inheritance of hypoxanthine-guanine phosphoribosyltransferase deficiency and detection of heterozygotes, *Fed. Proc.* **27**:1085–1086 (1968).

140. Henderson, J. F., *Regulation of Purine Biosynthesis*, American Chemical Society (1973).

141. Henderson, J. F., Brox, L. W., Kelley, W. N., Rosenbloom, F. M., and Seegmiller, J. E., Kinetic studies of hypoxanthine-guanine phosphoribosyltransferase, *J. Biol. Chem.* **243**:2514 (1968).

142. Henderson, J. F., and Paterson, A. R. P., *Nucleotide Metabolism*, Academic Press, New York (1973).

143. Henderson, J. F., Kelley, W. N., Rosenbloom, F. M., and Seegmiller, J. E., Inheritance of purine phosphoribosyltransferases in man, *Am. J. Hum. Genet.* **21**:61–70 (1969).

144. Henderson, J. F., and LePage, G. A., Utilization of host purines by transplanted tumors, *Cancer Res.* **19**:67–71 (1959).

145. Henderson, J. F., McCoy, E. E., and Fraser, J. H., Purine nucleotide synthesis, interconversion and catabolism in human leukocytes, *Advan. Exp. Med. Biol.* **41A**:113–116 (1974).

146. Henderson, J. F., Rosenbloom, F. M., Kelley, W. N., and Seegmiller, J. E., Variations in purine metabolism of cultured skin fibroblasts from patients with gout, *J. Clin. Invest.* **47**:1511–1516 (1968).

147. Herbert, V., Streiff, R. R., Sullivan, L. W., and McGeer, P. L., Deranged purine metabolism manifested by aminoimidazolecarboxamide excretion in megaloblastic anaemias, haemolytic anaemia and liver disease, *Lancet* **2**:45–46 (1964).

148. Hershko, A., Hershko, C., and Mager, J., Increased formation of 5-phosphoribosyl-1-pyrophosphate in red blood cells of some gouty patients, *Israel Med. J.* **4**:939–944 (1968).

149. Hershko, A., Razin, A., and Mager, J., Regulation of the synthesis of 5-phosphoribosyl-1-pyrophosphate in intact red blood cells and in cell free preparations, *Biochim. Biophys. Acta* **184**:64–76 (1969).

149a. Heynen, G., Andrien, J. M., Dodnival, P., and Franchimont, P., Observations cliniques: Un cas de syndrome de Lesch–Nyhan, *Acta Clin. Belg.* **26**:357–365 (1971).

150. Hockstadt-Ozer, J., The regulation of purine utilization in bacteria. IV. Role of membrane-localized and pericytoplasmic enzymes in the mechanism of purine nucleoside transport across *E. coli* membranes, *J. Biol. Chem.* **247**:2419 (1972).

151. Hoefnagel, D., The syndrome of athetoid cerebral palsy, mental deficiency, self mutilation and hyperuricemia, *J. Ment. Defic. Res.* **9**:69–74 (1965).

152. Hoefnagel, D., Andrew, E. D., Mireault, N. G., and Berndt, W. O., Hereditary choreoathetosis, self mutilation, and hyperuricemia in young males, *New Engl. J. Med.* **273**:130–135 (1965).

153. Holmes, E. W., McDonald, J. A., McCord, J. M., Wyngaarden, J. B., and Kelley, W. N., Human glutamine phosphoribosylpyrophosphate amidotransferase: Kinetic and regulatory properties, *J. Biol. Chem.* **248**:144–150 (1973).

154. Holmes, E. W., Pehlke, D. M., and Kelley, W. N., Human IMP dehydrogenase: Kinetics and regulatory properties, *Biochim. Biophys. Acta* **364**:209–217 (1974).

155. Holmes, E. W., Wyngaarden, J. B., and Kelley, W. N., Human glutamine phosphoribosylpyrophosphate amidotransferase: Two molecular forms interconvertible by purine ribonucleotides and phosphoribosylpyrophosphate, *J. Biol. Chem.* **248**:6035–6040 (1973).

156. Holmes, E. W., Jr., Wyngaarden, J. B., and Kelley, W. N., Human glutamine phosphoribosylpyrophosphate (PP-ribose-P) amidotransferase: Kinetic, regulation and configurational changes, *Advan. Exp. Med. Biol.* **41A**:177–185 (1974).

157. Hösli, P., De Bruyn, C. H. M. M., and Oei, T. L., Development of a micro HG-PRT activity assay: Preliminary complementation studies with Lesch–Nyhan cell strains, *Advan. Exp. Med. Biol.* **41B**:811–815 (1974).

158. Hooft, C., Van Nevel, C., and DeSchaepdryver, A. F., Hyperuricosuric encephalopathy without hyperuricemia, *Arch. Dis. Childh.* **43**:734–737 (1968).

159. Jacob, F., and Monod, J., On the regulation of gene activity, *Cold Spring Harbor Symp. Quant. Biol.* **26**:193 (1961).

160. Jerushalmy, Z., Sperling, O., Pinkhas, J., Krynska, M., and de Vries, A., Enzymes of purine metabolism in platelets: Phosphoribosylpyrophosphate synthetase and purine phosphoribosyltransferases, *Advan. Exp. Med. Biol.* **41A**:159–162 (1977).

161. Johnson, M. G., Rosenzweig, S., Switzer, R. L., Becker, M. A., and Seegmiller, J. E., Evaluation of the role of 5-phosphoribosyl-α-1-pyrophosphate synthetase in congenital hyperuricemia and gout: A simple isotopic assay and an activity stain for the enzyme, *Biochem. Med.* **10**:266–275 (1974).

162. Juene, M., Hermier, M., Rosenberg, D., Michel, M., Collombel, D., and Collombel, C., Encéphalopathie familiale avec hyperuricémie: À propos d'une observation, *Pediatrie* **21**:663–675 (1966).

163. Kaufman, J. M., Greene, M. L., and Seegmiller, J. E., Urine uric acid to creatinine ratio: A screening test for inherited disorders of purine metabolism, *J. Pediat.* **73**:583–592 (1968).

164. Kelley, W. N., Biochemistry of the X-linked uric aciduria-enzyme defect and its genetic variants, *Arch. Intern. Med.* **130**:199–206 (1972).

165. Kelley, W. N., Hypoxanthine-guanine phosphoribosyltransferase in the Lesch–Nyhan syndrome and gout, *Fed. Proc.* **27**:1047 (1968).

166. Kelley, W. N., Pathophysiology of purine metabolism in man, *Enzyme* **18**:161–175 (1974).

167. Kelley, W. N., and Arnold, W. J., Human hypoxanthine-guanine phosphoribosyl-

transferase: Studies on the normal and mutant forms of the enzyme, *Fed. Proc.* **32**:1656–1659 (1973).

168. Kelley, W. N., Beardmore, T. D., Fox, I. H., and Meade, J. C., Effect of allopurinol and oxipurinol on pyrimidine synthesis in cultured human fibroblasts, *Biochem. Pharmacol.* **20**:1471–1478 (1971).

169. Kelley, W. N., Fox, I. H., Beardmore, T. D., and Meade, J. C., Allopurinol and oxipurinol: Alteration of purine and pyrimidine metabolism in cell culture, *Ann. N.Y. Acad. Sci.* **179**:588–595 (1971).

170. Kelley, W. N., Fox, I. H., and Wyngaarden, J. B., Regulation of purine biosynthesis in cultured human cells. I. Effects of orotic acid, *Biochim. Biophys. Acta* **215**:512–516 (1970).

171. Kelley, W. N., Fox, I. H., and Wyngaarden, J. B., Essential role of phosphoribosylpyrophosphate (PRPP) in regulation of purine biosynthesis in cultured human fibroblasts, *Clin. Res.* **18**:457 (1970).

172. Kelley, W. N., Greene, M. L., Fox, I. H., Rosenbloom, F. M., Levy, R. I., and Seegmiller, J. E., Effects of orotic acid on purine and lipoprotein metabolism in man, *Metabolism* **19**:1025–1035 (1970).

173. Kelley, W. N., Greene, M. L., Rosenbloom, F. M., Henderson, J. F., and Seegmiller, J. E., Hypoxanthine-guanine phosphoribosyltransferase deficiency in gout: A review, *Ann. Intern. Med.* **70**:155–206 (1969).

174. Kelley, W. N., and Meade, J. C., Studies on hypoxanthine-guanine phosphoribosyltransferase in fibroblasts from patients with the Lesch–Nyhan syndrome: Evidence for genetic heterogeneity, *J. Biol. Chem.* **246**:2953–2958 (1971).

175. Kelley, W. N., Meade, J. C., and Evans, M. C., Studies on the adenine phosphoribosyltransferase enzyme in human fibroblasts lacking hypoxanthine-guanine phosphoribosyltransferase, *J. Lab. Clin. Med.* **77**:33–38 (1971).

176. Kelley, W. N., Rosenbloom, F. M., Henderson, J. F., and Seegmiller, J. E., Xanthine phosphoribosyltransferase in man: Relationship to hypoxanthine-guanine phosphoribosyltransferase, *Biochem. Biophys. Res. Commun.* **28**:340–345 (1967).

177. Kelley, W. N., Rosenbloom, F. M., Henderson, J. F., and Seegmiller, J. E., A specific enzyme defect in gout associated with overproduction of uric acid, *Proc. Natl. Acad. Sci. U.S.A.* **57**:1735–1739 (1967).

178. Kelley, W. N., Rosenbloom, F. M., Miller, J., and Seegmiller, J. E., An enzymatic basis for variation in response to allopurinol, *New Engl. J. Med.* **278**:287–293 (1968).

179. Kelley, W. N., Rosenbloom, F. M., and Seegmiller, J. E., The effect of azathioprine (Imuran) on purine synthesis in clinical disorders of purine metabolism, *J. Clin. Invest.* **46**:1518–1529 (1967).

180. Kelley, W. N., and Wyngaarden, J. B., Effects of allopurinol and oxipurinol on purine synthesis in cultured human cells, *J. Clin. Invest.* **49**:602–609 (1970).

181. Kelley, W. N., and Wyngaarden, J. B., The Lesch–Nyhan syndrome, in: *The Metabolic Basis of Inherited Disease,* 3rd ed. (J. B. Stanbury, J. B. Wyngaarden, and D. S. Fredrickson, eds.), pp. 969–991, McGraw-Hill, New York (1972).

182. Klinenberg, J. R., Goldfinger, S. E., and Seegmiller, J. E., The effectiveness of the xanthine oxidase inhibitor, allopurinol, in the treatment of gout, *Ann. Intern. Med.* **62**:639–647 (1965).

183. Klinger, H. P., and Shin, S. I., 1974, Modulation of the activity of an avian gene transferred into a mammalian cell by cell fusion, *Proc. Natl. Acad. Sci. U.S.A.* **71**:1398.

184. Kogut, M. D., Donnell, G. N., Nyhan, W. L., and Sweetman, L., Disorder of purine metabolism due to partial deficiency of hypoxanthine-guanine phosphoribosyltransferase, a study of a family, *Am. J. Med.* **48**:148–161 (1970).
185. Krenitsky, T. A., Elion, G. B., Strelitz, R. A., and Hitchings, G. H., Ribonucleosides of allopurinol and oxoallopurinol: Isolation from human urine, enzymatic synthesis and characterization, *J. Biol. Chem.* **242**:2675–2682 (1967).
186. Krenitsky, T. A., Papainnou, R., and Elion, G. B., Human hypoxanthine phosphoribosyltransferase. I. Purification, properties, and specificity, *J. Biol. Chem.* **244**:1263–1270 (1969).
187. Labrune, B., Cartier, P., Bonnenfant, F., Ribierre, M., and Mallet, R., Encéphalopathie familiale avec hyperuricémie: Étude du métabolisme des purines essals thérapeutiques, *Arch. Fr. Pediat.* **26**:139–154 (1969).
188. Lampert, P. W., and Seegmiller, J. E., Unpublished observation.
189. Lajtha, L. G., and Vane, J. R., Dependence of bone marrow cells on the liver for purine supply, *Nature (London)* **182**:191–192 (1958).
190. LePage, G. A., and Jones, M., Purinethiols as feedback inhibitors of purine synthesis in ascites tumor cells, *Cancer Res.* **21**:642 (1961).
191. Lepercq, G., Poupinet, S., Steinschneider, R., and Weller, C., Lithiase urinaire révélatrice d'un syndrome de Lesch–Nyhan, *Nouv. Presse Med.* **2**:1571–1574 (1973).
192. Lesch, M., and Nyhan, W. L., A familial disorder of uric acid metabolism and central nervous system function, *Am. J. Med.* **36**:561–570 (1964).
193. Levenberg, B., Melnick, I., and Buchanan, J. M., Biosynthesis of the purines. XV. The effect of aza-L-serine and 6-diazo-5-oxo-L-norleucine on inosinic acid biosynthesis *de novo*, *J. Biol. Chem.* **225**:163–176 (1957).
194. Lever, J. E., Nuki, G., and Seegmiller, J. E., Expression of purine overproduction in a series of 8-azaguanine resistant diploid human lymphoblast lines, *Proc. Natl. Acad. Sci. U.S.A.* **71**:2679–2683 (1974).
195. Littlefield, J. W., The inosinic acid pyrophosphorylase activity of mouse fibroblasts partially resistant to 8-azaguanine, *Proc. Natl. Acad. Sci. U.S.A.* **50**:568–576 (1963).
196. Littlefield, J. S., Selection of hybrids from matings of fibroblasts *in vitro* and their presumed recombinants, *Science* **145**:709–710 (1964).
197. Lommen, E. J. P., De Abreu, R. A., Trijbels, J. M. F., and Schretlen, E. D. A. M., The IMP dehydrogenase catalyzed reaction in erythrocytes of normal individuals and patients with hypoxanthine guanine phosphoribosyltransferase deficiency, *Acta. Paediat. Scand.* **63**:140–142 (1974).
198. Lommen, E. J. P., Vogels, G. D., Van der Zee, S. P., Trijbels, J. M. F., and Schretlen, E. D. A. M., Concentrations of purine nucleotides in erythrocytes of patients with the Lesch–Nyhan syndrome before and during oral administration of adenine, *Acta Paediat. Scand.* **60**:642–646 (1971).
199. Lowry, B. A., and Lerner, M. H., Role of liver adenosine in the renewal of the adenine nucleotides of human and rabbit erythrocytes, *Advan. Exp. Biol. Med.* **41A**:129–139 (1974).
200. Lyon, M. F., Gene action in the X-chromosome of the mouse (*Mus musculus* L.), *Nature (London)* **190**:372–373 (1961).
201. McBride, O. W., and Ozer, H. L., Transfer of genetic information by purified metaphase chromosomes, *Proc. Natl. Acad. Sci. U.S.A.* **70**:1258 (1973).
202. McCollister, R. J., Gilbert, W. R., Jr., Ashton, D. M., and Wyngaarden, J. B., Pseudofeedback inhibition of purine synthesis by 6-mercaptopurine ribonucleotide and other purine analogues, *J. Biol. Chem.* **239**:1560–1563 (1964).

203. McDonald, J. A., and Kelley, W. N., Lesch–Nyhan syndrome: Altered kinetic properties of mutant enzyme, *Science* **171**:689–691 (1971).
204. McDonald, J. A., and Kelley, W. N., Lesch–Nyhan syndrome: Absence of the mutant enzyme in erythrocytes of a heterozygote for both normal and mutant hypoxanthine-guanine phosphoribosyltransferase, *Biochem. Genet.* **6**:21–26 (1972).
205. McDonald, J. A., and Kelley, W. N., Hypoxanthine-guanine phosphoribosyltransferase deficiency: Altered kinetic properties of a specific mutant form of the enzyme, *Advan. Exp. Med. Biol.* **41A**:167 (1974).
206. McInnes, R., Lamm, P., Clow, C. L., and Scriver, C. R., A filter paper sampling method for the uric acid:creatinine ratio in urine: Normal values in the newborn, *Pediatrics* **49**:80 (1972).
207. McKeran, R. O., Howell, A., Andrews, T. M., Watts, R. W. E., and Arlett, C. F., Observations on the growth *in vitro* of myeloid progenitor cells and fibroblasts from hemizygotes and heterozygotes for "complete" and "partial" hypoxanthine-guanine phosphoribosyltransferase (HGPRT) deficiency, and their relevance to the pathogenesis of brain damage in the Lesch–Nyhan syndrome, *J. Neurol. Sci.* **22**:183 (1974).
208. Manzke, H., Hyperuricamie mit Cerebralparese—Syndrome eines hereditaren Purinstoffwechselleidens, *Helv. Paediat. Acta* **22**:258 (1967).
209. Manzke, H., Unpublished observation.
210. Manzke, H., Harms, D., and Dörner, K., Zur Problematik der Behandlung der Kongenitalen Hyperurikämie, *Monatsschr. Klinderheilkd.* **119**:424–428 (1971).
211. Marie, J., Royer, P., and Rappaport, R., Hyperuricémie congénitale avec troubles neurologiques, rénaux et sanguins, *Arch. Fr. Pediat.* **24**:501 (1967).
212. Marks, J. F., Baum, J., Keele, D. K., Jacob, L. K., and MacFarlen, A., Lesch–Nyhan syndrome treated from the early neonatal period, *Pediatrics* **42**:357 (1968).
213. Marks, J. F., Baum, J., Kay, J. L., Taylor, W., and Curry, L., Amniotic fluid concentrations of uric acid, *Pediatrics* **42**:359 (1968).
214. Metzger-Freed, L., Effect of ploidy and mutagens on bromodeoxyuridine resistance in haploid and diploid frog cells, *Nature New Biol.* **235**:245–246 (1972).
215. Michener, W. M., Hyperuricemia and mental retardation with athetosis and self mutilation, *Am. J. Dis. Childh.* **113**:195 (1967).
216. Migeon, B. R., Der Kaloustian, V. M., Nyhan, W. L., Young, W. J., and Childs, B., X-linked hypoxanthine-guanine phosphoribosyl transferase deficiency: Heterozygote has two clonal populations, *Science* **160**:425 (1968).
217. Migeon, B. R., X-linked hypoxanthine-guanine phosphoribosyl transferase deficiency: Detection of the heterozygotes by selective medium, *Biochem. Genet.* **4**:377 (1970).
218. Miller, O. J., Cook, P. R., Meera Khan, P., Shin, S., and Siniscalco, M., Mitotic separation of two human X-linked genes in man–mouse somatic cell hybrids, *Proc. Natl. Acad. Sci. U.S.A.* **68**:116–120 (1971).
219. Milunsky, A., Littlefield, J. W., Kanfer, J. N., Kolodny, E. H., Shih, V. E., and Atkins, L., Prenatal genetic diagnosis, *New Engl. J. Med.* **283**:1370–1381, 1441–1447, 1498–1504 (1970).
220. Mizuno, T., Segawa, M., Kurumada, T., Maruyama, H., and Onisawa, J., Clinical and therapeutic aspects of the Lesch–Nyhan syndrome in Japanese children, *Neuropaediatrie* **2**:38–52 (1970).
221. Mizuno, T.-I., and Yugari, Y., Self-mutilation in the Lesch–Nyhan syndrome, *Lancet* **1**:761 (1974).
222. Monkus, E. S. J., Nyhan, W. L., Fogel, B. J., and Yankow, S., Concentrations of

uric acid in the serum of neonatal infants and their mothers, *Am. J. Obstet. Gynecol.* **108**:91–97 (1970).

223. Müller, M. M., Allopurinolmedikation und der Enzymdefekt der Hypoxanthin-guanin-phosphoribosyltransferase bei primärer Gicht, *Z. Klin. Chem. Klin. Biochem.* **3**:283 (1971).

224. Müller, M. M., Die Isoenzyme der Purin-Phosphoribosyltransferasen im Erythro-cyten bei Lesch–Nyhan Syndrom, *Z. Klin. Chem. Klin. Biochem.* **12**:28–32 (1974).

225. Müller, M. M., and Debrovitz, A., A simple and rapid method for separation and characterization of hypoxanthine guanine phosphoribosyltransferase enzyme, *Prep. Biochem.* **2**: 375 (1972).

226. Müller, M. M., and Stemberger, H., Immunological studies of hypoxanthine-guanine phosphoribosyltransferase in Lesch–Nyhan syndrome, *Advan. Exp. Med. Biol.* **41A**:187–194 (1974).

227. Müller, M. M., and Stemberger, H., Biochemische und immunologische Untersu-chungen der Hypoxanthin-Guanin-Phosphoribosyltransferase in den Erythrozyten von Lesch-Nyhan-Patienten, *Wien. Klin. Wochenschr.* **86**:127–131 (1974).

228. Munsat, T. L., Klinenberg, J., Carrel, R. E., and Menkes, J., Defects in purine metabolism and neurologic disease, *Bull. Los Angeles Neurol. Soc.* **33**:101–112 (1968).

229. Murray, A. W., The biological significance of purine salvage, *Ann. Rev. Biochem.* **40**:811 (1971).

230. Nabholz, M., Miggiano, V., and Bodmer, W., Genetic analysis with human–mouse somatic cell hybrids, *Nature (London)* **223**:358 (1969).

231. Nadler, H. L., Prenatal detection of genetic defects, *J. Pediat.* **74**:132–143 (1969).

232. Naylor, E. W., Personal communication.

233. Newcombe, D. S., Shapiro, S. L., Sheppard, G. L., and Dreifuss, F. E., Treatment of X-linked primary hyperuricemia with allopurinol, *J. Am. Med. Assoc.* **198**:315–317 (1966).

234. Newcombe, D. S., The urinary excretion of aminoimidazolecarboxamide in the Lesch–Nyhan syndrome, *Pediatrics* **46**:508–512 (1970).

235. Newcombe, D. S., and Willard, J. M., A spectrophotometric assay for guanine phosphoribosyl transferase, *Anal. Biochem.* **43**:454–459 (1971).

236. Nissim, S., Ciompi, M. L., Barzan, L., and Pasero, G., Behavioral changes during adenine therapy in Lesch–Nyhan syndrome, *Advan. Exp. Med. Biol.* **41B**:677–679 (1974).

237. Nuki, G., Lever, J. E., and Seegmiller, J. E., Biochemical characteristics of 8-azaguanine resistant human lymphoblast mutants selected *in vitro*, *Advan. Exp. Med. Biol.* **41A**:255–267 (1974).

238. Nuki, G., Astrin, K., and Seegmiller, J. E., In preparation.

239. Nyhan, W. L., Personal communication.

240. Nyhan, W. L., Summary of clinical features in seminars on Lesch–Nyhan syndrome, *Fed. Proc.* **27**:1034–1041 (1968).

241. Nyhan, W. L., Purine metabolism and abnormal behavior in children, in: *Brain Chemistry and Mental Disease* (B. T. Ho and W. M. McIsaac, eds.), pp. 281–301, Plenum Press, New York (1971).

242. Nyhan, W. L., Clinical features of the Lesch–Nyhan syndrome, *Arch. Intern. Med.* **130**:186–192 (1972).

243. Nyhan, W. L., The Lesch–Nyhan syndrome, *Ann. Rev. Med.* **24**:41–60 (1973).

244. Nyhan, W. L., Bakay, B., Connor, J. D., Marks, J. F., and Keele, D. K., Hemizygous expression of glucose-6-phosphate dehydrogenase in erythrocytes of

heterozygotes for the Lesch–Nyhan syndrome, *Proc. Natl. Acad. Sci. U.S.A.* **65:**214–218 (1970).

245. Nyhan, W. L., James, J. A., Teberg, A. J., Sweetman, L., and Nelson, L. G., A new disorder of purine metabolism with behavioral manifestations, *J. Pediat.* **74:**20–27 (1969).

246. Nyhan, W. L., Pesek, J., Sweetman, L., Carpenter, D. G., and Carter, C. H., Genetics of an X-linked disorder of uric acid metabolism and cerebral function, *Pediat. Res.* **1:**5–13 (1967).

247. Nyhan, W. L., Sweetman, L., Carpenter, D. G., Carter, C. H., and Hoefnagel, D., Effects of azathioprine in a disorder of uric acid metabolism and cerebral function, *J. Pediat.* **72:**111–118 (1968). .

248. Oei, T. L., and De Bruyn, C. H. M. M., Studies on metabolic cooperation using different types of normal and hypoxanthine-guanine phosphoribosyltransferase (HG-PRT) deficient cells, *Advan. Exp. Med. Biol.* **41A:**237–243 (1974).

249. Olney, J. W., Brain lesions, obesity and other disturbances in mice treated with monosodium glutamate, *Science* **164:**719–721 (1969).

250. Olsen, A. S., and Milman, G., Chinese hamster hypoxanthine-guanine phosphoribosyltransferase: Purification, structural, and catalytic properties, *J. Biol. Chem.* **249:**4030 (1974).

251. Olsen, A. S., and Milman, G., Subunit molecular weight of human hypoxanthine-guanine phosphoribosyltransferase, *J. Biol. Chem.* **249:**4038 (1974).

252. Ozer, H. L., Purine pyrophosphorylase as a selective genetic marker in a mouse lymphoma, P388, in cell culture, *J. Cell Physiol.* **68:**61–67 (1966).

253. Parker, W. C., and Bearn, A. G., Application of genetic regulatory mechanisms to human genetics, *Am. J. Med.* **34:**680 (1963).

254. Partington, M. W., and Hennen, B. K. E., The Lesch–Nyhan syndrome: Self-destructive biting, mental retardation; neurological disorder and hyperuricaemia, *Dev. Med. Child. Neurol.* **9:**563 (1967).

255. Partsch, G., Altmann, H., and Eberl, R., Purine salvage in spleen cells, *Advan. Exp. Med. Biol.* **41A:**103 (1974).

256. Pehlke, D. M., McDonald, J. A., Holmes, E. W., and Kelley, W. N., Inosinic acid dehydrogenase activity in the Lesch–Nyhan syndrome, *J. Clin. Invest.* **51:**1398 (1972).

257. Peters, J. F., Caffeine toxicity in starved rats, *Toxicol. Appl. Pharmacol.* **9:**390 (1966).

258. Proctor, P., and McGinness, J. E., Levodopa side-effects and the Lesch–Nyhan syndrome, *Lancet* **2:**1367 (1970).

259. Raivio, K. O., and Seegmiller, J. E., Genetic diseases of metabolism, *Ann. Rev. Biochem.* **41:**543 (1972).

260. Raivio, K. O., and Seegmiller, J. E., Adenine, hypoxanthine, and guanine metabolism in fibroblasts from normal individuals and from patients with hypoxanthine phosphoribosyltransferase deficiency, *Biochim. Biophys. Acta* **299:**273 (1973).

261. Raivio, K. O., and Seegmiller, J. E., Role of glutamine in purine synthesis and in guanine nucleotide formation in normal fibroblasts and in fibroblasts deficient in hypoxanthine phosphoribosyltransferase activity, *Biochim. Biophys. Acta* **299:**283 (1973).

262. Reed, W. B., and Fish, C. H., Hyperuricemia with self-mutilation and choreoathetosis: Lesch–Nyhan syndrome, *Arch. Dermatol.* **94:**194 (1966).

263. Reem, G. H., Regulation of *de novo* purine synthesis in the Lesch–Nyhan syndrome, *Advan. Exp. Med. Biol.* **41A:**245 (1974).

264. Reem, G. H., *De novo* purine biosynthesis by two pathways in Burkitt lymphoma cells and in human spleen, *J. Clin. Invest.* **51**:1058 (1972).

265. Richardson, B. J., and Cox, D. M., Rapid tissue culture and microbiochemical methods for analyzing colonially grown fibroblasts from normal, Lesch–Nyhan and Tay–Sachs patients and amniotic fluid cells, *Clin. Genet.* **4**:376 (1973).

266. Richardson, B. J., Ryckman, D. L., Komarnicki, L. M., and Hamerton, J. L., Heterogeneity in the biochemical characteristics of red blood cell hypoxanthine-guanine phosphoribosyltransferase from two unrelated patients with the Lesch–Nyhan syndrome, *Biochem. Genet.* **9**:197 (1973).

267. Riley, I. D., Gout and cerebral palsy in a three year old boy, *Arch. Dis. Childh.* **35**:293 (1960).

267a. Rockson, S., Stone, R., Van Der Weyden, M., and Kelley, W. N., Lesch–Nyhan syndrome: Evidence for abnormal adrenergic function, *Science* **186**:934–935 (1974).

268. Rosenberg, A. L., Bergstrom, L., Troost, B. T., and Bartholomew, B. A., Hyperuricemia and neurologic deficits, a family study, *New Engl. J. Med.* **282**:992 (1970).

269. Rosenberg, D., Monnet, P., Mamelle, J. C., Colombel, M., Salle, B., and Bovier-Lapierre, M., Encéphalopathie avec troubles du métabolisme des purines: Observation familiale, *Presse Méd.* **76**:2333 (1968).

270. Rosenbloom, F. M., Henderson, J. F., Caldwell, I. C., Kelley, W. N., and Seegmiller, J. E., Biochemical bases of accelerated purine biosynthesis *de novo* in human fibroblasts lacking hypoxanthine-guanine phosphoribosyltransferase, *J. Biol. Chem.* **243**:1166 (1968).

271. Rosenbloom, F. M., Kelley, W. N., Henderson, J. F., and Seegmiller, J. E., Lyon hypothesis and X-linked disease, *Lancet* **2**:305 (1967).

272. Rosenbloom, F. M., Kelley, W. N., Miller, J., Henderson, J. F., and Seegmiller, J. E., Inherited disorder of purine metabolism: Correlation between central nervous system dysfunction and biochemical defects, *J. Am. Med. Assoc.* **202**:175 (1967).

273. Rosenblum, W. I., Rosenbloom, F., and Seegmiller, J. E., Unpublished observation.

274. Roy, K. L., and Ruddle, F. H., Microscale isoelectric focusing studies of mouse and human hypoxanthine-guanine phosphoribosyltransferase, *Biochem. Genet.* **9**:175–185 (1973).

275. Rubin, C. S., Balis, M. E., Piomelli, S., Berman, P. H., and Dancis, J., Elevated AMP pyrophosphorylase activity in congenital IMP pyrophosphorylase deficiency (Lesch–Nyhan disease), *J. Lab. Clin. Med.* **74**:732 (1969).

276. Rubin, C. S., Dancis, J., Yip, L. C., Nowinski, R. C., and Balis, M. E., Purification of IMP: Pyrophosphate phosphoribosyltransferase, catalytically incompetent enzymes in Lesch–Nyhan syndrome. *Proc. Natl. Acad. Sci. U.S.A.* **68**:1461 (1971).

277. Ruddle, F. H., Linkage analysis using somatic cell hybrids, *Advan. Hum. Genet.* **3**:173 (1972).

278. Ruddle, F. H., Assignment of genes to human chromosomes by somatic cell genetics, in: *The Use of Long-Term Lymphocytes in the Study of Genetic Diseases* (D. Bergsma, L. G. Smith, and A. Bloom, eds.), pp. 188–194, The National Foundation, New York (1973).

279. Ruddle, F. H., Linkage analysis in man by somatic cell genetics, *Nature (London)* **242**:165 (1973).

280. Ruddle, F. H., Chapman, V. M., Ricciuti, F., Murnane, M., Klebe, R., and Meera

Khan, P., Linkage relationships of seventeen human gene loci as determined by man–mouse somatic cell hybrids, *Nature New Biol.* **232:**69 (1971).

281. Rundles, R. W., Wyngaarden, J. B., Hitchings, G. H., Elion, G. B., and Silberman, H. R., Effects of a xanthine oxidase inhibitor on thiopurine metabolism, hyperuricemia, and gout, *Trans. Assoc. Am. Physicians* **76:**126 (1963).

282. Salzmann, J., DeMars, R., and Benke, P., Single-allele expression at an X-linked hyperuricemia locus in heterozygous human cells, *Proc. Natl. Acad. Sci. U.S.A.* **60:**545 (1968).

283. Sass, J. K., Itabashi, H. H., and Dexter, R. A., Juvenile gout with brain involvement, *Arch. Neurol.* **13:**639 (1965).

284. Sato, S., Slesinski, R. S., and Littlefield, J. W., Chemical mutagenesis at the phosphoribosyltransferase locus in cultured mammalian lymphoblasts, *Proc. Natl. Acad. Sci. U.S.A.* **69:**1244 (1972).

285. Schulman, J. D., Greene, M. L., Fujimoto, W. Y., and Seegmiller, J. E., Adenine therapy for Lesch–Nyhan syndrome, *Pediat. Res.* **5:**77 (1971).

286. Schwartz, A. G., Cook, P. R., and Harris, H., Correction of a genetic defect in a mammalian cell, *Nature New Biol.* **230:**5 (1971).

287. Sciaky, N., Razin, A., Gazit, B., and Mager, J., Regulatory aspects of the synthesis of 5-phosphoribosyl-1-pyrophosphate in human red blood cells, *Advan. Exp. Med. Biol.* **41A:**87 (1974).

288. Seegmiller, J. E., Pathology and pathologic physiology in: Seminars on Lesch–Nyhan syndrome, *Fed. Proc.* **27:**1042 (1968).

289. Seegmiller, J. E., Lesch–Nyhan syndrome—Management and treatment: Seminars on Lesch–Nyhan syndrome, *Fed. Proc.* **27:**1019 (1968).

290. Seegmiller, J. E., Amniotic fluid and cells in the diagnosis of genetic disorders, in: *Amniotic Fluid: Physiology, Biochemistry, and Clinical Chemistry* (S. Natelson, A. Scommegna, and M. B. Epstein, eds.), pp. 291–316, Wiley, New York (1974).

291. Seegmiller, J. E., 1972, The Lesch–Nyhan syndrome, in: *Antenatal Diagnosis* (A. Dorfman, ed.), pp. 137–144, University of Chicago Press, Chicago (1972).

292. Seegmiller, J. E., Diseases of purine and pyrimidine metabolism, in: *Duncan's Diseases of Metabolism*, 7th ed. (P. K. Bondy and L. E. Rosenberg, eds.), pp. 655–774, Saunders Co., Philadelphia (1974).

293. Seegmiller, J. E., Biochemical and genetic studies of an X-linked neurological disease (the Lesch–Nyhan syndrome), *Harvey Lect.* **65:**175 (1969/1970).

294. Seegmiller, J. E., Metabolic aberrations in gout, *Clin. Orthoped.* **71:**87 (1970).

295. Seegmiller, J. E., New prospects for understanding and control of genetic diseases, *Arch. Int. Med.* **130:**181 (1972).

296. Seegmiller, J. E., Molecular aspects of the Lesch–Nyhan syndrome, *Biochimie* **54:**703 (1972).

297. Seegmiller, J. E., Lesch–Nyhan syndrome and the X-linked uric acidurias, *Hosp. Pract.* **7:**79 (1972).

298. Seegmiller, J. E., Metabolic basis of renal lithiasis from overproduction of uric acid: Urinary calculi, in: *Proceedings of the International Symposium on Renal Stone Research, Madrid, 1972*, pp. 89–95, Karger, Basel (1973).

299. Seegmiller, J. E., Unpublished observation (1975).

300. Seegmiller, J. E., Klinenberg, J. R., Miller, J., and Watts, R. W. E., Suppression of glycine-^{15}N incorporation into urinary uric acid by adenine-8-^{13}C in normal and gouty subjects, *J. Clin. Invest.* **47:**1193 (1968).

301. Seegmiller, J. E., Rosenbloom, F. M., and Kelley, W. N., Enzyme defect

associated with a sex-linked human neurological disorder and excessive purine synthesis, *Science* **155**:1682 (1967).

302. Seegmiller, J. E., Siniscalco, M., Klinger, H. P., Eagle, H., Koprowski, H., and Fujimoto, W. Y., Intergenomic complementation of two X-linked genes by hybridization of mutant human fibroblasts, *Trans. Assoc. Am. Physicians* **82**:239 (1969).

303. Shin, S., Nature of mutations conferring resistance to 8-azaguanine in mouse cell lines, *J. Cell Sci.* **14**:235 (1974).

304. Shin, S.-I., Khan, P. M., and Cook, P. R., Characterization of hypoxanthine-guanine phosphoribosyl transferase in man–mouse somatic cell hybrids by an improved electrophoretic method, *Biochem. Genet.* **5**:91 (1971).

305. Silvers, D. N., Cox, R. P., Balis, M. E., and Dancis, J., Detection of the heterozygote in Lesch–Nyhan disease by hair-root analysis, *New Engl. J. Med.* **286**:390 (1972).

306. Siniscalco, M., Somatic cell hybrids as tools for genetic studies in man, *Symp. Int. Soc. Cell Biol.* **9**:205 (1971).

307. Siniscalco, M., Klinger, H. P., Eagle, H., Koprowski, H., Fujimoto, W. Y., and Seegmiller, J. E., Evidence for intergenic complementation in hybrid cells derived from two human diploid strains, each carrying an X-linked mutation, *Proc. Natl. Acad. Sci. U.S.A.* **62**:793 (1969).

308. Skaper, S., and J. E. Seegmiller, The role of ammonia in metabolism of human lymphoblasts, in preparation (1975).

309. Smith, M. G., Bland, J. H., Kelley, W. N., and Seegmiller, J. E., Unpublished observation.

310. Snyder, F., and Hershfield, M., Unpublished procedure.

311. Skyler, J. S., Neelon, F. A., Arnold, W. J., Kelley, W. N., and Lebovitz, H. E., Growth retardation in the Lesch–Nyhan syndrome, *Acta Endocrinol.* **75**:3 (1974).

312. Sokoloff, L., and Seegmiller, J. E., Unpublished observation.

313. Sorenson, L. B., Suppression of the shunt pathway in primary gout by azathioprine, *Proc. Natl. Acad. Sci. U.S.A.* **55**:571 (1966).

314. Sorenson, L. B., in: Proceedings of seminars on the Lesch–Nyhan syndrome, *Fed. Proc.* **27**:1055 (1968).

315. Sorenson, L. B., Mechanism of excessive purine biosynthesis in hypoxanthine-guanine phosphoribosyltransferase deficiency, *J. Clin. Invest.* **49**:968 (1970).

316. Sorenson, L. B., and Benke, P. J., Biochemical evidence for a distinct type of primary gout, *Nature (London)* **213**:1122 (1967).

317. Sorenson, L. B., Kawahara, F., Chow, D., Benke, P. J., and Coben, L., Excessive purine synthesis and neurologic dysfunction in children, *Arthritis Rheum.* **13**:835 (1970).

318. Spector, T., and Johns, D. G., Stoichiometric inhibition of reduced xanthine oxidase by hydroxypyrazolo-[3,4-*d*]-pyrimidines, *J. Biol. Chem.* **245**:5079 (1970).

319. Sperling, O., Boer, P., Persky-Brosh, S., Kanarek, E., and de Vries, A., Altered kinetic property of erythrocyte phosphoribosylpyrophosphate synthetase in excessive purine production, *Rev. Eur. Etud. Clin. Biol.* **17**:703 (1972).

320. Sperling, O., Boer, P., and de Vries, A., Properties of erythrocyte purine phosphoribosyltransferases in partial hypoxanthine-guanine phosphoribosyltransferase deficiency, *Advan. Exp. Med. Biol.* **41A**:211 (1974).

321. Sperling, O., de Vries, A., and Wyngaarden, J. B., eds., *Purine Metabolism in*

Man: Enzymes and Metabolic Pathways, Vol. 41A of *Advances in Experimental Medicine and Biology*, Plenum Press, New York (1974).

322. Sperling, O., Eilam, G., Persky-Brosh, S., and de Vries, A., Accelerated erythrocyte 5-phosphoribosyl-1-pyrophosphate synthesis: A familial abnormality associated with excessive uric acid production and gout, *Biochem. Med.* **6**:310 (1972).

323. Sperling, O., Persky-Brosh, S., Boer, P., and de Vries, A., Mutant phosphoribosyl-pyrophosphate synthetase in two gouty siblings with excessive purine production, *Advan. Exp. Med. Biol.* **41A**:299 (1974).

324. Srivastava, S. K., and Beutler, E., Purification and kinetic studies of adenine phosphoribosyltransferase from human erythrocytes, *Arch. Biochem. Biophys.* **142**:426–434 (1971).

325. Subak-Sharpe, H., Bürk, R. R., and Pitts, J. D., Metabolic cooperation by cell to cell transfer between genetically different mammalian cells in tissue culture, *Heredity (London)* **21**:342–343 (1966).

326. Subak-Sharpe, H., Bürk, R. R., and Pitts, J. D., Metabolic cooperation between biochemically marked mammalian cells in tissue culture, *J. Cell Sci.* **4**:353–367 (1969).

327. Sweetman, L., Urinary and cerebrospinal fluid oxypurine levels and allopurinol metabolism in the Lesch–Nyhan syndrome, *Fed. Proc.* **27**:1055–1059 (1968).

328. Sweetman, L., and Nyhan, W. L., Excretion of hypoxanthine and xanthine in genetic disease of purine metabolism, *Nature (London)* **215**:859–860 (1967).

329. Sweetman, L., and Nyhan, W. L., Detailed comparison of the urinary excretion of purines in a patient with the Lesch–Nyhan syndrome and a control subject, *Biochem. Med.* **4**:121–134 (1970).

330. Sweetman, L., and Nyhan, W. L., Further studies of the enzyme composition of mutant cells in X-linked uric aciduria, *Arch. Intern. Med.* **130**:214–220 (1972).

331. Szybalski, W., Szybalska, E. H., and Ragni, G., Genetic studies with human cell lines, *Natl. Cancer Inst. Monogr.* **7**:75–89 (1962).

332. Szybalska, E. H., and Szybalski, W., Genetics of human cell lines. IV. DNA-mediated heritable transformation of a biochemical trait, *Proc. Natl. Acad. Sci. U.S.A.* **48**:2026–2034 (1962).

333. Tatibana, M., and Shigesada, K., Two carbamyl phosphate synthetases of mammals: Specific roles in control of pyrimidine and urea biosynthesis, *Advan. Enz. Regul.* **10**:249–271 (1972).

334. Thomas, C. B., Arnold, W. J., and Kelley, W. N., Human adenine phosphoribosyl-transferase: Purification, subunit structure, and substrate specificity, *J. Biol. Chem.* **248**:2529–2535 (1973).

335. Thomas, C. B., Arnold, W. J., and Kelley, W. N., Human adenine phosphoribosyl-transferase: Purification, subunit structure and substrate specificity, *Advan. Exp. Med. Biol.* **41A**:23–32 (1974).

336. Tomkins, G. M., and Martin, D. W., Hormones and gene expression, *Ann. Rev. Genet.* **4**:91–106 (1970).

337. Van Bogaert, L., Van Damme, J., and Verschueren, M., Sur un syndrome progressif d'hypertonie extrapyramidale avec osteoarthropathies goutteuses chez deux frères: Première observation chez l'adulte, *Rev. Neurol. (Paris)* **114**:15 (1966).

338. Van der Zee, S. P., Lommen, E. J. P., Trijbels, J. M. F., and Schretlen, E. D. A. M., The influence of adenine on the clinical features and purine metabolism in the Lesch–Nyhan syndrome, *Acta Paediat. Scand.* **59**:259–264 (1970).

339. Van der Zee, S. P., Monnens, L. A., and Schretlen, E. D. A. M., Een hereditaire purine stofwisselingsstoornis met een cerebrale aandoening en megaloblastaire

anemia (syndroom van Lesch en Nyhan), *Ned. Tijdschr. Geneeskd.* **112:**1475–1481 (1968).

340. Van der Zee, S. P. M., Schretlen, E. D. A. M., and Monnens, L. A., Megaloblastic anaemia in the Lesch–Nyhan syndrome, *Lancet* **1:**1427 (1968).

341. Van Heeswijk, P. J., Blank, C. H., Seegmiller, J. E., and Jacobson, C. B., Preventive control of the Lesch–Nyhan syndrome, *Obstet. Gynecol.* **40:**109–113 (1972).

342. Wada, Y., Arakawa, T., and Koizumi, K., Lesch–Nyhan syndrome: Autopsy findings and *in vitro* study of incorporation of ^{14}C-8-inosine into uric acid, guanosine-monophosphate and adenosine-monophosphate in the liver, *Tohoku J. Exp. Med.* **95:**253–260 (1968).

343. Watson, B., Gormley, I. P., Gardner, S. E., Evans, H. J., and Harris, N., Reappearance of murine hypoxanthine guanine phosphoribosyltransferase activity in mouse A9 cells after attempted hybridization with human cell lines, *Exp. Cell Res.* **75:**401–409 (1972).

343a. Watts, R. W. E., McKeran, R. O., Brown, E., Andrews, T. M., and Griffiths, M. I., Clinical and biochemical studies on treatment of Lesch–Nyhan syndrome, *Arch. Dis. Child.* **49:**693–702 (1974).

344. Windhorst, D. B., Holmes, B., and Good, R. A., A newly defined X-linked trait in man with demonstration of the Lyon effect in carrier females, *Lancet* **1:**737–739 (1967).

345. Wood, A. W., Becker, M. A., Minna, J. D., and Seegmiller, J. E., Purine metabolism in normal and thioguanine-resistant neuroblastoma, *Proc. Natl. Acad. Sci. U.S.A.* **70:**3880 (1973).

346. Wood, A. W., Becker, M. A., and Seegmiller, J. E., Purine nucleotide synthesis in lymphoblasts cultured from normal subjects and a patient with Lesch–Nyhan syndrome, *Biochem. Genet.* **9:**261–274 (1973).

347. Wood, S., and Pinsky, L., Lesch–Nyhan syndrome: Rapid detection of heterozygotes, *Clin. Genet.* **1:**216–219 (1970).

348. Wood, A. W., and Seegmiller, J. E., Properties of 5-phosphoribosyl-1-pyrophosphate glutamine amidotransferase from human lymphoblasts, *J. Biol. Chem.* **248:**138–143 (1973).

349. Wyngaarden, J. B., and Kelley, W. N., Gout, in: *The Metabolic Basis of Inherited Disease* 3rd ed. (J. B. Stanbury, J. B. Wyngaarden, and D. S. Fredrickson, eds.), pp. 889–968, McGraw-Hill, New York (1972).

350. Yip, L. C., Dancis, J., and Balis, M. E., Immunochemical studies of AMP: pyrophosphate phosphoribosyltransferase from normal and Lesch–Nyhan subjects, *Biochim. Biophys. Acta* **293:**359–369 (1973).

351. Yip, L. C., Dancis, J., Mathieson, B., and Balis, M. E., Age-induced changes in adenosine monophosphate: pyrophosphate phosphoribosyltransferase and inosine monophosphate: pyrophosphate phosphoribosyltransferase from normal and Lesch–Nyhan erythrocytes, *Biochemistry* **13:**2558–2561 (1974).

352. Yu, T.-F., Balis, M. E., Krenitsky, T. A., Dancis, J., Silvers, D. N., Elion, G. B., and Gutman, A. B., Rarity of X-linked partial hypoxanthine-guanine phosphoribosyltransferase deficiency in a large gouty population, *Ann. Intern. Med.* **76:**255–264 (1972).

353. Zoref, E., Sperling, O., and DeVries, A., Stabilization by PRPP of cellular purine phosphoribosyltransferases against inactivation by freezing and thawing: Study of normal and hypoxanthine-guanine phosphoribosyltransferase deficient human fibroblasts, *Advan. Exp. Med. Biol.* **41A:**15 (1974).

Chapter 3

Hereditary Hemolytic Anemia Due to Enzyme Defects of Glycolysis

Sergio Piomelli

Division of Pediatric Hematology
New York University School of Medicine
New York, New York

and

Laurence Corash

Hematology Service, Clinical Pathology Department
Clinical Center, National Institutes of Health
Bethesda, Maryland

INTRODUCTION

In view of our present knowledge of the genetic control of protein synthesis, it seems logical to assume that occasional mutations should give rise to specific defects of individual enzymes in the chain which controls glycolysis in the red cells.[87] Indeed, it is an easy prophecy, today, that in the very near future individuals deficient in each of the glycolytic enzymes will be clearly identified. On the other hand, it is extraordinary to reflect that the first specific enzymatic defect responsible for chronic hemolytic anemia—a deficiency of pyruvate kinase—was postulated and described less than 15 years ago.[201,251] This discovery came 5 years after the demonstration that a deficiency of glucose-6-phosphate dehydrogenase in the red cells is responsible for the genetically determined sensitivity to acute hemolysis upon exposure to certain drugs.[45]

The most common and classical form of chronic hemolysis, hereditary spherocytosis, has been known to hematologists since the early 1900s.[52] This syndrome, which had been considered *the* congenital hemolytic anemia by antonomasia, is characterized by small densely staining red cells, chronic hemolysis, splenomegaly, and dominant inheritance. Generations of hematologists have been familiar with the concept that these odd-shaped (spherical) red cells cannot travel through the capillary maze of the spleen. Hence once the spleen is removed surgically, the same odd-shaped cells persist but the clinical symptoms of the individual disappear. The true molecular basis for hereditary spherocytosis is today still largely unexplained, but this disorder remains by far the most common form of hereditary hemolytic anemia.[109] The prominent position of hereditary spherocytosis in hematology explains the need for the awkward jargon "nonspherocytic congenital hemolytic anemia" initially used to describe those rare cases of chronic hemolysis where neither spherocytic appearance of the red cells nor dominant inheritance could be found.[59,62] The techniques applicable to the study of hereditary spherocytosis were used by analogy to study the nonspherocytic congenital hemolytic anemias. In 1954, Selwyn and Dacie[218] noticed that when red cells from these patients were incubated under sterile conditions at 37°C they exhibited the same (or greater) tendency to hemolysis as red cells from individuals with hereditary spherocytosis (autohemolysis). However, a few differences became apparent: in some cases the hemolysis upon incubation was reduced by the previous addition of glucose (type I nonspherocytic congenital anemia), while in other cases it was either unaffected or even increased (type II nonspherocytic congenital anemia). The autohemolysis test then provided at least a rudimentary tool for a tentative classification of these syndromes. Robinson *et al.*[201] in 1961 undertook the study of phosphorylated compounds in the red cells of type II patients and discovered a decreased amount of ATP and an increased amount of 2, 3-DPG. Since it was also clear from the results of the autohemolysis that these red cells had difficulty utilizing glucose, these authors postulated a specific defect of a glycolytic enzyme somewhere in the chain after 2,3-DPG synthesis. Within the same year, 1961, Valentine *et al.*,[251] applying classical techniques of enzymology, demonstrated that a specific enzymatic defect was indeed present in three type II patients: a greatly decreased level of pyruvate kinase. The following years have seen the description of several

specific defects of glycolytic enzymes associated with chronic hemolysis, and sometimes also with symptoms related to other organs and
systems.[20,245] It has been shown that most type I patients also have a
defect in a glycolytic enzyme.[61] Some, however, have inherited a
mutant of glucose-6-phosphate dehydrogenase, with different biochemical characteristics than the usual mutants responsible for drug-induced
hemolysis.[20,117,199] Specific defects of enzymes outside the main glycolytic chain have also been described in association with congenital
nonspherocytic anemia.[246] Enzymatic defects of the red cells which do
not result in chronic hemolysis[32,206] have been observed, a situation
analogous to that of "characters in search of an author"[196] or, to
remain in the scientific field, of "viruses in search of disease."[96]
Specific enzymatic defects in the red cells, on the other hand, have
been observed in hereditary metabolic defects in which the primary
effect is in different organs. Classical examples of this situation are the
defects in hypoxanthine-guanine phosphoribosyltransferase[217] (Lesch–
Nyhan syndrome) and in adenosine deaminase.[82,148] In both of these
conditions, the lack of a specific enzyme leaves the red cell unaffected,
presumably since the involved pathway is nonessential to red cell
survival. The search for specific enzymatic defects of the red cells has
been so intensive that at least one type of deficiency—glutathione
reductase—was found in individuals with disorders as diverse as
hemoglobin C disease, thrombocytopenia, and chronic diseases.[20,254]
Later studies showed that this enzyme is activated when bound to
flavin adenine dinucleotide and that reduced activity of glutathione
reductase in the red cells can be rapidly corrected by the oral
administration of riboflavin[83,227]; thus a supposedly genetic disorder
proved to be an acquired nutritional problem.[19]

   The picture of the congenital hemolytic anemias secondary to
enzymatic defects of the red cells is at present fragmentary and largely
anecdotal. Most of these defects have been described only recently and
the number of patients and families studied remains very small (Table
I), the only exception being pyruvate kinase deficiency, which is the
most common congenital hemolytic disorder after hereditary spherocytosis.[231] The rarity of these syndromes is compounded by the
complexity of the techniques necessary to diagnose a specific enzymatic defect. Only very few laboratories can routinely perform all the
required enzymatic assays. It is not surprising that the largest number
of specific red cell enzymatic defects were discovered by (or in

TABLE I. Enzymatic Defects of Red Cell Glycolysis Associated with Hemolysis

Enzyme	Abbreviation	Number of propositi	References
Hexokinase	HK	4	113, 161, 166, 248
Glucosephosphate isomerase	GPI	19	5, 10, 22, 25, 50, 54, 98, 132, 135, 155, 156, 170, 180, 182, 214, 215
Phosphofructokinase	PFK	4	129, 160, 237, 255
Triosephosphate isomerase	TI	7	2, 89, 120, 209, 210, 250
Glyceraldehyde-3-phosphate dehydrogenase	PGAD	2[a]	86, 177
Diphosphoglycerate mutase	DPGM	1[a]	47
Phosphoglycerate kinase	PGK	7	3, 48, 92, 121, 123, 157, 247
Enolase	ENO	1[a]	228
Pyruvate kinase	PK	>150	231
Lactate dehydrogenase	LDH	1	158
Enzymes for which *no defect* has been described			
Aldolase	ALD		
Diphosphoglycerate phosphatase	DPGP		
Phosphoglucomutase	PGM		

[a] Uncertain demonstration.

cooperation with) the laboratory of Valentine and coworkers,[10,247,248,250] the same group that originally described the specific defect of pyruvate kinase.[251] It is a tribute to the ingenuity of the workers in this field that in such a short period of time the study of these rare syndromes has contributed to the understanding of such disorders and to other related scientific fields. Careful investigation of a single family permitted Valentine *et al.*[247] to postulate the X linkage of phosphoglycerate kinase, which was later confirmed by classical segregation studies of electrophoretic mutants in humans[53] and by genetic studies with man–mouse and man–hamster somatic cell hybrids.[116] Detailed metabolic studies by Keitt[112] of a single pyruvate kinase deficient family provided an elegant biochemical explanation for the efficacy of splenectomy and placed on firm scientific ground the apparently iconoclastic concept that an increase (rather than a decrease) in reticulocytes after splenectomy reflects improved red cell survival. The episodic study of individual families sometimes suggested correlations that later turned out to be only sporadic associations; among these are the concomitance of Fanconi's anemia and hexokinase deficiency[138] and of the *cri-du-chat* syndrome with triosephosphate isomerase deficiency.[223] Paradoxically, it was shown recently that in some cases a red cell enzymatic defect may simulate the classical presentation of hereditary spherocytosis, as in a case of glucosephosphate isomerase deficiency described by Oski and Fuller.[170] This observation suggests that scientific research also undergoes *courses* and *recourses*, as does history.[253]

A detailed description of all of the individual enzymatic defects hitherto reported would be primarily descriptive and, at the present state of the art, would rapidly become incomplete even before publication. For these reasons, a discussion of red cell glycolytic metabolism and its interrelationship with cell functions and the aging process follows a table in which most, if not all, cases of specific glycolytic enzymatic defects presently reported are listed (Table I). Defects in hexokinase, glucosephosphate isomerase, phosphofructokinase, phosphoglycerate kinase, and pyruvate kinase will be discussed in detail as these disorders appear at present to be the best understood and the most frequently observed. Chronic hemolytic anemia associated with glucose-6-phosphate dehydrogenase deficiency has been recently discussed in this series.[118] Chronic hemolytic anemias associated with disorders of glycolysis have also recently been reviewed, primarily from a clinical hematological viewpoint.[17,145,149,176,245,246]

GLUCOSE UTILIZATION BY THE RED CELL

The mature red cell depends almost entirely on the utilization of glucose for its energy metabolism. The mature red cell lacks nucleus, mitochondria, or endoplasmic reticulum, so that most of its metabolic activities take place in a homogeneous cytoplasm, without any compartmentation to subcellular organelles. As the mature red cell has no appreciable tricarboxylic acid cycle, respiration, or glycogenesis, energy metabolism rests on the process of conversion of 1 mole of glucose into 2 moles of lactate (Fig. 1). Since the initial substrate (glucose) and the terminal products (pyruvate and lactate) are in equilibrium with the plasma, the entire process may be seen as a futile

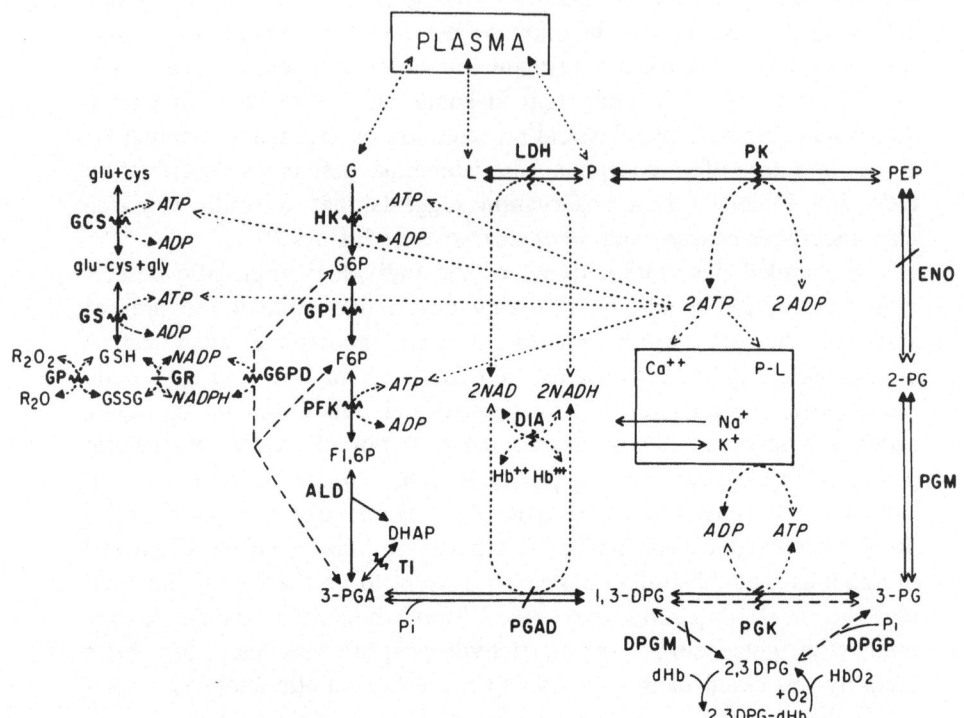

Fig. 1. Scheme of glycolysis. ---, Alternate pathway; →, direction of equilibrium; {, demonstrated deficiency; /, uncertain demonstration of defect. Enzymes (bold type): GCS, glutamyl cysteine synthetase; GS, glutathione synthetase; GP, glutathione peroxidase; GR, glutathione reductase; G6PD, glucose-6-phosphate dehydrogenase (other enzymes of pentose pathways are not shown; for details of these, see Piomelli[188]); DIA, diaphorase; other enzyme abbreviations as in Table I. Substrates: glu, glutamic acid; cys, cysteine; gly, glycine; R_2O_2, peroxide; R_2O, reduced peroxide; GSH, glutathione, reduced; GSSG, glutathione, oxidized; G, glucose; G6P, glucose-6-phosphate; F6P, fructose-6-phosphate; F1,6P, fructose-1,6-diphosphate; DHAP, dihydroxyacetone phosphate; 3-PGA, 3-phosphoglyceraldehyde; 1,3-DPG, 1,3-diphosphoglycerate; 3-PG, 3-phosphoglycerate; 2-PG, 2-phosphoglycerate; 2,3-DPG, 2,3-diphosphoglycerate; PEP, phosphoenolpyruvate; P, pyruvate; L, lactate. Cofactors (italics): ATP, adenosine triphosphate; ADP, adenosine diphosphate; NAD, nicotinamide adenine dinucleotide; NADH, reduced NAD; NADP, nicotinamide adenine dinucleotide phosphate; NADPH, reduced NADP. Miscellaneous abbreviations: P_i, inorganic phosphate; Hb^{2+}, hemoglobin with reduced Fe; Hb^{3+}, methemoglobin; dHb, deoxyhemoglobin; HbO_2, oxyhemoglobin; Na^+, sodium ion; K^+, potassium ion; Ca^{2+}, calcium ion; O_2, oxygen; P-L, phospholipids. Boxed area represents cell membrane.

effort to secrete pyruvate and lactate into plasma. The metabolic importance of glucose utilization, however, resides in a series of by-products generated at various points in the chain of reactions. The utilization of glucose to form lactate may be arrested, accelerated more than tenfold, or diverted to shunt pathways depending on changing needs of the cell. In this sense, the metabolic flow of the red cell can be seen as a stream of energy which can be channeled into different paths and activate several independent wheels, through a series of self-regulating relays which open or close individual cataracts.

Overall Regulation of Glycolysis

The rate of glycolysis in the red cell obviously cannot depend on feedback control by the final two products (pyruvate and lactate), since both readily diffuse into plasma. In a complex enzymatic pathway such as glycolysis, the potential activity of an individual enzyme exceeds its actual activity severalfold, sometimes even a thousandfold.[90] It is more efficient for the overall level of activity of the enzymatic system to be less than the potential of its individual steps, so that a demand for increased production can be satisfied before the least active step becomes rate limiting.

In fact, red cell glycolysis exhibits several regulatory mechanisms interrelated to provide a flexible means of control.[114,150,202,203,224] Through these, the rate of metabolic flow can be adjusted to the cell's needs and individual segments may be shunted through alternate pathways.

Since hexokinase, the first enzyme of the chain, is also the least active by several orders of magnitude, it has been suggested that this may be the single rate-limiting step.[51,198] However, if hexokinase were the only limiting step, no intermediate products of glycolysis should be found inside the cells.[151] In fact, all intermediate products can be found in different proportions in the red cell. This observation suggests that regulatory mechanisms exist at multiple sites throughout the glycolytic chain. Indeed, the primary regulation appears to operate through the ratio of reduced/oxidized coenzymes (NADH/NAD, NADPH/NADP) and of phosphorylated/unphosphorylated coenzymes (ATP/ADP), as well as through the generation of side-products (2,3-DPG). These regulatory mechanisms operate through a complex interlocking of modulator, inhibitor, and derepressor by-products. These alternately function as clutches to direct the metabolic flow—slowing down, accelerating, or even bypassing specific steps to suit the cells' immediate needs. Reductions in the rate of individual reactions may cause an upstream accumulation and a downstream depletion of intermediates. Accumulation of intermediates in the initial part of glycolysis causes a decrease in overall metabolism.

There are four main products of glycolysis; two of these, ATP and NADH, are products of the mainstream pathway and two are shunt products: NADPH of the pentose phosphate shunt and 2,3-DPG of the Rapaport–Luebering shunt.

The ATP/ADP Ratio

The ATP/ADP ratio represents the state of the primary pool of energy-rich compounds in the red cell. In the initial reaction of glycolysis (hexokinase) as well as in the third reaction (phosphofructo-kinase), one molecule of ATP is converted to ADP. In the later steps of the pathway, two ADP molecules are phosphorylated into ATP at the 3-phosphoglycerate kinase reaction and two more at the pyruvate kinase step. The conversion of each molecule of glucose into two molecules of lactate thus ultimately results in the net generation of two ATP molecules. However, if the 2, 3-DPG shunt is utilized, then the phosphoglycerate kinase reaction is bypassed, and no net generation of ATP takes place; instead, two molecules of 2,3-DPG are produced. The two steps at which ATP is generated, phosphoglycerate kinase and pyruvate kinase, are not functionally equivalent. It has been shown that phosphoglycerate kinase is anatomically related to the membrane at the site where active energy in the form of ATP is necessary for cation transport.[185] Thus the ATP produced by phosphoglycerate kinase is primarily committed to this function while the ATP produced by pyruvate kinase is available for a variety of cell needs. The red cell maintains an elevated concentration of K^+ and a low concentration of Na^+ by an active transport mechanism. This balance is obtained by the action of a membrane "cation pump" which is, in essence, a Na^+- and K^+-activated adenosine triphosphatase.[114] Transfer of the γ-terminal phosphate group of ATP to an intermediate is stimulated by Na^+; the removal of this phosphate group as inorganic phosphate is stimulated by K[+].[66] Ouabain and other glycosides inhibit this reaction and thus block the "cation pump." Since ouabain inhibition also decreases glycolysis, it is apparent that the activity of the cation pump has a regulatory effect.[152] Inhibition by ouabain results in an accumulation of intermediates above the phosphoglycerate kinase step, except for ADP. Parker and Hoffman[185] have suggested on the basis of this finding that the cation pump and phosphoglycerate kinase derive their ATP from a separate pool of ADP and that the size of this pool controls the flow of glycolysis. Schrier[211] demonstrated in fact that phosphoglycerate kinase separates with the red cell stroma upon centrifugation. These observations suggest that generation of ATP to maintain the intracellular cation concentration occurs at the cell membrane. Cation transport is such an essential cellular function that glycolytic rates may be adjusted to meet this requirement.

The ATP/ADP ratio may be decreased by inhibition of glycolysis with compounds such as iodoacetate (which inhibits glyceraldehyde-3-phosphate dehydrogenase) or fluoride (which inhibits enolase)[70] or by glucose depletion.[69] In ATP-depleted red cells, a selective leak of K[+] occurs, leading to loss of intracellular water ("Gardos effect")[78]; ATP-depleted cells thus undergo a process of osmotic shrinkage, known as "desicytosis."[165] The exact mechanism of this effect of ATP depletion is not known. It has been suggested that Ca^{2+} and possibly "a mediator" may be necessary.[24] The ATP/ADP ratio controls the ionic strength of the red cell by its effect on both cation pump and K[+] leak. Thus water content is conserved and with it the appropriate membrane tension to maintain the biconcave shape. A further function of intracellular ATP in maintaining the red cell shape has been recently described: ATP appears necessary to chelate Ca^{2+} and prevent excessive membrane rigidity. This effect may be mediated by several mechanisms: the existence of a contractile membrane protein with Ca^{2+}-activated adenosine triphosphatase activity,[204] the operation of a specific Ca^{2+} pump (non-oubain-inhibited and presumably independent of the Na^+-K^+ pump),[207] or the direct chelation of Ca^{2+} [125] to prevent interaction with membrane phospholipids.[220] ATP is also necessary for the orderly turnover of the red cell membrane phospholipids. Shohet *et al.*[221] demonstrated that 2% of the total membrane phospholipids are regenerated per hour, at the apparent metabolic cost of approximately 5% of the total energetic output of glycolysis. Since ATP is necessary in the first and third steps of glycolysis, a portion of the ATP produced in the later steps is utilized to reinitiate this cycle.

Inorganic phosphate concentration plays an important controlling role in the generation of ATP, by facilitating the phosphofructokinase reaction and directly participating in the glyceraldehyde-3-phosphate dehydrogenase reaction.[203] In fact, in patients with severe phosphate depletion markedly decreased ATP levels are observed, with the expected effects on membrane rigidity, and clinical hemolysis.[240]

The picture of the key importance of ATP in red cell metabolism would not be complete without mentioning that ATP is also an essential cofactor in the two-step synthesis of glutathione from glutamic acid, cysteine, and glycine.[153] To accommodate these various functions, ATP production is the primary function of glycolysis and the ATP/ADP ratio is one of the fundamental controlling mechanisms of glucose utilization. When ATP production is defective, as in pyruvate kinase deficiency, red cell survival is rapidly curtailed and spiny desiccated cells with rigid membranes appear in the circulation.[175]

The NADH/NAD Ratio

The NADH/NAD ratio in the red cell is maintained by the generation of NADH at the glyceraldehyde-3-phosphate dehydrogenase step and its reoxidation in the lactic dehydrogenase reaction. The NADH/NAD ratio is also dependent on the plasma lactate/pyruvate ratio. Since both lactate and pyruvate diffuse freely across the red cell membrane, it is possible to rapidly offset any increased utilization of NADH for intracellular needs. NADH is the essential cofactor for NADH diaphorase, an enzyme which in the presence of cytochrome b_5 converts methemoglobin to hemoglobin and thus maintains heme Fe in the reduced state.[97] A slow continuous oxidation of hemoglobin to methemoglobin occurs in the red cells; thus individuals deficient in NADH diaphorase have considerable elevation of methemoglobin concentration.[216] The necessary NADH for the function of the diaphorase is supplied by the glyceraldehyde-3-phosphate dehydrogenase reaction,[68] although it has recently been suggested that part of it may be supplied by the sorbitol pathway, which is also operative in the red cell.[239]

The NADPH/NADP Ratio

A high ratio of NADPH/NADP is essential to the maintenance of cell integrity, to protect the cell membrane and other essential components, including hemoglobin itself, from the oxidizing effect of peroxides and peroxide-generating agents. This protection is mediated through the coupled action of glutathione reductase and glutathione peroxidase, which utilize NADPH as a hydrogen donor.[55,107] NADPH is not directly generated through the mainstream of glycolysis, but it is produced through the diversion of significant amounts of glucose through the pentose phosphate pathway. For each molecule of glucose completely converted to CO_2 through repeated turns of this cycle, 12 molecules of NADPH are generated.

A very precise mechanism exists in the red cell to allow an enormous amount of glucose to be diverted through the pentose phosphate pathway. In the steady state, the first enzyme of the pentose phosphate pathway, glucose-6-phosphate dehydrogenase, is in its monomeric subactive form[199] and is inhibited by high concentrations of NADPH.[260] In response to oxidative stimulation, NADPH is oxidized to NADP through the glutathione cycle, and the NADPH/NADP ratio decreases.[107] The decrease in NADPH eliminates the inhibition of glucose-6-phosphate dehydrogenase and the increased concentration of NADP results in the conversion of the enzyme from its monomeric subactive form to its dimeric active form.[199] As a result of the sudden increase in glucose-6-phosphate dehydrogenase activity, the intracellular concentration of glucose-6-phosphate decreases. Since the primary controlling mechanism of the activity of hexokinase is the end-product inhibition by glucose-6-phosphate,[202] a decreased level of glucose-6-phosphate causes the derepression of this enzyme. Additional glucose is then phosphorylated to glucose-6-phosphate, and the pentose phosphate pathway cycling is maintained. This chain of events permits a sudden, almost explosive, diversion of glucose metabolism toward the pentose phosphate shunt and increases the NADPH/NADP ratio, which in turn permits the neutralization of peroxide.[55] Individuals deficient in glucose-6-phosphate dehydrogenase cannot activate the pentose phosphate shunt adequately and are therefore subject to extreme cell damage when exposed to oxidizing stimuli.[188] This is the basis for the drug-induced hemolysis observed in glucose-6-phosphate dehydrogenase deficiency.[45]

The 2,3-DPG Cycle

The primary function of the red cell is to act as a carrier of oxygen through the specific oxygen-carrying protein, hemoglobin. Although the oxygen-carrying function does not *per se* require energy, it is interrelated with cell metabolism since it is greatly influenced by increased or decreased generation of the compound 2,3-DPG from glucose metabolism.[12] The 2,3-DPG is not a direct product of the mainstream of glycolysis, but it may be generated through a shunt which bypasses the 3-phosphoglycerate kinase reaction. This bypass, as mentioned above, results in a decreased generation of ATP and in this sense is an energy expenditure. The production of 2,3-DPG is very precisely regulated by a balance which responds to anoxic stimulation. In case of decreased oxygen concentration, a greater proportion of the hemoglobin is in the deoxygenated state which has an increased affinity for 2,3-DPG. Benesch and Benesch[13] have shown that 2,3-DPG binds with great avidity to deoxyhemoglobin with 1:1 stoichiometry (one molecule of 2,3-DPG per hemoglobin tetramer) and profoundly modifies its oxygen affinity. The site of 2,3-DPG binding, in the central cavity of the β-chain, has also been recently clarified.[4] Increased levels of 2,3-DPG greatly decrease the oxygen affinity of hemoglobin and thus facilitate the "unloading" of oxygen at the tissue level. By this mechanism, greater quantities of oxygen are delivered to the tissues in hypoxic situations; thus an increase in 2,3-DPG provides a physiological compensatory mechanism for hypoxia. The concentration of 2,3-DPG is consistently increased in most types of anemia; by this effect, nearly normal amounts of oxygen may be delivered to the tissues despite a decreased hemoglobin level in most situations.[71] Genetic disorders of glycolysis in the red cells may influence 2,3-DPG levels in the opposite direction; defects above the 2,3-DPG shunt will result in decreased levels and below the 2,3-DPG shunt in increased levels. In cases of anemia secondary to enzymatic defects of glycolysis, the site of the metabolic block thus greatly influences the clinical symptomatology of the patient. Delivoria-Papadopoulos *et al.*[63] showed that patients with hexokinase deficiency have a decreased level of 2,3-DPG and thus an unfavorable oxygen dissociation curve while patients with pyruvate kinase deficiency have greatly increased 2,3-DPG levels with a much more favorable oxygen dissociation curve.

For this reason, at an equally low level of hemoglobin, hexokinase-deficient patients are clinically greatly hampered while pyruvate kinase deficient patients tolerate the anemia remarkably well.

The ratio 2,3-DPG/3-PG is maintained constant by the participation of these compounds as cofactors in the reactions that control their synthesis. 3-PG is a cofactor for 2,3-diphosphoglycerate mutase and at the same time the product of the inhibitor of 2,3-diphosphoglycerate phosphatase. Hence an increased level of 3-PG will automatically induce a rise in 2,3-DPG by both accelerated synthesis and decreased catabolism. On the other hand, 2,3-DPG is a cofactor for 3-phosphoglycerate mutase.[171] Elevated concentrations of 2,3-DPG accelerate the conversion of 3-PG to 2-PG; the reduced concentration of 3-PG in turn decreases the synthesis and accelerates the catabolism of 2,3-DPG.[112] By these balancing effects, the concentration of 2,3-DPG and the 2,3-DPG/3-PG ratio are maintained constant in the cytoplasm. However, the overall cell concentration of 2,3-DPG is affected by the 2,3-DPG bound to deoxyhemoglobin, which is unavailable to metabolic turnover as well by the postulated existence of another compartment of 2,3-DPG attached to the cell membrane.[174] Hypoxia further increases the synthesis of 2,3-DPG, by raising intracellular pH. This stimulates the 2,3-diphosphoglycerate mutase and inhibits the 2,3-diphosphoglycerate phosphatase. Production of additional 2,3-DPG lowers intracellular pH and reverses the process.[12]

Mass Action Ratio

The multiple control mechanisms by which the concentration of products and cofactors regulates the rate and direction of metabolic flow provide several independent and yet interlocked regulatory steps in overall cell glycolysis. Analysis of the concentration of glycolytic intermediates by steady-state mass action ratios has indicated that most glycolytic reactions approach equilibrium, with the exception of hexokinase, phosphofructokinase, and pyruvate kinase, which have the greatest free energy changes (ΔF) and appear thus to be the key points in regulation of metabolism.[151] It is clear that none of these three steps is the exclusive site of regulation, although each may be viewed as a pivotal step in red cell glycolysis.

EFFECT OF CELL AGE ON METABOLISM

Studies of red cell metabolism are based on results obtained by analysis of samples from circulating blood. These are in reality a mixture of cells of various ages, with great differences in metabolic activities. Since the human red cell has a finite life span of 120 days[114] and nearly no cells are lost at random, a peripheral blood sample contains equal proportions of cells of increasing age from day 0 to day 120. The life span of the red cell may be divided into three separate stages: normoblast, reticulocyte, and mature red cell. In the bone marrow, during the normoblast stage, there is active synthesis of cell structures and hemoglobin as well as of the enzymatic machinery necessary for cell metabolism. After the nucleus is extruded, the red cell enters the circulation as a reticulocyte, retaining limited synthetic capacity as well as active mitochondria only for the first 24–48 hr in the circulation. The mature red cell is devoid of any capacity for protein synthesis and has to rely for all of its metabolic function on the survival of a preformed machinery. The journey of the red cell has been estimated at 175 miles[88]; this cannot be considered smooth sailing, but rather as a series of obstacle courses. Passage through highly specialized capillary circulations, such as in the spleen and liver, is the ultimate test of cell viability. A certain amount of "polishing" (removal of redundant membrane) occurs in the spleen throughout the cell life span,[114] but when the membrane becomes rigid the cell is incapable of the deformability necessary for safe passage through the capillary circulation. The energy metabolism of the red cell is spent repairing wear and tear on the membrane phospholipids pumping cations in and out, and preserving membrane flexibility and structural integrity. However, there is no mechanism to revitalize the wear and tear on the metabolic machinery itself.

Marks and Johnson[141] first demonstrated that certain enzyme activities progressively decline with aging of the red cell. Their studies introduced the concept of "age-dependent enzymes" and suggested that enzymatic activities may decline in aging red cells to a level incompatible with cell survival. Analysis of the rate of decline of metabolic activities of the red cell requires the isolation of discrete fractions of cells of different mean age for cross-sectional measurements. The initial observations were obtained utilizing the different osmotic resistance of cells of different ages; this technique suffers from the disadvantage that old red cells cannot be isolated intact, but only in the form of dilute hemolysates, and several enzymes become inactivated in dilute solutions.[142] Better separation of intact cells of different age may be obtained by centrifugation, after the initial observation by Key[115] that reticulocytes tend to concentrate in the upper part of the red cell column. Studies with ^{59}Fe-labeled red cells have confirmed that young red cells are lighter.[31] The difference in specific gravity with cell age can be best exploited by equilibrium centrifugation using density gradients.[58,133,190] Both continuous[133] and discontinuous[58,190] gradients have been utilized for this purpose. Discontinuous gradients appear preferable, since remixing of the cell layers during removal can be prevented by slicing the tube through clear cell-free bands.[57,58,190] The adherence of the red cells to the tube walls prevents the use of conventional tube piercing for fraction collection. In our laboratories, discontinuous gradients have been used extensively for separation of cells of progressively increasing age for metabolic studies. Dating of red cells with glycine-2-^{14}C (a nonreutilized label) has indicated that a progressive increase in cell density occurs throughout the cell life span and it is not only limited to the transition from reticulocyte to mature red cell.[190] However, it must be considered that techniques of separation cannot yield groups of cells 100% homogeneous with regard to age but only fractions with a shifted proportion of cells of any given age. Absolute separation is not possible using any physical characteristic of the red cells since these emerge from the bone marrow as a normally distributed population. With regard to density, newly formed red cells also exhibit normal distribution; the mean density increases with age, but the variance remains constant. In every fraction isolated by difference in density, there is therefore a predictable overlap of cells of varying ages. It is possible to correlate mathematically the position of each cell fraction in the gradient with its mean cell age. Values obtained in several fractions of progressively increasing age thus provide a slope of decline of age-dependent parameters from which sensible extrapolation to theoretical values at 0 and 120 days is possible.[189]

By use of this technique, the rate of decline of glycolytic enzymes was systematically studied (Fig. 2). It is apparent that all glycolytic enzymes progressively lose activity with aging of the cells; however, in most cases the loss of activity is negligible and 120-day-old red cells still have more than half the activity of 0-day-old red cells. The three

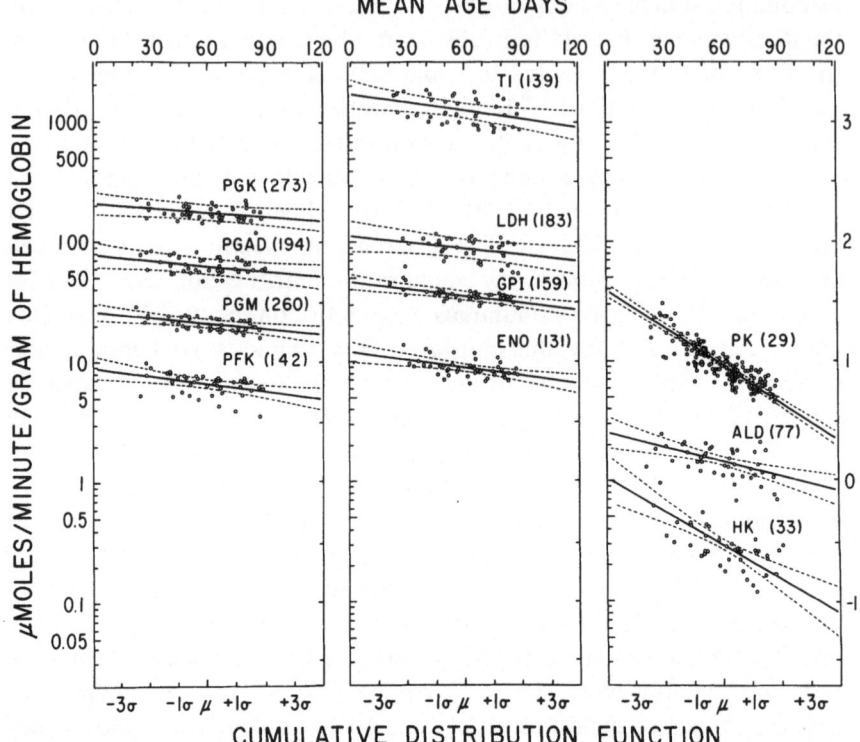

Fig. 2. Rates of decline of enzymatic activity of glycolysis with red cell age. Abbreviations as in Table I, number in parentheses indicates *in vivo* $t_{1/2}$. Cell separation according to Piomelli et al.[190]; correlation with cell age according to Piomelli et al.[189] From S. Piomelli, C. Seaman, and S. Wyss (manuscript in preparation).

glycolytic enzymes which exhibit a marked rate of decline are hexokinase and pyruvate kinase, with a $t_{1/2}$ of approximately 30 days each, and aldolase, with a $t_{1/2}$ of 77 days.[194]

Rates of decline of enzymatic activities measured by *in vitro* assays do not necessarily reflect changes in true intracellular metabolism. In fact, the assays are performed in optimal conditions, at substrate concentrations which permit maximal enzyme velocity (V_{max}). Within the cell, the interplay of concentrations of substrates, inhibitors, and activators may reduce actual enzyme activity to only a fraction of its maximal potential. Individual enzymes act within the cell only as an integral part of the entire system. For these reasons—for instance, in the case of pyruvate kinase—although the potential activity may decrease tenfold between day 0 and day 120, it always remains several times greater than the maximal flow of the glycolytic system. A better estimate of changes in metabolic capacity with cell aging is thus obtained by studies of actual utilization of glucose and production of lactate, partially shown in Fig. 3. A significant reduction in glucose utilization to a value approximately one-fourth of the initial rate is apparent in 120-day-old cells. This decreased metabolic rate does not necessarily imply metabolic failure, since the minimum rate of glucose consumption required for cell survival is unknown. Of greater significance, however, is the observation that "stressed glycolysis" (measured in the presence of either methylene blue, which stimulates primarily the pentose phosphate shunt, or increased P_i, which stimulates the main glycolytic pathway) decreases at a faster rate. As a

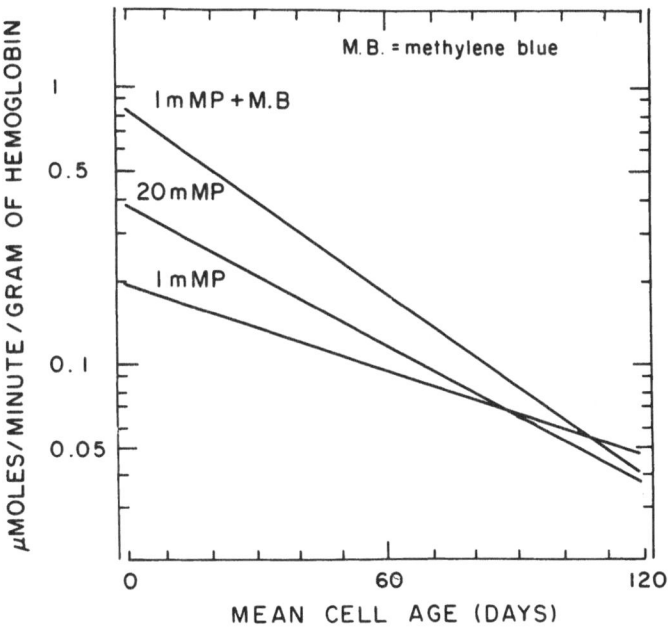

Fig. 3. Rates of decline of glucose comsumption with red cell age. Cell separation according to Piomelli et al.[190]; correlation with cell age according to Piomelli et al.[189] 1 mM P, normal rate of glycolysis; 20 mM P, glycolysis stimulated by high phosphate; 1 mM P + MB, pentose phosphate pathway stimulated by methylene blue. From S. Piomelli, C. Seaman, and S. Wyss (manuscript in preparation).

consequence, while young red cells may increase their glucose utilization up to tenfold in response to stress, old red cells with a fixed low basal metabolic rate have lost most metabolic flexibility.[194] The mechanism for this defect probably resides in the rate of decline of hexokinase. In 120-day-old red cells, the actual metabolic rates and the maximal hexokinase activity are of the same order of magnitude. In this situation, hexokinase becomes the true limiting step in overall cell metabolism. The loss in metabolic flexibility with aging may not *per se* cause the death of the red cell but greatly limits its ability to survive energy-requiring stresses.

Several other metabolic differences between young and old red cells are described and have recently been reviewed by Bunn.[41] Among the differences directly related to the reduction in glycolysis is a progressive decline in ATP[39] and 2,3-DPG levels.[85] The metabolic decline is reflected in a greatly decreased deformability. LaCelle and Weed[125] elegantly demonstrated that old red cells are more rigid and thus presumably more easily entrapped in the capillary circulations of spleen and liver.

Since younger red cells have increased metabolic activity, the mean age of the cells should be taken into consideration when comparing metabolic rates to "normal" levels. A classic example of this effect was the demonstration that in hexokinase-deficient patients the enzyme level itself may be in the normal range if compared to red cells of normal age, but it is in reality greatly decreased when compared to that of red cells from individuals with a comparable degree of hemolysis (and equally younger cell population).[248]

Cell age may also be decreased, in enzyme-deficient individuals, by the concomitant presence of an inherited or acquired independent hemolytic defect. For instance, glucose-6-phosphate dehydrogenase deficiency is encountered with great frequency among individuals with sickle cell anemia, since both traits are peculiar to individuals of West African origin.[139] In these individuals, since glucose-6-phosphate dehydrogenase of the type A⁻ is extremely age dependent, the red cell enzymatic level may be in the normal range because of the age shift caused by sickle cell anemia.[191] A correct diagnosis of enzyme deficiency may be obtained when enzyme levels from these individuals are correlated with those of individuals with reticulocytosis. Alternatively, the enzyme deficiency may be demonstrated by the ratio of the activity of glucose-6-phosphate dehydrogenase over the activity of another age-dependent enzyme (pyruvate kinase[192] or hexokinase[21]).

Enzyme levels are usually measured in red cell hemolysates; activity is expressed in international units, correlated to grams of hemoglobin.[257] This method of expression is used primarily for reasons of convenience, since hemoglobin is simpler to quantitate than red cell number and it can be measured in the same hemolysate used for enzyme assay. However, measurements of enzyme activity in I.U./g Hb are meaningful only when the red cells are of normal size. For instance, in the case of thalassemia trait, in which the red cells are smaller,[74] enzyme levels per g Hb may seem to be elevated. In one study, however, in which enzyme activities in individuals with thalassemia trait were calculated also in terms of I.U./number of red cells, the apparently elevated level of glucose-6-phosphate dehydrogenase observed in I.U./g Hb was shown to be spurious.[192] The amount of enzyme synthesized for each individual red cell is a constant, regardless of cell size.

MOLECULAR GENETIC MECHANISMS OF ENZYME DEFICIENCY

There are two possible basic molecular explanations for enzyme deficiency: quantitative synthetic failure ("quantitative defect") and synthesis of a qualitatively defective gene product ("qualitative defect").[119] These two mechanisms are distinguishable by the absence or presence, respectively, of a protein coded for by a specific gene as measured by quantitative biochemical or quantitative immunological measurements. The proof of total lack of a long-lived catalytic protein is made technically difficult because, even under normal conditions, the absolute amount of enzyme protein synthesized is miniscule. This is further complicated in the red cell because 33% of the cell wet weight consists of a single protein—hemoglobin. Under these conditions, even the purification of a normal enzyme becomes a monumental task. For example, Yoshida[259] started his purification process for glucose-6-phosphate dehydrogenase with 15 liters of whole blood and terminated with a final purified protein yield of 15 mg. On a weight basis, this is one part purified protein to 150,000 parts total protein: thus in this case the normal enzyme represents only 0.0007% of the total protein. If one had to purify an enzyme which was decreased to 1% of normal, one would be searching for one part in 15 million. By comparison, absent synthesis of the β-chain of hemoglobin can be assumed with techniques of much less sensitivity.[74]

Enzyme proteins can be detected in minute quantities by advantageous use of their catalytic activity. On the other hand, failure to demonstrate catalytic activity is not sufficient evidence of the absence of a gene product.

The use of immunological techniques can provide evidence for the existence of a catalytically silent gene product. The most classical application of this technique in humans is the demonstration of an inert gene product in hemophilia A.[95] This has been shown by the presence of immunological cross-reactive material (CRM$^+$) in the absence of procoagulant function. The foundation of the CRM methodology is once again the preparation of a highly purified normal enzyme from which the antibody is prepared. For these reasons, proof of the total lack of a red cell glycolytic enzyme has not been technically feasible to date and the absence of a gene product as a mechanism of enzyme defect may be only inferentially postulated. It was shown for human catalase that acatalasic individuals lack an immunologically detectable product (such patients are designated as CRM$^-$).[167] Even in this case, however, two alternate explanations of the CRM$^-$ state remain possible: the amount of gene product may be below the threshold sensitivity of the test or the catalytically defective gene product may also be antigenetically inert. Because of the multiplicity of antigenic sites in the size of proteins under consideration, the latter case would be highly unlikely. It appears reasonable from the above considerations that absent synthesis is a theoretical mechanism of red cell glycolytic enzyme deficiency. However, in most cases synthesis is only decreased.

Failure of synthesis is not the only possible mechanism; qualitative defects are also possible and may be divided into three categories: synthesis of a nonfunctional product, synthesis of a kinetically abnormal product, and synthesis of an *in vivo* unstable product. The demonstration of a totally nonfunctional product rests on the presence of cross-reactive material with absent catalytic function as discussed above. The last two mechanisms alone or combined appear to be most commonly operative in red cell glycolytic enzymopathies based on currently available data. A severe hemolytic defect may be associated with kinetically abnormal products which have a greater activity *in vitro* than in the cell itself. Kirkman[117] emphasized that enzymatic assays *in vitro* are performed in hemolysates under ideal conditions at concentrations of substrates and cofactors entirely different from those actually present in the cell. Thus enzymes with abnormal kinetics may appear to have significant activity in optimal conditions and yet lack function intracellularly. The affinity for the substrate (expressed by the K_m) is a better measure of the functional impairment caused by the structural mutation than is the maximum potential velocity (expressed by the V_{max}). Different intracellular efficiencies of various mutants may explain the discrepancies between clinical manifestations. The severe congenital hemolytic anemia observed in some cases of glucose-6-phosphate dehydrogenase deficiency is often associated with kinetically aberrant enzymes.[117] For instance, individuals with the common type of enzyme deficiency, Gd^{Mediterranean}, have no symptoms (except for drug-induced hemolysis) in the steady state, although their enzyme level is extremely low (1–3% of normal). This low activity is still adequate for red cell survival, since in the steady state the rate of activity of glucose-6-phosphate dehydrogenase in normal red cells is less than 0.1% of its maximal potential activity.[35] Thus red cell life span is nearly normal[15] despite a greatly decreased enzyme level. In individuals with chronic hemolysis due to mutants with abnormal substrate affinity (high K_m), there may be almost total lack of enzyme activity within the cell, where substrate concentration is low, despite apparently adequate activity in the assay.[117] However, in some cases of chronic hemolytic anemia secondary to glucose-6-phosphate dehydrogenase deficiency, no kinetic abnormalities could be demonstrated with available techniques. It has been postulated that these enzymes may be nonfunctional in the monomeric subactive state which occurs in the cells at extremely low NADP concentration[199]; for other mutants, an increased sensitivity to NADPH inhibition has been shown.[260] Presently available evidence indicates that a variety of kinetic abnormalities may cause intracellular failure of activity. The effect of *in vivo* enzyme instability on red cell deficiency will be discussed in the next section.

It must be noted that the majority of red cell enzymopathies are partial deficiencies in which even the cells of patients with significant hemolysis retain some residual activity. The mature red cell, devoid of mitochondria, is totally dependent on glycolysis. Total deficiency of a glycolytic enzyme such as hexokinase would be lethal. Only in the case of pyruvate kinase deficiency are there individuals whose red cells have no enzyme activity. Their viability is made possible by the existence of a population of young red cells with mitochondria, possessing oxidative phosphorylation capacity, which survive in the circulation for at least a few days.

EXPRESSION OF ENZYME DEFECTS IN THE RED CELL AND OTHER TISSUES

The presence of a given enzymatic deficiency in the red cells may not necessarily indicate a defect in all tissues. An enzyme defect may be observed solely in the red cells when a single genetically determined mutant enzyme has a different functional expression in different cell lines or when there is separate genetic control for different isozymes present in various tissues.

A unique functional expression of a mutant enzyme may become apparent only in the red cells because of their peculiar metabolic characteristics. For instance, it is clearly established that only one isozyme of glucose-6-phosphate dehydrogenase is present in all tissues of homozygous males.[117] In several well-studied mutants, the defect is limited to the red cells while the white cells and other tissues exhibit either normal (Gd^{A-}) or slightly decreased (Gd^{Mediterranean}) activity.[140] This apparent dichotomy reflects different degrees of instability of the various mutants. Since red cells are incapable of protein synthesis, lost enzymatic activity is not replaced. Because of the long life span of the red cell, an unstable enzyme reaches extremely low levels much before the cell is removed from the circulation. On the other hand, in the white cells (and other tissues) loss of enzyme protein may be partly compensated. Residual activity may be present when the $t_{1/2}$ of the mutant enzyme, although reduced, is long by comparison with the relatively short life span of the cell. In this case, there is not enough time for the instability of the enzyme to produce a significant decrease of activity. In the case of the two most common mutants of glucose-6-phosphate dehydrogenase, the half-lives ($t_{1/2}$) of the enzymes are reflected not only in red cells but also in white cells and other tissues.

In the case of $Gd^{Mediterranean}$, the enzyme $t_{1/2}$ is a few hours and thus enzyme activity in the long-lived red cells is nearly absent; the white cells exhibit reduced activity, since the $t_{1/2}$ of the enzyme is also shorter than the life span of these cells. In the case of Gd^{A-}, the enzyme $t_{1/2}$ is 13 days; thus enzyme activity is decreased only in the red cells, since the white cells life span itself is shorter than the $t_{1/2}$ of the enzyme. By this relationship, instability of the enzyme may produce apparently normal levels in the white cells, while the red cells appear defective.

The observation of normal level of enzyme activity in the white cells does not therefore necessarily imply a different genetic control. On the other hand, when equally decreased levels of enzyme activity are observed in both white and red cells, this is a clear indication of single genetic control. In this case, the mechanism is usually decreased production, although it is not possible to exclude an extremely increased instability or an equivalent qualitative defect.

There are other situations in which, however, lack of activity in the red cells and normal activity in the white cells result from a different genetic control for various isozymes in different tissues. For instance, in the case of individuals with defects in red cell pyruvate kinase, enzymatic activity of the white cells is normal since this is controlled by a different unaffected isozyme.[231] It is known that two distinct isozymes are present in blood, with different electrophoretic mobility, one in the red cells and one in the white cells and only the red cell isozyme is affected by the mutation.[23,195]

Enzymatic defects of the red cells, on the other hand, may reflect a generalized defect in other tissues: the glycolytic pathway is active in all tissues and the effect of the deficiency may be functionally variable depending on the metabolic capacities of various organs to replace glycolysis by alternate pathways. An example of this situation is observed in the defect of triosephosphate isomerase, which produces not only hemolysis of the red cells but also impairment of nervous tissue and muscle function.[145] An example of metabolic compensation can be seen in the lack of effect of pyruvate kinase deficiency on the hepatocyte. This defect results in a deficiency of the isozyme which is common to both red cells and hepatocytes.[231] Liver function is not directly impaired, however, presumably because mitochondrial metabolism generates adequate amounts of ATP, thus obviating the primary effect of pyruvate kinase deficiency.[112]

Spurious involvement of the neurological system may occur with many congenital hemolytic anemias. This may be due to the neurological damage secondary to extreme hyperbilirubinemia in the perinatal period and consequent kernicterus. These neurological abnormalities are preventable by removing the hemolysis-prone red cells with exchange transfusion, and thus they are unrelated to the direct effect of the metabolic deficiency.

Since enzyme activity may be normal in the white cells (and platelets) and decreased in the red cells, through one of the mechanisms discussed above, quantitative measurements of red cell activity requires careful total removal of all other cell types. The activity of most glycolytic enzymes in normal blood is 200- to 300-fold higher in white cells and platelets than in red cells, per unit volume. When the red cells are defective, the differences may be more than a thousand-fold greater. Therefore, assays of enzyme activity in red cells heavily contaminated with white cells or platelets may fail to detect deficiency. Contamination by platelets may be even more significant in those patients who have been splenectomized and exhibit an increased platelet count. The problem of contamination is of additional importance in the purification of defective tissues. Even minute amounts of normal white cells and platelet enzymes may significantly contaminate purified and concentrated enzyme preparations derived from red cell suspensions from patients with extremely decreased activity. This contamination may explain the spurious observation of defective pyruvate kinases with greater affinity for the substrate than even the normal enzyme.[169,226] In reality, these abnormal characteristics correspond to those of the unaffected white cell and platelet isozyme carried over through the purification step.

The commonly used method for removal of white cells and platelets is the aspiration of the "buffy coats." In our laboratories, aspiration of "buffy coats" from packed cell suspensions has been found to be an inefficient method for the removal of white cells and platelets because of trapping of the latter elements and the overlapping densities of granulocytes, platelets, and red cells.[57] Additionally, substantial reticulocyte loss occurs. A simpler and more efficient method to completely remove placelets and white cells is defibrination of whole blood followed by filtration through filter paper. This technique provides a nearly pure suspension of red cells without loss of reticulocytes.[190]

HEXOKINASE DEFICIENCY

Hexokinase catalyzes the phosphorylation of glucose to glucose-6-phosphate, the initial step of glycolysis. Given the limited metabolic alternatives of the anucleate erythrocyte, it is not surprising that even modest reductions in hexokinase activity may result in shortened *in vivo* red cell survival. The relative lethality of this genetic defect is reflected perhaps in the paucity of hexokinase mutants reported to date (Table II). In contrast, the benign nature of the heterozygous state has not brought these individuals to the attention of the physician-geneticist.

Clinical Spectrum

The scanty available information about hexokinase deficiency of the red cell is derived from a limited number of case reports. Valentine et al.,[248] Keitt, [113]Necheles et al.,[166] and Moser et al.[161] have reported a total of six cases from four families of red cell hexokinase deficiency resulting in hemolytic anemia (Table II). These patients had partial red cell enzyme deficiency, generally mild hemolysis with reticulocytosis from 5 to 20%, type I autohemolysis, and decreased exercise tolerance which is disproportionate to the level of anemia.[63,173] Splenectomy has generally ameliorated the severity of anemia. A second unique syndrome associated with red cell hexokinase deficiency has been described by Löhr et al.[136–138] Three subjects had moderate red cell hexokinase deficiency accompanying a Fanconi's anemia-like syndrome with concomitant pancytopenia and chromosomal abnormalities. Hemolysis was also reported to be part of this clinical picture. It is not clear if these cases reflect a primary or a secondary manifestation of hexokinase deficiency. In other patients with Fanconi's anemia who have been investigated, however, enzyme deficiency has not been observed.[145]

Biochemical Considerations

The biochemical effects of hexokinase deficiency must be considered in light of the properties of the normal enzyme and its role in red

TABLE II. Hexokinase Deficiency: Clinical and Biochemical Aspects[a]

Ref	Age	Sex	Hb	Retics	Enzyme activity		Electrophoretic mobility[c]	Other[d]
					RBC[b]	WBC		
248, 249	11	F	9.4	13.4	62.5	—	I	
113	38	F	12	6.1	80	NL	I, II, III	**
166	—	F	12	2–4	76	↓[f]		
	2	M	6.5	5	67(2)[e]	↓	I, II	
	—	M	15	3–4	152(10)			
161	19	—	10	17–60	50	—	—	***
137, 138	18	M	14.3	11	70	→		—****
	21	M	7.5	15	35	→		—****
	24	M	—	—	88	→		—****
1	—	—	NL	NL	100	—	II, III, IV	Hematologically normal

[a] Abbreviations: Ref, reference; Age (in years); M, male; F, female; Hb, hemoglobin (g/dl); Retics, reticulocytes in % (normal 1–2%); Enzyme activity, expressed in % of control at V_{max} conditions; —, not available; ↓, decreased, value not given; NL, normal. First case in each reference is propositus; others are sibs or parents.

[b] Enzyme activity must be referred to values of individuals with reticulocytosis in order to appreciate the reduction.

[c] Electrophoresis according to Altay et al.[1]

[d] Symbols: **, normal autohemolysis; ***, abnormal autohemolysis; ****, Fanconi's anemia, abnormal K_m glucose and K_{mATP}.

[e] Value in parentheses obtained at low glucose.

[f] WBCs deficient only at low glucose.

cell metabolism. Because it is the initiator of red cell glycolysis and is less active by several orders of magnitude than other glycolytic enzymes, it has been hypothesized that hexokinase is the rate-limiting step in glycolysis and the arbiter of cell senescence.[168,198]

Valentine et al.[248] demonstrated the important relationship between red cell hexokinase activity and cell age and emphasized the necessity to consider mean cell age when interpreting data derived from whole blood biochemical assay. Hexokinase is always the most age-dependent red cell glycolytic enzyme.[194] It is also important that hemolysates be prepared free from leukocytes, which contain 300-fold greater hexokinase activity[113] and may contribute separate electrophoretic isoenzyme patterns.[1]

Hexokinase activity is controlled by multiple regulators. Extracellular glucose concentration does not, however, influence its rate. Intact cell incubation experiments in which glucose is exhausted[113] demonstrate that normal cells can maintain their intracellular glucose-6-phosphate levels as long as the glucose concentrations are higher than 50 μM. Only below this level does intracellular glucose-6-phosphate concentration precipitously drop, lactate production fall, and pyruvate increase as glycolysis slows to a halt. It is unlikely that red cells are ever exposed to environments with such low extracellular glucose concentration. A mutant hexokinase was described[113] where glucose consumption measured in the intact cell system became nonlinear at 200 μM. This point of malfunction is below plasma glucose levels (5.5 mM) and well below the lowest reported glucose levels (1.1 mM) in massively enlarged spleens.[166] Therefore, even though these experiments may be of theoretical importance to demonstrate abnormal kinetics of mutant enzymes, they indicate that there is no physiological condition where glucose concentration is limiting for the enzyme. Thus the hypothesis[166] that regional splenic hypoglycemia may critically impair the metabolism of hexokinase-deficient red cells appears untenable. The metabolic failure of the hexokinase-deficient cell seems to be due to the absolute low activity and loss of metabolic reserve (Fig. 3) rather than to the aberrant enzyme kinetics.

Hexokinase activity becomes suboptimal when the concomitant phosphofructokinase inhibition results in the accumulation of glucose-6-phosphate, which in turn further inhibits hexokinase.[197] The ATP/ADP ratio is another regulator of hexokinase activity; as the ratio decreases, the enzyme is inhibited.[113] In the hexokinase-deficient red cells, metabolic activity is reduced to the point where the normal distal regulators (glucose-6-phosphate, ATP/ADP ratio, and 2,3-DPG) never attain concentrations adequate for inhibitory effects.[37,113] Thus, unlike the normal enzyme, which is inhibited to one-tenth its maximum potential, the defective enzyme functions at nearly maximum capacity. Although the defective enzyme V_{max} is greatly decreased, the basal metabolic rate of the cell is thus not grossly compromised. However, the deficient cells are devoid of any potential metabolic reserve. In this sense, a hexokinase-deficient red cell is prematurely aged and is severely limited in its capacity for survival.

In view of the special metabolic characteristics of the anucleate erythrocyte and of the critical location of hexokinase, several special features which are tentatively significant in the premature senescence of deficient cells should be mentioned.Decreased hexokinase results in lowered glucose-6-phosphate, which curtails pentose phosphate shunt activity; the deficient production of NADPH should result in decreased resistance to oxidative stress. However, spontaneous Heinz body formation has not routinely been observed in cases of hexokinase deficiency associated with chronic hemolysis. This has been explained as due to preferential preservation of shunt activity.[248] It is surprising therefore to note that Heinz bodies were found by Löhr et al.[138] in their patients with red cell hexokinase deficiency associated with Fanconi's anemia. Hexokinase itself contains sulfhydryl groups which may be susceptible to oxidative denaturation. Low as well as normal glutathione levels are described for hexokinase-deficient cells.[16,122,161,198]

Hexokinase deficiency also lowers the level of two other important glycolytic intermediates: ATP and 2,3-DPG.[19] The ATP concentration of deficient cells was found in one case to be 1.08 μmoles per milliliter of cells (normal is 1.40 $\pm$ 0.14 μmoles per milliliter of cells); the 2,3-DPG level was 2.4 μmoles per milliliter of cells (normal is 4.39 $\pm$ 0.45 μmoles per milliliter of cells). The reduced 2,3-DPG concentration exerts a secondary influence on the hemoglobin–oxygen affinity curve. Low 2,3-DPG levels cause a shift in the affinity curve which decreases the release of oxygen at tissue levels[63] The net result for these patients is exercise intolerance disproportionate to the level of anemia. Failure to maintain adequate ATP levels also results in failure to maintain intracellular–extracellular ionic gradients with subsequent osmotic lysis.

Biochemical characterization of hexokinase mutants has been

complicated by several factors. Contamination of hemolysates by leukocytes and platelets contributes significantly to enzyme activity. Electrophoresis of pure leukocyte and platelet extracts[1] demonstrates discrete electrophoretic patterns which may be the source of confusion concerning variable zymograms of red cell hexokinase contaminated with other cellular elements.

Biochemical characterization of mutant enzymes was attempted, using crude lysates. Under these conditions, the accurate determination of Michaelis constants is uncertain. In fact, there is considerable variation among normal red cell hexokinase K_m values measured in hemolysates. Keitt[113] noted his difficulties in biochemical characterization of one mutant hexokinase and pointed up the problems associated with "broken cell systems." Enzyme activity is rapidly labile under certain conditions; thus lysates are not a true reflection of internal cellular enzyme kinetics. Shifts in mean cell age significantly affect whole blood enzyme activity; therefore, comparison of whole blood biochemical assays from different individuals must take into account variations in mean cell age. This may be important not only for comparison of maximal velocities but also for determination of Michaelis constants. Mutant hexokinases with increased *in vivo* lability may exhibit different kinetics as a result of the mean age of the cell sample.

By use of crude cell lysates, steady-state kinetics are unattainable. It is established that multiple isozymes exist simultaneously in normal blood[1] and may operate with different kinetics.[1,111] In view of this, it is difficult to interpret the multiple kinetics reported by some investigators[166] for normal and defective enzymes. Where biochemical characterization of mutant glycolytic enzymes from cell lysates is difficult, the determination of glycolytic intermediates may be much more descriptive of mutant enzymes and more efficient in the detection of the asymptomatic heterozygote.[113]

Review of the variable biochemical data attempting to delineate the molecular defect of mutant hexokinases reveals the limited conclusions possible at this time. The heterogeneity of enzyme kinetics suggests at first glance that genetic polymorphism is present. However attractive this statement is, the data are in no way sufficient to permit a definitive conclusion. The mutant hexokinases thus far described appear to be quantitatively defective, but the lack of purified preparations of any of these mutant proteins causes one to be very cautious about the nature of the molecular defect.

Genetic Considerations

Family studies based on hematological data (phenotypic expression and "broken cell" enzyme characterizations) suggest that the defect is transmitted in an autosomal recessive fashion. Heterozygotes, with the exception of the propositus' father in one case,[166] are hematologically unaffected. Heterozygotes are not easily detectable by biochemical assay; in this respect, measurements of the pattern of glycolytic intermediates could be more sensitive (low levels of glucose-6-phosphate).

Electrophoretic analyses (Fig. 4) indicate that there are four hexokinase bands(I, II, III, IV) in the red cells. Of these, types II, III, and IV are specific to red cells and may be absent in hexokinase deficiency.[1] Type I appears to be shared in common with leukocytes and platelets. Altay[1] described a mutant hexokinase which lacked band I but retained bands II, III, and IV and full red cell hexokinase activity.

Discrete bands after electrophoresis are not synonymous with true isozymes, unless confirmed by studies of genetic segregation. Electrophoresis of purified bands will be necessary before concluding that bands I, II, III, and IV are true isozymes. Population surveys of normal individuals will be useful to provide the necessary family studies to corroborate whether these qualitative differences are indeed the result of genetic segregation of isozymes and not of *in vitro* degradation altering electrophoretic distributions, as has been the case for other glycolytic enzymes.[64] This appears possible in the case of hexokinase. For instance, a mutant enzyme was reported which was rapidly labile in the absence of glucose but could be partly activated by the addition of mercaptoethanol: thus oxidative denaturation of sulfhydryl groups could lead to the formation of spurious isozymes.[113]

Combined red cell, leukocyte, and platelet hexokinase deficiency were reported in association with three cases of Fanconi's anemia.[136-138] In view of the unique clinical syndrome, these reports are difficult to correlate with the other cases and stand only as a peculiar observation. The deficiency of leukocyte enzyme in another family

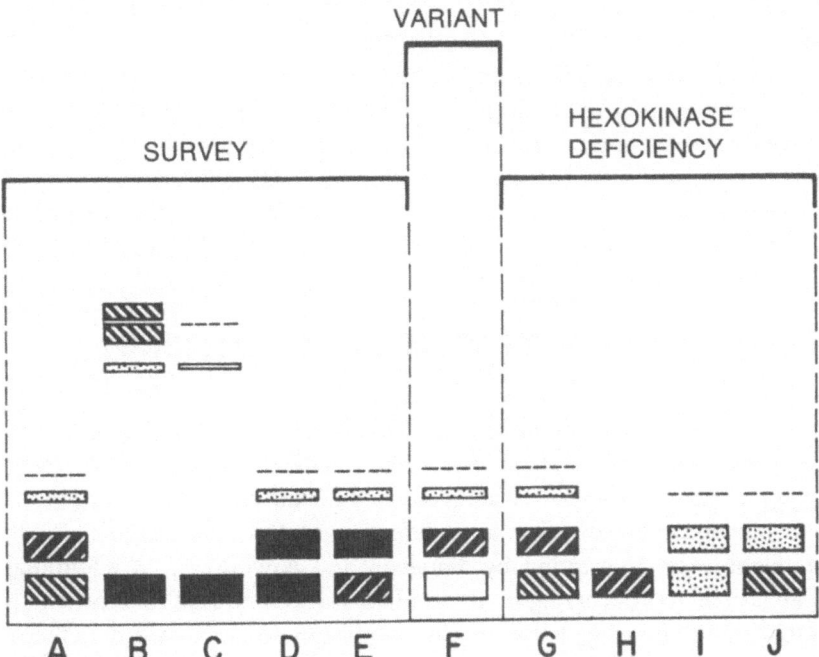

Fig. 4. Diagram of various hexokinase patterns obtained by electrophoresis in agarose gel at pH 7.86. Left to right, patterns are (A) normal hemolysate, (B) white blood cell lysate, (C) platelet lysate, (D) hemolysate from patient with sickle cell anemia, (E) hemolysate from newborn infant or from patient with hereditary spherocytosis, (F) hemolysate from normal subject with decreased band 1, (G) hemolysate from normal members of N family, (H) hemolysate from proposita of N family, (I) hemolysate from brother of proposita, and (J) hemolysate from father and paternal grandmother of proposita. Intensity of bands in decreasing order, shown by complete black, diagonal wide black stripes, diagonal narrow black stripes, stippling, clear areas, and dashed lines. From Altay et al.[1] by permission of Grune and Stratton.

with chronic hemolysis was manifest only at low glucose levels in a single experiment and it is difficult to definitely conclude that the leukocytes were truly deficient. The only possible conclusions about leukocyte hexokinase at this time are that there is a band electrophoretically identical to one of the red cell bands but that no clinical correlation with a leukocyte defect can be reached.

One critical experiment which might shed some light on the qualitative versus quantitative aspect of mutant enzymes would be to examine the in vivo decay rates of normal and deficient hexokinases.

The data of Valentine *et al.*[248,249] and Necheles *et al.*[166] suggest that for a given degree of reticulocytosis the cellular content of hexokinase is low. Age-dependent separation of red cells, devoid of white cells and platelets, may help to delineate a biologically labile protein defect as opposed to a deficient rate of synthesis. If the former is the case, the nucleated red cells should contain enzyme activity approaching normal cell levels. Of course, the ultimate proof would require determination of hexokinase synthetic rates measured in protein synthesis systems.

GLUCOSEPHOSPHATE ISOMERASE DEFICIENCY

Following glucose-6-phosphate dehydrogenase and pyruvate kinase deficiency, glucosephosphate isomerase deficiency has been the most frequently reported cause of clinically significant congenital nonspherocytic hemolytic anemia due to a defective erythrocyte enzyme. Since the initial case description by Baughan and coworkers, 24 additional cases (Table III) occurring in 19 families have been described in which the causal relationship between glucosephosphate isomerase deficiency and hemolytic anemia has been solidly established. Investigation of family pedigrees for abnormal glucosephosphate isomerase enzymes, partial biochemical characterization of semipurified enzyme, *in vitro* whole red cell metabolic studies, and population surveys of electrophoretic variants have contributed to our understanding of the mode of inheritance, the metabolic consequences for the defective red cell, and the possible molecular genetic basis of the defect.

Clinical Spectrum

The usual mode of presentation for most patients with clinically significant glucosephosphate isomerase deficiency is as an undiagnosed congenital hemolytic anemia. The severity of hemolysis and the degree of hepatosplenomegaly may be variable. The autohemolysis is type I. It is of note that contrary to the classic dichotomy which separated the spherocytic from the nonspherocytic congenital anemias, Oski and Fuller[170] have described a case in which spherocytes were prominent and osmotic fragility increased. They astutely comment that glucose-

TABLE III. Glucosephosphate Isomerase Deficiency: Clinical and Biochemical Aspects[a]

Ref	Age	Sex	Hb	Retics	Enzyme activity RBC	Enzyme activity WBC	Electrophoretic mobility[b]	Designation and other
10	16	M	9.8	28.3	19	26.7	9–10	GPI Seattle
180	13	F	8.0	72.1	15.9	6.6	SS	GPI Whitley County
	12	M	7.6	42.3	13.7	10.3	SS	GPI Whitley County
	2	M	6.0	70.5	30.4	5.2	SS	GPI Whitley County
98	2	F	4–5	20	30–50	—	NL	*c
98	1	M	5.2	32	30–50	→	NL	
50	5	M	—	—	40	73	NL	
5	24	M	12.3	11	25	—	PHI 9	GPI Espelen
	21	M	—	—	23	—	PHI 9	
214	18	M	9–12	7.5–20	24.2	—	PHI 9	Hemizygous G6PD deficient
170	12	M	—	—	10	10	—	Spherocytes
25	1	M	7.4	33.6	14	22	VS	GPI LA/GPI(−)
135	26	F	11.1	33.1	29	NA	SS	GPI Winnepeg
156	9	F	7.0	16.2	15	35	S	GPI Recklinghausen
155	22	M	7.3	10.1	40	→	F[d]	GPI Narita
22	24	F	8.6	6.5	38	→	NL	GPI Matsumoto; acid shift pH optimum
215	13	F	4–13	0.2–51	14.2	—	S	GPI Elyria
132	1	M	8.5	45–60	22	39	F	GPI Nordhorn
	10	F	—	—	50	—	—	Elliptocytosis
182	—	F	—	—	50	—	—	
182	2	—	—	—	22	—	—	
	6	M	11	25	23	—	—	
54	9	M	10	20	15	—	—	
183	14	F	9–10	15–20	25	100	NL	GPI Valle Hermoso

[a] Abbreviations as in Table II.

[b] SS, slightly slower than normal; VS, very slow compared to normal; F, faster than normal. See specific author for method; reference system is that of Detter et al.[64]

[c] Related to GPI Whitley County.

[d] Parents resemble PHI 7-1.

phosphate isomerase deficiency must be considered in the differential diagnosis of hereditary spherocytosis.

It has been a general clinical pattern that the degree of hemolysis was exacerbated during times of biological stress: infections, general anesthesia, or exposure to drugs. Almost all patients have had significant splenomegaly and the majority have undergone splenectomy resulting in clinical improvement. An increased reticulocytosis is noted in postsplenectomy glucosephosphate isomerase deficients similar to that observed in pyruvate kinase deficiency.[143,147] Presumably the same mechanism is operative: very severely affected cells which would have been trapped in the spleens are now free to circulate. Reticulocytes are more prone to splenic entrapment, and once their mitochondrial mechanism fails in the relatively anaerobic, hypoglycemic splenic environment the glucosephosphate isomerase deficient cell would be unable to survive. Morphological analysis of spleens from splenectomized patients shows selective reticulocyte phagocytosis.[143]

Therapy with pentose phosphate shunt stimulants, ascorbic acid, or methylene blue, in an attempt to bypass the metabolic block, has not ameliorated the hemolysis[5,20,182] A trial of inorganic phosphate infusion directed to stimulate phosphofructokinase was transiently beneficial in one case.[5]

There is one case report of simultaneous glucosephosphate isomerase deficient induced hemolysis and mild glucose-6-phosphate dehydrogenase deficiency.[214] This patient exhibited one severe drug-related hemolytic crisis; however, episodic increased hemolysis has also been described in isolated glucosephosphate isomerase deficiency.[5] There has not been a large-scale study to date which investigates the concomitant gene frequency of glucosephosphate isomerase alleles with other erythrocyte enzyme mutations.

Biochemical Considerations

Glucosephosphate isomerase occupies a crucial crossroads in the energy metabolism of the mature, anucleate red cell. Since it facilitates the reversible interconversion of glucose-6-phosphate and fructose-6-phosphate, it is a common step to both the pentose pathway and the glycolytic cascade. Under normal conditions, more than 90% of glucose entering the red cell is catabolized via the Embden–Meyerhof pathway while only a fraction enters the pentose phosphate shunt.[35] However, fructose-6-phosphate is a product of shunt catabolism and via glucosephosphate isomerase may recycle through the shunt, as evidenced by studies of glucose-^{14}C labeled in the C-2 position.[35,170,180] The ability to recycle shunt products increases the capacity of the shunt to generate reduced nucleotides which participate via the glutathione reductase and glutathione peroxidase reactions in the removal of peroxides from the red cell environment. This provides the red cell with protection against the oxidative denaturation of hemoglobin, the formation of precipitates of mixed disulfides, and Heinz body formation, which shorten red cell life span.

Glucosephosphate isomerase deficient red cells demonstrate apparent increased glucose consumption and lactate production: 160% and 190% respectively, compared to normal cells.[10] However, in reality this augmented metabolic capacity is spuriously elevated due to a lower mean red cell age in glucosephosphate isomerase deficient patients as compared to controls. In addition to the augmented metabolic capacity, reticulocytes possess mitochondria and thus have an alternate pathway for ATP production. When the total energy production capacity of glucosephosphate isomerase deficient erythrocytes is adjusted for mean cell age differences, these deficient cells lack the ability to maintain normal ATP or 2,3-DPG concentrations.[155,156,214]

Metabolism of glucose via the pentose phosphate shunt is also disturbed. Baughan et al.[10] have shown that the resting-state pentose phosphate shunt metabolism of glucosephosphate isomerase deficient erythrocytes, as measured by evolution of $^{14}CO_2$ from glucose-1-^{14}C, is twice normal. Once again, this augmented catabolic rate is the result of a younger mean cell age in deficient cells. Of greater interest is the observation[10] that methylene blue stimulation of the pentose phosphate shunt causes an equivalent or lesser increase of shunt metabolism for glucosephosphate isomerase deficient cells than for normal red cells, but always lower than anticipated on the basis of cell age.

When glucose-2-^{14}C is the substrate, the evolution of $^{14}CO_2$ is a measure of the cell's ability to recycle through the shunt. Various groups[10,170,180] have shown that glucosephosphate isomerase deficient erythrocytes when stimulated by methylene blue are able to recycle only 10% or less substrate as compared to normal cells. The obvious result of this recycling deficiency is decreased availability of reduced pyridine nucleotides during periods of increased oxidative stress.

The crucial location of glucose phosphate isomerase in both the Embden–Meyerhof pathway and the pentose phosphate shunt is manifest by the combined clinical picture of chronic hemolysis (because of glycolytic defect) and episodic hemolytic crisis (the result of failure to recycle actively through the shunt).

Biochemical characterization of mutant glucosephosphate isomerase enzymes has been conducted for the most part in hemolysates and in one case[6] on a 20,000-fold purified preparation. With one possible exception,[10] the K_{mF6P} of leukocyte and erythrocyte enzymes has been normal. Purification of mutant enzymes is complicated because many deficients are heterozygotes with two distinct mutant proteins and possibly a third hybrid as well. The most consistent biochemical characteristic of the mutant glucosephosphate isomerase is increased thermal lability at 48°C.[5,22,25,54,98,135,182,215] There is a single case report of a mutant enzyme manifesting an acid-shifted pH optimum.[155]

Simplified fractionation of glucosephosphate isomerase deficient red cells into relatively "young"-reticulocyte-rich and "old"-reticulocyte-poor subpopulations[7,135,215] shows an accelerated *in vivo* decline of enzyme activity as compared to controls. These observations have been obtained for three separate glucosephosphate isomerase mutants and suggest that the molecular defect of red cell glucosephosphate isomerase deficiency may often be a qualitatively labile enzyme which is quantitatively equivalent to the normal. Also of note is the observation that crude hemolysate K_{mF6P} is the same for old and young cells. However, definitive evidence—normal enzyme activity in pure populations of young cells—is not available. The finding of increased thermal lability has been emphasized as a corollary to the *in vivo* situation; and indeed this appears to be a common characteristic of mutant glucosephosphate isomerases. Attempts to simulate cell aging with *in vitro* systems have also shown an increased decline in glucosephosphate isomerase activity from deficient cells compared to normal controls. Additionally, whole cell incubation experiments have demonstrated the decline of general metabolic function for the deficient cell[7]—decreased lactate production and lowered intracellular ATP concentration. Of interest is the preservation of mannose-dependent lactate production in the glucosephosphate isomerase deficient cell, suggesting independent genetic control for mannose phosphate isomerase. Thermal lability studies and *in vitro* aging are empirical observations made in artificial systems and as such are of limited value for extrapolation to the *in vivo* situation. Careful fractionation of glucose-phosphate isomerase deficient red cells on an age-dependent basis and comparison with other age-dependent glycolytic enzymes—hexokinase or pyruvate kinase—may give more definitive data as to *in vivo* enzyme half-life and perhaps yield cell fractions with full enzyme activity to definitively establish the absence of a quantitative defect.

Genetic Considerations

Starch gel electrophoresis has been a useful tool in the characterization of genetic polymorphism of glucosephosphate isomerases. Using this method, Detter *et al.*[64] showed the existence of heterozygote mutants. Corroborative information about alterations in net charge was also recently found from isoelectric focusing.[6,25]

Although the starch gel system is cumbersome and complicated by poor resolution with frequent appearance of minor bands, it has provided information about the molecular structure of normal and variant enzymes.

Among 3397 individuals tested by Detter *et al.*,[64] 3377 had a similar pattern designated PHI 1 (Fig. 5) composed of a major band and two minor bands. Subsequent variants from this "wild-type" zymogram were designated PHI 2-1 through PHI 10-1, band 1 being common to all patterns. Family studies indicated that in the heterozygote a triplet isozyme pattern is observed. These observations led to the hypothesis that the enzyme is a dimer composed of identical subunits and recombination of subunits gives two homogeneous and one hybrid isozyme. The triplet isozyme pattern has been observed by other investigators.[46,162,235] No evidence to date has been presented to indicate whether these hybrids exist *in vivo*. Detter *et al.*[64] did not attempt to make artificial hybrids *in vitro* from lysates of two different variants. Most heterozygous individuals who have the type 1 band are hematologically normal. Types 3-1 (the most frequent electrophoretic variant), 5-1, and 6-1 are associated with normal red cell enzyme activity. Types 3-3, 5-5, and 6-6 have not been described to date. Types 9-1 and 10-1 are associated with decreased activity. These two types were initially described in the parents of a child with hemolytic anemia due to glucosephosphate isomerase deficiency with type 9-10 electrophoretic pattern. Subsequently, three other cases of hemolytic anemia have been described in individuals with type 9-9 electrophoretic pattern.[5,214] These findings suggest that the electrophoretic pattern 9 is the expression of a functionally defective enzyme. Additional cases have been reported of patients who are heterozygotes for two different defective mutants.[10,22,25,215] On the other hand, glucosephosphate isomerase deficiency hemolytic anemia has been clearly documented in individuals with a normal electrophoretic pattern. These observations indicate that glucosephosphate isomerase deficiency may result from the inheritance of a double dose of one of several mutant alleles coding for defective enzymes, associated with abnormal or normal electrophoretic pattern. It is therefore possible to be glucosephosphate isomerase deficient by homozygosity for one mutant allele or by heterozygosity for two different mutant alleles. Paglia et al[180] have described a family in which both parents' zymograms appeared normal while an affected offspring had an abnormal pattern. They postulated that the defective protein is masked by the normal enzyme component in the parents but is evident in the homozygous proband. Family

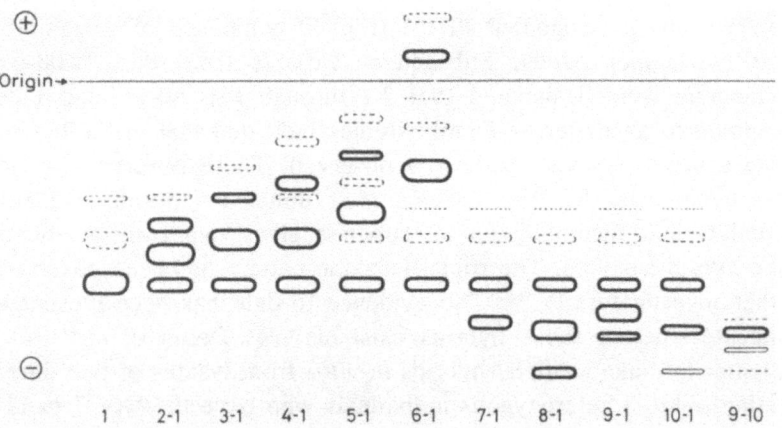

Fig. 5. Diagram showing the PHI isozymes in individuals of the common phenotype, PHI 1, and several rare phenotypes. Solid lines indicate main components; broken lines indicate minor components. The patterns of 9-1, 10-1, and 9-10 are those obtained from white cell lysates: pattern 9-10 is from a patient with hemolytic anemia secondary to GPI deficiency; patterns 9-1 and 10-1 are from mother and father, respectively. The 5-1 pattern shown is that observed in "aged" red cell lysates. From Detter et al.[64] by permission of Cambridge University Press.

studies demonstrate that the inheritance is clearly of autosomal recessive type.

Analysis of glucosephosphate isomerase isozyme pattern for heart, liver, kidney, and brain shows identity with red cells.[186] With one isolated exception,[182] white cells have always been defective in glucosephosphate isomerase deficiency of the red cells (see Table III). Confirmatory data for a single enzyme in all tissues[162] have been shown for a mutant enzyme in liver, spleen, and muscle. The identity of the enzyme in fibroblast cultures and their utility for diagnosis have been described by Krone et al.[124] The sole piece of evidence against a single genetic determinant for all tissues is the report by Paglia and Valentine[182] of normal leukocyte enzyme in the presence of erythrocyte glucosephosphate isomerase deficiency. The bulk of evidence to date from crude enzyme extracts and purified preparations[46,215,244] is also in favor of a single genetic determinant for glucosephosphate isomerase in all tissues.

The minor bands described by Detter and others are probably the result of in vitro enzyme degradation, as shown by the aging of hemolysates or the presence of conformational isomers.[64]

Detter's survey[64] clearly demonstrates the genetic variation of glucosephosphate isomerase. The frequency of mutant glucosephosphate isomerase phenotypes has been variable in different laboratories. Löhr[135] found no heterozygous deficients in a survey of 350 subjects. (Whole blood biochemical assays are not sufficient for the detection of heterozygotes for normal-activity mutants such as PHI 3-1, 5-1, and 6-1 types.) Paglia and Valentine[182] found only two heterozygotes in 1000 subjects. A fourth large survey by Fitch et al.[72] of 1650 individuals revealed nine heterozygotes, of whom five had the same zymogram. Glucosephosphate isomerase deficiency has been observed in association with other red cell defects. Leger et al.[132] reported a case with concomitant elliptocytosis. Schröter et al.[214] reported a case of homozygous glucosephosphate isomerase deficiency concomitant with an unspecified type of glucose-6-phosphate dehydrogenase deficiency; siblings who were heterozygotes for both defects [glucosephosphate isomerase (+/−)/G6PD(+/−)] were hematologically normal. A similar combination has also been reported in Thailand, with normal hematological findings.[205] Schröter postulates that G6PD deficiency may ameliorate glucosephosphate isomerase deficiency by elevating the levels of G6P. Yet the proband has almost 70% of normal G6PD activity,[214] a level of deficiency probably of no physiological relevance.

PHOSPHOFRUCTOKINASE DEFICIENCY

To date, eight cases of documented red cell phosphofructokinase deficiency occurring in six unrelated families have been reported. The defect is rare and the associated chronic hemolysis, if present, is moderate without episodic hemolytic crises. Information as to the biochemical and genetic nature of the defect is derived largely from case reports, a limited number of normal enzyme purification studies, and biochemical genetic experiments in nonhuman mammalian species. Because of the small number of symptomatic cases, the frequency of mutation is unknown and the postulated genetics are derived largely from the limited family studies.

Clinical Spectrum

Red cell phosphofructokinase deficiency has been associated with four clinically distinct syndromes (Table IV). The first is characterized by severe myopathy and moderate, compensated hemolysis.[129,237] Muscle phosphofructokinase activity is virtually absent, while red cell activity is partially reduced. The second patient group exhibits moderate hemolysis with partial red cell enzyme deficiency[160,255,256]; these individuals do not have the myopathic syndrome and ischemic exercise tolerance tests show normal lactate production. Unfortunately, muscle phosphofructokinase activity has not been directly assayed in any patient with this clinical presentation. One patient with myopathy, reduced red cell enzyme, but no hemolysis is also reported.[219] The fourth type is totally asymptomatic, presenting solely with the biochemical finding of decreased red cell phosphofructokinase activity.[32] There are two minor variants from the first syndrome. One patient[238] had severe myopathy (6% muscle phosphofructokinase activity) but no evidence of hemolysis even of a subclinical degree. Another individual[219] exhibited an atypical myopathic syndrome, hepatic glycogenesis, and no description of anemia. In this patient, there was decreased red cell phosphofructokinase activity and muscle phosphofructokinase

TABLE IV. Phosphofructokinase Deficiency: Clinical and Biochemical Aspects[a]

Ref	Age	Sex	Hb	Retics	Enzyme activity RBC	Enzyme activity Muscle	Hemolysis[b]	Myopathy[b]	Other[c]
237	20	F	—		29	1	+	+	*
	23	M	—	4–6	48	1	+	+	*
	27	M	—		42	1	+	+	*
129	18	M	—	4	50	2	+	+	*
238	20	M	17	—	—	6	0	+	*·
219	37	M	—	—	17	0	0	+	*d
255	24	M	16	4–41	50	—	++	0	**e
160	38	F	13	7–14	8.3	—	++	0	**e
32	—	M	15	1.5	28	—	0	0	

[a] Abbreviations as in Table II.
[b] Indicates severity from 0 to ++++.
[c] Symbols: *, decreased anaerobic lactate production; **, normal anaerobic lactate production.
[d] Atypical myopathic syndrome and hepatic glycogenesis.
[e] ^{51}Cr $t_{1/2}$ markedly decreased.

activity was completely absent. To summarize, red cell phosphofructo-kinase deficiency may be seen with myopathy and moderate hemolysis, without myopathy but with moderate hemolysis, with myopathy but without hemolysis, and without evidence of myopathy or hemolysis. The heterogeneity of clinical syndromes has given rise to several possible molecular genetic theories.

Biochemical Considerations

Phosphofructokinase irreversibly catalyzes the conversion of fructose-6-phosphate (F6P) to fructose-1,6-diphosphate with the consumption of 1 mole of ATP per mole F6P. ATP is a co-substrate and potent inhibitor of phosphofructokinase activity. The enzyme exhibits allosteric kinetics at pH 7.2 with fructose-6-phosphate as the substrate; cyclic AMP has been shown to overcome the ATP inhibition.[131,256] At physiological intracellular pH and substrate levels, phosphofructokinase is a rate-limiting reaction in the red cells' glycolytic pathway and functions under inhibitory conditions.[131,150,151] Phosphofructokinase may be bypassed by means of the pentose phosphate pathway. Measurement of glycolytic intermediates in phosphofructokinase-deficient red cells has revealed normal levels of glucose-6-phosphate, fructose-6-phosphate, and fructose-1,6-diphosphate but slightly decreased ATP and 2,3-diphosphoglycerate concentrations.[160,256] Total lactate formation was normal when adjusted for mean cell age. It was shown also that phosphofructokinase-deficient red cells are capable of maintaining normal intracellular potassium and sodium concentrations.[256] The mild clinical syndrome probably reflects the low level of phosphofructokinase activity required for the red cell to maintain an intact glycolytic pathway. It also may indicate, however, the ability of the red cell to bypass the metabolic defect through the pentose shunt. There is no evidence of increased pentose phosphate pathway metabolism of phosphofructokinase-deficient cells, although this would seem a feasible escape route from the metabolic blockade. Qualitative defects for mutant red cell phosphofructokinase have been described: elevated K_{mF6P}, increased in vitro lability, and an increased sensitivity to ATP inhibition.[256] Because of the limited number of case reports and difficulties of purifying mutant enzymes, there is little kinetic data to suggest a uniform qualitative defect.

Genetic Considerations

Useful data about the structure of muscle and red cell phosphofructokinase have been derived from electrophoresis and DEAE chromatography. It has been shown that the red cell and muscle enzymes are chromatographically and electrophoretically distinct.[126,131,236] Normal muscle and red cell phosphofructokinase enzymes migrate as distinct single, cathodal bands at pH 7.0.[131] Both enzymes are eluted from DEAE-cellulose as single peaks, although the red cell enzyme is more diffuse. DEAE chromatography of human leukocytes, platelets, thyroid, and brain phosphofructokinase suggested the existence of four distinct isoenzymes.[126] Platelets show two isozymes unrelated to either muscle or red cells.[126]

In light of the existence of separate red cell and muscle isozymes, the observation that patients with complete absence of muscle phosphofructokinase catalytic activity have only a 50% reduction of red cell activity led to the hypothesis that there may be a common subunit for muscle and red cell phosphofructokinase.[129] An antibody prepared against normal muscle phosphofructokinase caused 50% neutralization of normal red cell phosphofructokinase activity. Reaction of this antimuscle antibody with phosphofructokinase-deficient muscle extract gave no immunoprecipitate nor did it neutralize the residual enzyme activity of the patient's red cells[129] These data led to the hypothesis that a subunit (designated the muscle or M component) was present in both isoenzymes and that muscle phosphofructokinase was composed solely of this M unit while red cell phosphofructokinase had a second specific subunit designated R.[128,129]

Based on findings with other tissues, it is postulated that the active form of phosphofructokinase exists as a tetramer.[179] Layzer and Rasmussen[128] hypothesized that muscle phosphofructokinase exists with the structure M_4 and red cell has the M_2R_2 structure. Thus lack of the M subunit would result in absent muscle activity with severe myopathy, but only partial red cell activity and moderate hemolysis; lack of the R subunits would result in hemolysis only. This hypothesis is theoretically supported by the observation that in myopathy the residual enzyme present in the red cell (R_4 type?) is not neutralized by anti-M antibody. The molecular genetic corollary to the common subunit theory was that the M and the R subunits were under separate genetic control and the genetic defect resulted from lack of synthesis of the M subunit. Failure to detect antigenic material in the patient's muscle extract was interpreted as evidence for the failure of synthesis of a given gene product.[128,129] Thus residual red cell activity was attributed to a partially functional pure R type molecule. However, in a subsequent patient who exhibited hemolysis without myopathy,[256] antimuscle antibody also failed to neutralize residual red cell catalytic activity. In order to fit the initial common subunit hypothesis,[129] the authors concluded that a qualitatively defective M unit was present which could be metabolically compensated for in muscle but was expressed in red cells and that the lack of antibody recognition was due to a structural alteration at the M subunit antigenic site.[256]

In Boulard's patient, there was no hemolysis or myopathy despite decreased red cell phosphofructokinase activity. Red cell phosphofruc-tokinase activity was neutralized by anti-M antibody, as was the control; this would imply the residual activity to be of M type with a defective R subunit. These complex observations suggest that this patient had a qualitative R unit defect with reduced enzymatic activity, because even after anti-M neutralization there was some residual phosphofructokinase activity. Since the patient was hematologically normal, the R subunit defect was a functionally insignificant impairment to cell survival. Furthermore, the mutant enzyme had a normal K_{mATP} but was very unstable *in vitro*.

By use of immunological cross-reaction, Layzer has attempted to substantiate his R, M hypothesis.[128] These studies must be interpreted with caution because cross-reactivity between proteins with similar catalytic function may produce unpredictable results. Cross-reactivity may in fact occur between isozymes as a result of antigenic identity between active sites without the presence of a postulated common subunit. Analogous cross-reactivity experiments with pyruvate kinase were interpreted to indicate an identity of subunit[233] but were later shown to be nonspecific.[44] The existence of a hybrid enzyme may be demonstrated only by the appearance of the predicted number of hybrid bands after the dissociation and reassociation of the native hybrid enzyme.

Such experiments have been conducted by Tsai and Kemp[241,242] with rabbit liver and muscle phosphofructokinase. They have shown that rabbit liver (B) and muscle (A) phosphofructokinases exist as tetramers composed of identical subunits—respectively, B_4 and A_4. Dissociation of a mixture of these tetramers in solution produces three hybrids in addition to the two native molecules. These hybrids are distinct by electrophoresis. Native adipose tissue demonstrates the presence of all five molecules: A_4, A_3B, A_2B_2, AB_3, and B_4. These authors have also shown that liver and red cell phosphofructokinases are identical. Moreover, antibody prepared against muscle phosphofructokinase was able to neutralize 32% of purified liver phosphofructokinase catalytic activity, although the converse was not true.[242] Thus it is well established that, in the rabbit, muscle and liver phosphofructokinases (the latter identical to red cell phosphofructokinase) are each composed of distinct identical subunits, yet share immunological cross-reactivity, and hybridization of these two isozymes yields the expected hybrid number concordant with this hypothesis. The analogous experiments remain to be done with human phosphofructokinase to substantiate Layzer's hypothesis, although it would seem likely that the situation for human phosphofructokinase would be the same as that of the rabbit—that the red cell phosphofructokinase is not a hybrid molecule. Definitive proof is awaited. In the case of human red cell phosphofructokinase, Layzer's experiments of dissociation and recombination failed to yield any hybrid molecules.[128] Furthermore, dissociation of the postulated red cell hybrid R_2M_2 and removal of the M subunit by anti-M antibody to yield a theoretical R_4 molecule could not be chromatographically demonstrated. A control experiment in which the native R_2M_2 molecule was dissociated in the presence of nonimmune sera failed to reveal the formation of new hybrid molecules.

A definitive unified molecular genetic explanation for red cell phosphofructokinase deficiency is currently not possible. The clinical dissociation of myopathic syndromes from hemolytic syndromes suggests separate tissue isozymes: however, this is not the only possible alternative. Examples of other red cell enzyme defects demonstrate that qualitative or quantitative variation of a mutant enzyme may be differentially expressed in separate tissues because of tissue-specific factors: cell half-life, compensatory protein synthesis, or metabolic alternatives to bypass critical steps. Biochemical studies do support the conclusion that red cell and muscle phosphofructokinases are isozymes, and as such may be under separate genetic control. If the experiments of Tsai and Kemp are applicable to the human enzyme, then muscle and red cell phosphofructokinases are each unique tetramers with shared antigenicity analogous to pyruvate kinase white cell and muscle isozymes. Although complete absence of muscle phosphofructokinase catalytic activity is apparent, the immunological data as to the absence of a nonfunctional gene product are inconclusive. Several cases involving a variety of red cell phosphofructokinase qualitative defects are reported but none with documented total synthetic failure.

Family studies indicate that the inheritance of mutant phosphofructokinase is by the autosomal recessive mode for both the myopathic and hemolytic syndromes.

Early reports that elevated red cell phosphofructokinase was found in trisomy 21 patients[9] led to the theory that the phosphofructokinase structural gene was located on chromosome 21.[8,14,56] Subsequent studies[127] have shown that increased red cell enzyme levels were not the result of a gene dosage effect since phosphofructokinase levels in other tissues with isozyme identity to that of red cells were not elevated.

PHOSPHOGLYCERATE KINASE DEFICIENCY

A defect in phosphoglycerate kinase in the red cells was described for the first time in 1968[123]; since then a total of seven unrelated

TABLE V. Phosphoglycerate Kinase Deficiency: Clinical and Biochemical Aspects[a]

Ref	Age	Sex	Hb	Retics	Enzyme activity		Other
					RBC	WBC	
247	12	M	10	18	6	5	
	4	M	10.3	15	0	—	
48	2/12	M	7	43	22	22	
157	4	M	8	38	10	13	*[b]
121	19	M	6–13	1–10	10	0	
	17	M	—	11	8	0	
92	26	M	7	—	9	—	
123	63	F	8	6–11	76	—	
3	62	F	9	5	42	—	

[a] Abbreviations as in Table II.
[b] Slow electrophoretic mobility; high K_{mPG}.

families have been reported. The patient in the first case reported was a female; however, five of the six subsequent reports have been of males (Table V).

Clinical Spectrum

The clinical feature of phosphoglycerate kinase deficiency consists of severe chronic hemolysis, associated in most cases with neurological abnormalities. The hemolysis is improved by splenectomy. The level of phosphoglycerate kinase in the red cells varies from 3% to 23% of normal; in the white cells, it was found to be absent in one family and decreased in another.

Biochemical Considerations

Phosphoglycerate kinase catalyzes the conversion of ADP to ATP and of 1,3-DPG to 3-PG. The physiological importance of the enzyme resides primarily in its close functional and anatomical proximity to the K$^+$-Na$^+$ cation pump.[185] The phosphoglycerate kinase reaction may be completely bypassed when 1,3-diphosphoglycerate is metabolized through the 2,3-DPG shunt. Therefore, the failure of the enzyme in the red cell should primarily result in a defect in cation transport, with secondary accumulation of 2,3-DPG on one hand and of upstream glycolytic intermediates on the other. The accumulation of 2,3-DPG and of glycolytic intermediates, in turn, should result in a decreased glycolytic rate. Measurements of glycolysis in phosphoglycerate kinase deficient red cells have, however, indicated nearly normal rates.[3,247] The intracellular concentration of ATP was found slightly decreased only when the younger cell age was taken into consideration.[247] It has been suggested that a sufficient flow of metabolism occurs in these red cells because of residual enzyme activity.

Recent studies have demonstrated in two separate families that a defect in phosphoglycerate kinase results in greatly increased levels of dihydroxyacetone phosphate in a range similar to that observed in the deficiency of triosephosphate isomerase.[3,121] The fact that accumulation of a precursor rather than failure of flow through the enzymatic step is of primary importance is supported by the consideration that in the case of triose phosphate isomerase the normal level of enzyme activity is over 1000 times greater than the level for hexokinase. Red cells with only 5% triose phosphate isomerase activity still have 50 times greater potential activity than required by the efficiency of the overall system. Triosephosphate isomerase may also be bypassed by diversion of metabolic flow through the pentose pathway shunt. Both phosphoglycerate kinase and triosephosphate isomerase deficiencies have in common a residual enzyme activity adequate for glycolysis and the possibility of bypass by shunt. Yet, a minor reduction in either of these enzymatic activities offsets the balance of metabolism and results in both cases in an enormous accumulation of dihydroxyacetone phosphate. It appears reasonable therefore to speculate that in both phosphoglycerate kinase and triosephosphate isomerase deficiencies the accumulation of dihydroxyacetone phosphate may represent the common denominator resulting, by a hitherto unexplained mechanism, in damage to both the red cell and the nervous tissue. This hypothesis would explain the peculiar association of chronic hemolysis and neurological disease observed in both genetic defects.

Genetic Considerations

Valentine et al.[247] in 1969 noticed for the first time in the study of a large Chinese kindred that the inheritance of the enzyme deficiency appeared to be X chromosome linked. They stressed as additional evidence for this hypothesis the fact that the mother and the grandmother of the propositus had greater phosphoglycerate kinase activity in the oldest rather than in the youngest red cells, as opposed to the pattern observed in normals, where there is a slight decrease in activity with cell aging. They interpreted these observations as evidence of X-linked mosaicism and postulated the existence of two different populations of red cells in these females: one normal and one enzyme deficient with decreased cell survival. Therefore, in the younger group of red cells there is a double population of normal and deficient cells, but all the older cells are homogeneously normal—hence the apparent increase in activity with cell aging.

The location of the structural gene for phosphoglycerate kinase on the X chromosome has been firmly established by two independent lines of evidence. Chen et al.[53] in 1971 demonstrated in a population study in New Guinea the existence of rare electrophoretic mutants of the enzyme, which appeared clearly to segregate as an X-linked trait by family studies. Yoshida and his group suggested on the basis of polypeptide mapping of the purified enzyme that the electrophoretically different mutant was the result of a single amino acid substitution (asparagine–threonine).[262] Khan et al.[116] in 1971 studying interspecies somatic cell hybrids demonstrated that phosphoglycerate kinase is retained or lost in constant association with two other well-known human X-linked markers, glucose-6-phosphate dehydrogenase and hypoxanthine-guanine phosphoribosyltransferase. Deys et al.[65] suggested that the entire human X chromosome can be involved in X inactivation. Subsequent studies have utilized phosphoglycerate kinase as a tool for the mapping of the human X chromosome.[222] Grzeschik et al.[84] used cell hybrids involving an X–autosome translocation for mapping the human X chromosome. The results obtained with this technique have led different laboratories to draw maps of the X chromosome conflicting on the location of different markers.[187] However, presently there appears to be at least a general agreement on the location of the PGK structural gene on the long arm of the X chromosome, although the position of other markers remains in dispute.

Recently, a mutant of phosphoglycerate kinase associated with hemolytic anemia has been shown to have a greatly decreased affinity (high K_m) for phosphoglycerate and an abnormal electrophoretic mobility and pH curve.[261]

There appears to be only one single isozyme of phosphoglycerate kinase in all tissues. Phosphoglycerate kinase shares with phosphoglucomutase the rare characteristic for glycolytic enzymes to occur as a single unit enzyme.[75] In fact, the molecular weight of phosphoglycerate kinase is approximately 50,000 daltons and the enzyme does not dissociate into smaller subunits by treatments *in vitro* which have caused dissociation of various other proteins.[262] These multiple arguments indicate that there is a single structural gene located on the X chromosome that controls synthesis of an apparently identical protein in all tissues. Red cells and white cells are always equally defective, although in different families the enzyme deficiency varies in degree. This fact suggests that the mutation may result from a variably expressed quantitative defect.

The reports of two females with hemolytic anemia associated with decreased activity of phosphoglycerate kinase appear peculiar for an X-linked trait.[3,123] Both females were in their 6th decade and in both cases enzyme activity was only slightly decreased, in the range expected for a heterozygote. It is therefore not possible to postulate that these were females with an extreme degree of inactivation of the normal X chromosome. It is possible, however, that these females may have been heterozygous for a mutant enzyme with abnormal kinetics (a situation analogous to what has been clearly observed in the case of pyruvate kinase deficiency). On the other hand, it is also possible to speculate that in heterozygous females a mild defect of phosphoglycerate kinase may be rendered more severe by the subsequent occurrence of other abnormalities of carbohydrate metabolism (diabetes?). This possibility is also suggested by the observation that in one of these two females the study of red cell glycolytic intermediates demonstrated a crossover between 3-phosphoglycerate and phosphoenolpyruvate.[3]

PYRUVATE KINASE DEFICIENCY

A defect in pyruvate kinase was the first identified cause of congenital nonspherocytic hemolytic anemia.[251] This is by far the most commonly observed form of red cell glycolytic defect associated with chronic hemolysis; all others are by comparison exceedingly rare. Since the original description, over 150 cases have been reported in the literature.[18,145,231,245] The number of cases observed is certainly much larger, since new cases are no longer described. By comparison, the next most common form of chronic hemolytic anemia, which is the type associated with kinetically aberrant mutants of glucose-6-phosphate dehydrogenase, is much less frequent; in a recent review of the world literature, approximately 80 cases were found to have been described.[199]

A defect of pyruvate kinase has been reported with greater frequency among Northern Europeans, but the syndrome has been observed in practically all races.[40,154,231,258,263] It is not clear whether the greater frequency of this defect among Northern Europeans is genetically based or only reflects the greater frequency of laboratories equipped for this type of study in the United States and Northern Europe.

A limited number of small surveys are available on the frequency of heterozygosity, at least for those defective mutants which result in a decreased level of activity in the heterozygote. In Germany, in two separate studies,[26,91] the frequency of heterozygosity has been found to range between 1% and 1.5%; estimates of homozygosity are between 0.005% and 0.0025%, corresponding to a frequency of 1:20,000–1:40,000 births. Even greater heterozygote frequencies have been observed among Chinese newborn infants[76] and a small group of Filipinos.[231]

Clinical Spectrum

The clinical features of pyruvate kinase deficiency consist of hemolytic anemia that may be extremely variable, ranging from mild chronic hemolysis to extreme hemolysis resulting in early death, preventable by splenectomy. Most patients have hemolysis of intermediate to severe degree; in this regard, pyruvate kinase deficiency hemolytic anemia is clinically more severe than hereditary spherocytosis. In most cases, the enzymatic defect is evident at birth, when accentuation of hemolysis results in severe jaundice, often requiring exchange transfusion. Later in life, the syndrome is manifested by severe chronic hemolysis, jaundice, and splenomegaly. Autohemolysis

of type II is almost invariably observed. The intense hyperproduction
of red cells may result in widening of the bone marrow spaces, with
consequent facial and roentgenographic abnormalities.[11,34] The intense
turnover of red cells with consequent hyperbilirubinemia results in the
early development of gallbladder stones.[231] A feature of pyruvate
kinase deficiency anemia common to most other glycolytic defects is
the favorable clinical response to splenectomy. In the most severe
cases, such as those observed in Amish kindreds in Pennsylvania, this
may be life saving.[34] Measurements of red cell survival with ^{51}Cr may
yield variable results, depending not only on the severity of the
syndrome but also on the existence of several cell subpopulations with
different life spans. The difference in cell survival between subpopulations may be so pronounced that the initial rapid decline due to
extremely defective cells is missed.[175] Although the site of cell damage
is the spleen, as evidenced by the beneficial effects of splenectomy,
surface counting after ^{51}Cr labeling indicates that the main site of cell
death is the liver.[164] Circulation through the spleen inflicts a fatal blow
on the red cells, but the liver is the main clearing organ.

Biochemical Considerations

Pyruvate kinase regulates one of the last glycolytic steps. The
primary metabolic importance of the pyruvate kinase reaction is the
generation of ATP. It must be noted that ATP is generated by
pyruvate kinase whether 1,3-DPG is metabolized through 3-phospho-
glycerate kinase or the 2,3-DPG shunt. The ATP generated in the
pyruvate kinase reaction is utilized by the cell for several functions
(Fig. 1) (maintenance of intracellular ionic equilibrium, exchange of
membrane phospholipids, chelation of Ca^{2+}, phosphorylation of glucose and of fructose-6-phosphate at the phosphofructokinase reaction),
in contrast to the ATP generated by the 3-phosphoglycerate kinase
reaction, which is primarily utilized for the cation pump.[211] The
reaction catalyzed by pyruvate kinase is not in equilibrium, suggesting
regulation of this enzymatic step by external modulations.[151]

Pyruvate kinase of the red cell is an enzyme which is subject to
activation by K^+ and Mg^{2+}, inhibition by ATP, and activation by
fructose-1,6-diphosphate. The saturation curve of pyruvate kinase with
regard to phosphoenolpyruvate has a sigmoidal shape which can be

converted to a hyperbole by minute (10^{-6} M) concentrations of fructose-1,6-diphosphate.[80,225] Several authors have postulated that pyruvate kinase is an allosteric enzyme with regulatory properties.[100,108,225] It has been recently pointed out that the sigmoid kinetics with regard to phosphenolpyruvate is observed only in the presence of ATP at physiological pH.[29] It has been suggested that ATP at higher concentration acts as an allosteric inhibitor and the inhibition is relieved by fructose-1,6-diphosphate. In the absence of ATP, or when the ATP is removed by an "ATP trap,"[134] the saturation curve with regard to phosphoenolpyruvate appears hyperbolic. However, at the concentration of ATP within the cell itself, pyruvate kinase would be almost inactive if it were not activated by fructose-1,6-diphosphate.[73] Fructose-1,6-diphosphate is produced upstream by the action of phosphofructokinase, the pivotal enzyme in glycolytic regulation. A physiological concentration of fructose-1,6-diphosphate is adequate to increase the affinity of pyruvate kinase for phosphoenolpyruvate to obtain a significant metabolic flow.[106] The inhibition of pyruvate kinase by ATP is also mediated by a different mechanism: chelation of Mg^{2+}, a divalent cation necessary for enzyme function.[94] Reynard et al.[200] have suggested that ATP and ADP may share one binding site and phosphoenolpyruvate and pyruvate a different one. The inhibition by ATP could thus be competitive, because of a common locus for their transferable phosphoryl group. The binding site for fructose-1,6-diphosphate appears to be separate; thus this compound seems to be a real effector.[42] The intracellular activity of pyruvate kinase is therefore regulated on the one hand by the flow of fructose-1,6-diphosphate through glycolysis and on the other by the concentration of ATP. The modulation of pyruvate kinase activity as a function of ATP concentration is further enhanced by the accumulation of 2,3-DPG which results from decreased activity of pyruvate kinase. Any slowdown of pyruvate kinase results in increased levels of its immediate upstream intermediates, 3- and 2-phosphoglycerate.[145] These compounds, through the mechanisms described before, divert the flow of glycolysis through the 2,3-DPG shunt by bypassing the phosphoglycerate kinase step and thus further reducing the generation of ATP. A reduction of activity of pyruvate kinase also results in a decreased generation of pyruvate; this reduces the activity of lactic dehydrogenase and consequently the reconversion of NADH to NAD, a cofactor necessary for the activity of glyceraldehyde-3-phosphate dehydrogenase. The ultimate result is an overall reduction of glycolysis, until the ATP concentration is reduced to a level that permits resumption of pyruvate kinase activity. These interlocking mechanisms provide a flexible system for the control of intracellular ATP levels.

The activity of pyruvate kinase in cell metabolism is so paramount that it is not surprising that failure of this enzyme is incompatible with red cell survival. Depending on the severity of the enzyme defect, upstream glycolytic intermediates may accumulate, all the way back through the glycolytic chain. The accumulation of extremely large amounts of 2,3-DPG in the red cell is so striking that it has been considered a significant hallmark of pyruvate kinase deficiency.[112] In more extreme cases, accumulation of glycolytic intermediates all the way back to glucose-6-phosphate has been observed.[49,145] The prospects for survival of the pyruvate kinase deficient cell are obviously very gloomy. The cell is loaded with glycolytic intermediates, incapable of effective glycolysis, nearly totally depleted of ATP, with a barely functioning cation pump, leaking K^+ through the "Gardos effect," incapable of regenerating phospholipids, and with a membrane made rigid by failure to chelate Ca^{2+}. In fact, on the peripheral smear of these patients, spiny, small red cells are present, which represent the morphological expression of "desicytosis," the extreme of water loss and membrane damage.[165] It is indeed surprising that, in the face of such a total metabolic failure, there are any circulating red cells. Metabolic studies of pyruvate kinase deficient blood samples, however, yield surprisingly significant ATP levels and, in certain cases, a nearly normal glycolytic rate; the only finding which is consistently in line with the anticipated effects of pyruvate kinase deficiency is the accumulation of glycolytic intermediates, mainly 2,3-DPG. These puzzling observations appeared contradictory to the disastrous predictable biochemical consequences until Keitt drew attention to the fact that maintenance of ATP levels in pyruvate kinase deficient red cells was totally independent from glucose and completely paralyzed by cyanide, in contrast to the situation in normal cells.[112] These observations indicated that ATP in pyruvate kinase deficient cells derives not from glycolysis but rather from the activity of the tricarboxylic acid cycle. Since the only red cells with an active tricarboxylic acid cycle are reticulocytes, Keitt reached the conclusion that only reticulocytes are capable of survival in severe pyruvate kinase deficiency, an observation consistent with the great elevation of reticulocytes observed in these patients. The metabolic studies by Keitt also explained why after splenectomy the reticulocyte percentage increases rather than decreases. An increase in reticulocytosis usually indicates an accentuation of hemolysis; such an increase appeared inconsistent with an improved level of hemoglobin and of the general clinical condition of the patient. After splenectomy, pyruvate kinase deficient patients exhibit reticulocyte counts as high as 80–90%; essentially all circulating red cells are reticulocytes. The demonstration by Keitt that reticulocytes are the only cells capable of maintaining ATP levels independently of glycolysis, coupled with the observation that reticulocytes in pyruvate kinase deficiency are preferentially retained by the spleen, explained both the clinical effects and the increase in reticulocytes induced by splenectomy. Removal of the spleen permits the passage into the circulation of a greater number of reticulocytes, that would have been otherwise trapped in the splenic circulation. The reticulocytes persist in the circulation for a period of only 2–3 days. Then, as soon as the mitochondria (and the tricarboxylic acid cycle) disappear, the metabolic failure of pyruvate kinase results in rapid disappearance of the cell. The resulting clinical situation remains one of severe chronic hemolysis; however, the severity is greatly diminished compared to the situation before splenectomy, when a large percentage of reticulocytes could not even remain in the circulation for 2 or 3 days.

The great accumulation of 2,3-DPG in pyruvate kinase deficient red cells results in a major clinical advantage for the patient, since this compound alters the oxygen affinity of hemoglobin and facilitates unloading of oxygen at tissue level.[63,77,172] For this reason, patients with pyruvate kinase deficiency have a much greater exercise tolerance than other patients with comparable degrees of anemia.[173]

Genetic Considerations

There are two aspects of the genetic variation of pyruvate kinase that have to be considered separately: the existence of different isozymes in various tissues, apparently under the genetic control of different loci, and the existence of defective mutants of the isozyme, which is characteristic of the red cells and responsible for the chronic hemolysis.

Tanaka et al.[233] first observed the existence of two different types of isozymes, one called L, predominant in liver tissue, and the other called M, present in muscle. These two enzymes not only have different electrophoretic mobility but also have entirely different kinetic characteristics. Further studies of the electrophoretic mobility of pyruvate kinase isozymes have demonstrated in most mammals three different pyruvate kinase isozymes[44,103,104]: according to the recommended nomenclature of the international committee on isozymes,[93] PK1, PK2, and PK3. PK1, the fastest-moving isozyme, corresponds to Tanaka's type L; PK2 corresponds to Tanaka's type M; PK3, the slowest-moving isozyme, is found in most other tissues, including kidney and adipose tissue, and is also present together with PK1 in liver extract. Van Berkel et al.[252] demonstrated that in the liver PK1 is found in the hepatocyte and PK3 in the Kupffer cells. [Their studies have been interpreted in light of more recent data that indicate that the slow enzyme present in liver is PK3 and not type M (PK2) as they had suggested.] The kinetic characteristics of PK1 (sigmoid curve of affinity for phosphoenolpyruvate and sensitivity to fructose-1,6-diphosphate) are different from those of PK2 (hyperbolic curve of affinity for phosphoenolpyruvate and no sensitivity to fructose-1,6-diphosphate). PK3 has intermediate kinetics. Immunological studies have demonstrated a common antigen between PK2 and PK3.[178,233] These observations led initially to the hypothesis that only two isozymes existed (PK1 and PK3) and that PK2 could represent a hybrid molecule.[105] However, Cardenas et al.[43,44] have obtained five distinct electrophoretic bands following dissociation and recombination of equivalent mixtures of PK1 and PK2 isozymes. These observations are consistent with a tetrameric structure for both PK1 and PK2, each composed of four identical discrete subunits, and rule out the possibility that PK2 may be the hybrid consisting of two pairs of dimers. Similarly, Ibsen and Krueger[99] have suggested that although five different bands can be demonstrated by electrofocusing these are in reality due to the presence of two "conformers" each for PK1 and PK3 (both allosteric enzymes) and one only for PK2 (the nonallosteric enzyme). On the basis of the present evidence, it appears that there are three independent genes for the three different isozymes and that in every tissue only a single isozyme is present.[44] The two different isozymes present in the liver extracts are in reality located in two different types of cells.[252] The only apparent exception is the kidney cortex, where besides the predominant PK3 a few minor components are observed;

these seem to consist of hybrids between PK1 and PK3, since dissociation and recombination of the intermediate band yield the expected five bands.[44] Since pyruvate kinase hybrids do not form spontaneously *in vivo*, Garnett et al.[79] suggested that their presence in the kidney extracts indicates that the two isozymes are synthesized in the same cell. Besides the hybrids PK1-2 and PK1-3 demonstrated by Cardenas et al.,[44] Sutor and Rutter[230] have formed the hybrid PK2-3. Thus *in vitro* all the theoretically possible hybrid sets have been observed that could be anticipated from three distinct isozymes, each one consisting of a tetramer of four identical subunits. Imamura et al.[105] suggested that the PK3 isozyme represents the "archetype" pyruvate kinase, from which the other two isozymes have evolved. PK1 and PK2 in fact appear only later in fetal life[79,178]; moreover, all three isozymes appear to have similar molecular weight and similar enough structure to hybridize with each other.[44]

The different kinetic characteristics of the pyruvate kinase isozymes suggest that more specialized PK1 and PK2 isozymes may have derived from the archetypal PK3. PK1, with its allosteric regulatory properties, appears particularly efficient in tissues which require regulation of glycolysis. PK2 with its hyperbolic kinetics appears best suited to tissue such as muscle with extremely active glycolysis but with little need for control at the pyruvate kinase step. On the other hand, PK3, of intermediate kinetics, may meet the various metabolic requirements of several tissues. The antigen shared by PK2 and PK3 appears to be nonspecies specific, since cross-reactivity existed between the corresponding human and rat isozymes.[104] Further evidence for the similarity of pyruvate kinase in animals has been given by the hybridization experiments of Cardenas et al.[44] between chicken PK2 and bovine PK1.

In normal human blood, two different types of pyruvate kinase exist, with distinct electrophoretic mobility and kinetic characteristics (Fig. 6). However, separation of different cell types indicates that one isozyme is characteristic of red cells while the other is found in white cells and platelets. The enzyme present in the red cells strongly resembles the PK1 isozyme present in liver, with regard to its allosteric kinetics.[225] The electrophoretic mobility of the red cell isozyme is identical to the mobility of PK1 liver isozyme on cellogel[195] (a medium insensitive to molecular sieving) but appears slightly different on thin layer acrylamide (a medium sensitive to molecular sieving).[163] On the

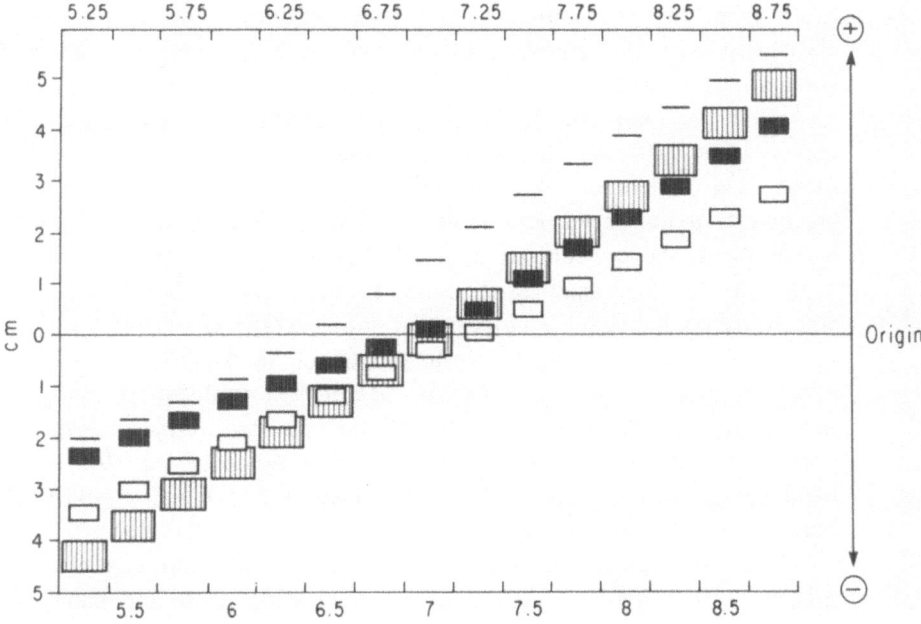

Fig. 6. Mobility of pyruvate kinase isozymes in normal blood at varying pH, on cellogel. ——, Tetrazolium reductase; shaded area, hemoglobin; dark area, PK_r (red cell isozyme); clear area, PK_w (white cell isozyme); horizontal axis, pH.

basis of this difference Imamura et al.[104] postulated that in the red cells a hybrid PK1-3 isozyme is present. The isozyme present in the white cells and platelets appears similar both electrophoretically and kinetically to PK3. Individuals deficient in pyruvate kinase lack only the red cell isozyme but have normal levels of the white cell isozyme. Studies of liver biopsies strongly suggest, however, identity between the red cell isozyme and the liver PK1, since only the PK3 but not the PK1 isozyme was found in liver extracts of deficient patients. The only exception was one patient in whom pyruvate kinase deficiency in the red cell was only partial (25% of normal) and resulted from a kinetically abnormal mutant.[163] The difference in electrophoretic mobility observed by Imamura and Tanaka[102] could also be explained by the presence of an allosteric conformer of the isozyme PK1 in their experimental conditions.

Study of the kinetics of red cell pyruvate kinase often has given contradictory results with regard to the allosteric or sigmoidal shape of the phosphoenolpyruvate saturation curve.[29,49,163] These differences result from the compounding effects of certain technical difficulties associated with the study of kinetics in crude hemolysates. Kinetic studies may in fact be performed in unpurified preparations only when no other reaction interferes with the enzyme studied. In crude hemolysates, however, the activity of adenylate kinase (which transforms two molecules of ADP into one each of ATP and AMP) profoundly modifies the kinetics of pyruvate kinase.[243] Thus, in crude hemolysates, the concentration of ADP is decreased and the concentration of ATP increased by adenylate kinase. Besides this effect, ATP concentration increases as a result of the reaction of pyruvate kinase itself. For these reasons, the results obtained in the kinetic study of pyruvate kinase in such hemolysates are at best doubtful. It has been noted, in fact, that the kinetics of the purified enzyme may be profoundly different from that of crude hemolysates.[30] On the other hand, conditions of purification may alter the original equilibrium between the allosterically active and inactive forms of the enzyme.

Studies of pyruvate kinase activity in the red cells can also be profoundly modified by contamination with white cells and platelets. The activity of pyruvate kinase in white cells and platelets is, per unit volume, 500–800 times greater than in red cells. Contamination with platelets may be particularly severe in splenectomized patients, who have elevated counts. If contaminating cells are not removed, the result may be failure to obtain a correct diagnosis of pyruvate kinase deficiency and the presence of even more significant artifacts in any attempt to purify residual enzyme activity in severely deficient patients.[27,169,234] Purification of small traces of enzyme activity may yield an apparently abnormal enzyme, with different enzyme mobility, paradoxically increased affinity for phosphoenolpyruvate (low $K_{m\mathrm{PEP}}$), and apparently great *in vitro* instability. In reality, these characteristics are those of the white cell and platelet isozyme. Several pyruvate kinase mutants with these characteristics have been reported, primarily in patients with greatly decreased red cell enzyme, and labeled as "kinetically abnormal."[27,36,169,226] It appears extremely unlikely that an enzyme with greater intracellular efficiency (low K_m) than the normal enzyme could result in a severe functional defect.[119]

Apart from these artifactual findings, it is clear the several defective mutant enzymes may be responsible for pyruvate kinase deficiency. In most families studied, a homozygous recessive pattern was observed, with the propositus exhibiting extremely decreased activity and both parents exhibiting intermediate levels.[34,232,245] However, in several kindreds in the standard assay one or both parents had normal and the propositus had significant residual enzymatic activity.[159,183,184] Further studies of the defective enzyme in these families have demonstrated that although the activity was superficially normal when measured *in vitro* at saturating concentrations of substrate the affinity for phosphoenolpyruvate was greatly decreased (high K_m).[34,181,183] These enzymes are nonfunctional at the low intracellular PEP concentration. This defect could not be attributed to increased sensitivity to ATP inhibition, since in most cases FDP activation did not occur.[146,184] Recently, abnormal electrophoretic mobility has been shown for at least two of these high K_{mPEP} mutants.[163] It will not be possible to categorize the number of defective PK mutants until the methods of biochemical characterization are standardized, as they have been for the study of glucose-6-phosphate dehydrogenase deficiency.[257]

At the present time, however, it appears clear that there are at least two classes of defective red cell pyruvate kinase mutants: one associated with greatly defective activity and another with kinetic abnormality (high K_{mPEP}). Thus individuals with pyruvate kinase deficiency hemolytic anemia may be either homozygotes for the same type of mutant or heterozygotes for two different mutant types.[231]

OTHER DEFECTS OF GLYCOLYTIC ENZYMES IN THE RED CELLS

Triosephosphate Isomerase Deficiency

Triosephosphate isomerase deficiency has been documented in eight different families; besides the propositi, the deficiency appears probably responsible for the early death of at least three additional sibs (Table VI). Genetic studies have suggested an autosomal recessive inheritance.

In another family, reduced (55% of normal) triosephosphate isomerase activity was observed in a female with the *cri-du-chat* syndrome (and partial deletion of chromosome 5).[223] However, the demonstration of normal triosephosphate isomerase levels in 13 additional cases of *cri-du-chat* syndrome, in which at least some of the

TABLE VI. Triosephosphate Isomerase Deficiency: Clinical and Biochemical Aspects[a]

Ref	Age	Sex	Hb	Retics	Enzyme activity		Other[b]
					RBC	WBC	
210	14/12	F^c	10.2	13	6	20	
	6/365	M^c	—	—	—	—	*
210	10/12	F^c	11.9	—	—	—	**
	1/365	M^c	—	—	—	—	**
	5	F^c	—	—	—	—	**
209	4	M	9	14.5	36	24	
210	3	F^c	10.7	17	7	9	
2	14	F^c	—	—	↓	—	
89	21	F	—	—	↓	↓	
120	5/365	—	—	—	↓	—	
123	—	F	NL	NL	55	—	***

[a] Abbreviations as in Table II.
[b] Symbols: *, case presumed, sib of previous patient; **, case presumed, because of relation with previous family; ***, presumed heterozygous, associated with cri-du-chat syndrome.
[c] Dead.

karyotypes were apparently indistinguishable from that in the previous case, suggests that the association may have been fortuitous.[38] The biochemical consequences of triosephosphate isomerase deficiency and their relationship to the clinical symptomatology are similar to those of phosphoglycerate kinase deficiency and have been discussed in a previous section. The deficiency appears responsible for early death: five of the eight propositi died before 15 months and one before 6 years of age. Only one case has been reported in an adult female, age 21 years of age; in this case, transfusion requirement ceased at puberty but neurological symptoms persisted.[89]

Glyceraldehyde-3-phosphate Dehydrogenase Deficiency

Glyceraldehyde-3-phosphate dehydrogenase deficiency has been briefly reported in a 40-year-old male with 55% of normal activity[177] and in a father and son with 20–30% of normal activity.[86] The latter finding excludes X-linked inheritance. In both studies, enzyme deficiency was established and greater sensitivity to iodoacetate inhibition of glycolysis was demonstrated. However, since glyceraldehyde-3-phosphate dehydrogenase is membrane bound,[144] it is not possible to rule out that the defect could have been secondary to membrane alterations, in the absence of supporting genetic and histochemical data.

2,3-Diphosphoglycerate Mutase Deficiency

2,3-Diphosphoglycerate mutase deficiency has been suspected in an infant with severe hemolysis who died at 3 months of age.[212] The evidence for the existence of this deficiency is, however, only indirect since the propositus could never be studied because of the transfusion requirement necessitated by the clinical status, and the defect was suspected only on the basis of decreased activity of the enzyme (approximately 50% in both parents and a sister). Three additional presumed heterozygotes have also been described by Cartier et al.[47]

Lactate Dehydrogenase Deficiency

Lactate dehydrogenase deficiency has been described in a diabetic Japanese in his sixth decade.[158] The defect appeared due to the complete absence of the H subunit of the enzyme in all tissues studied. Accumulation of triosephosphates was found in the red cells, suggesting a failure of the regeneration of NAD by lactic dehydrogenase, with consequent reduction in efficiency of glyceraldehyde-3-phosphate dehydrogenase. It is not, however, clear whether these abnormalities would have resulted in chronic hemolysis, without the coexistence of diabetes.

ACKNOWLEDGMENTS

Dr. Sergio Piomelli is a Career Scientist of the New York City Health Research Council (I-383). The work reported in this chapter

has been partly supported by Grant AM-HL 09274-10 from the
National Institures of Health, Bethesda, Maryland. The authors are
indebted to Ms. Carol Seaman for constructive criticism and help in
the preparation of the manuscript.

BIBLIOGRAPHY

1. Altay, C., Alper, C. A., and Nathan, D. G., Normal and variant isoenzymes of human blood cell hexokinase and the isoenzyme patterns in hemolytic anemia, *Blood* **36**:219 (1970).
2. Angelman, M., Brain, M. C., and MacIver, J. E., A case of triosephosphate isomerase deficiency with sudden death, *Proc. 13th Int. Congr. Hematol., Munich,* p. 122 (1970).
3. Arese, P., Bosia, A., Grallo, E., Mazza, U., and Pesearmona, G. P., Red cell glycolysis in a case of 3-phosphoglycerate kinase deficiency, *Eur. J. Clin. Invest.* **3**:86 (1973).
4. Arnone, A., X-ray diffraction study of binding of 2,3-diphosphoglycerate to human deoxyhaemoglobin, *Nature (London)* **221**:618 (1972).
5. Arnold, H., Blume, K. G., Busch, D., Leikeit, V., Löhr, G. W., and Lubs, E., Klinische und biochemische Untersuchungen zur Glucose-phosphatisomerase menschlicher Erythrocyten und bei Glucose phosphatisomerase Mangel, *Klin. Wochenschr.* **48**:1299 (1970).
6. Arnold, H., Blume, K. G., Engelhardt, R., and Löhr, G. W., Glucosephosphate isomerase deficiency: Evidence for *in vivo* instability of an enzyme variant with hemolysis, *Blood* **41**:691 (1973).
7. Arnold, H., Blume, K. G., Löhr, G. W., Schröter, W., Koch, H. H., and Wonneberger, B., Glucosephosphate isomerase deficiency with congenital nonspherocytic hemolytic anemia: a new variant (type Nordhorn). II. Purification and biochemical properties of the defective enzyme, *Pediat. Res.* **8**:26 (1974).
8. Baikie, A. G., Loder, P. B., deGruchy, G. C., Pitt, D. B., Phosphohexokinase activity of erythrocytes in mongolism: Another possible marker for chromosome 21, *Lancet* **I**:412 (1965).
9. Bartels, S., and Kruse, K., Enzymbestimmungen in Erythrocyten bei Kindern mit Down-Syndrom, *Humangenetik* **5**:305 (1968).
10. Baughan, M. A., Valentine, W. N., Paglia, D. E., Ways, P. O., Simon, E. R., and DeMarsh, Q. B., Hereditary hemolytic anemia associated with glucosephosphate isomerase (GPI) deficiency—A new enzyme defect of human erythrocytes, *Blood* **32**:232 (1968).
11. Becker, M. H., Genesier, N. B., and Piomelli, S., The radiology of pyruvate kinase deficiency hemolytic anemia, in: *Blood, Birth Defects, Original Article Series VIII: II,* The National Foundation, New York (1972).
12. Bellingham, A. J., The red cell in adaptation to anemic hypoxia, *Clinics Hematol.* **3**:577 (1974).
13. Benesch, R., and Benesch, R. E., Intracellular organic phosphates as regulators of oxygen release by haemoglobin, *Nature (London)* **221**:618 (1969).
14. Benson, P. F., Linacre, B., and Taylor, A. I., Erythrocyte ATP: D-Fructose-6-phosphate phosphotransferase (phosphofructokinase) activity in children with nor-

mal/G trisomosaic Down's syndrome and in normal and Down's syndrome controls, *Nature (London)* **220:**1235 (1968).

15. Bernini, L., Latte, B., Siniscalco, M., Piomelli, S., Spada, U., Adinolfi, M., and Mollison, P. L., Survival of ^{51}Cr-labelled red cells in subjects with thalassemia-trait or G6PD deficiency or both abnormalities, *Br. J. Haematol.* **10:**171 (1964).

16. Bethenod, M., and Kissin, C., Déficit en hexokinase intra-erythrocytaire, *Ann. Pediat. (Paris)* **50:**825 (1967).

17. Beutler, E., *Hereditary Disorders of Erythrocyte Metabolism*, Grune and Stratton, New York (1968).

18. Beutler, E., Genetic disorders of red cell metabolism, *Med. Clin. North Am.* **53:**813 (1969).

19. Beutler, E., Glutathione reductase: Stimulation in normal subjects by riboflavin supplementation, *Science* **165:**613 (1969).

20. Beutler, E., Abnormalities of the hexose monophosphate shunt, *Semin. Hematol.* **8:**311 (1971).

21. Beutler, E., Johnson, C., Powars, D., and West, C., Prevalence of glucose-6-phosphate dehydrogenase deficiency in sickle-cell disease, *New Engl. J. Med.* **290:**826 (1974).

22. Beutler, E., Sigalove, W. H., Muir, W. A., Matsumoto, F., and West, C., Glucosephosphate-isomerase (GPI) deficiency: GPI-Elyria, *Ann. Intern. Med.* **80:**730 (1974).

23. Bigley, R. H., Stenzel, P., Jones, R. T., Campos, J. D., and Koler, R. D., Tissue distribution of human pyruvate kinase isozymes, *Enzym. Biol. Clin.* **9:**10 (1968).

24. Blum, R. M., and Hoffman, J. F., Carrier mediation of Ca-induced K transport and its inhibition in red blood cells, *Fed. Proc.* **29:**663 (1970).

25. Blume, K. G., Hyrniuk, W., Powars, D., Trinidad, F., West, C., and Beutler, E., Characterization of two new variants of glucose-phosphate-isomerase deficiency with hereditary nonspherocytic hemolytic anemia, *J. Lab. Clin. Med.* **79:**942 (1972).

26. Blume, K. G., Löhr, G. W., Praetsch, O., Rudiger, H. W., and Wendt, G. G., Beitrag zur Populationsgenetik der Pyruvatekinase menschlicher Erythrocyten, *Humangenetik* **6:**261 (1968).

27. Boivin, P., and Galand, C., Constante de Michaelis anormale pour le phospho-enol-pyruvate au cours d'un déficit en pyruvate kinase erythrocytaire, *Rev. Fr. Etud. Clin. Biol.* **4:**372 (1967).

28. Boivin, P., Galand, C., and DeMartial, M. C., Coexistence de deux types de pyruvate-kinase cinétiquement differents dans les globules rouges humains normaux, *Nouv. Rev. Fr. Hematol.* **12:**159 (1972),

29. Boivin, P., Galand, C., and DeMartial, M. C., Études sur la pyruvate kinase erythrocytaire. I. Quelque propriétés de l'enzyme humaine normal, *Pathol. Biol.* **20:**583 (1972).

30. Boivin, P., Galand, C., and DeMartial, M. C., Études sur la pyruvatekinase erythrocytaire. II. Hétérogeneité enzymologique des déficits: Études à propos de 28 cas avec anémie hémolytique congénitale, *Nouv. Rev. Fr. Hematol.* **12:**569 (1972).

31. Borun, E. A., Figueroa, M., and Perry, S. M., The distribution of Fe^{59} tagged human erythrocytes in centrifuged specimens as a function of cell age, *J. Clin. Invest.* **36:**676 (1957).

32. Boulard, M. R., Meienofer, M. C., Bois, M., Reviron, M., and Najean, Y., Red cell phosphofructokinase deficiency, *New Engl. J. Med.* **291:**978 (1974).

33. Bowman, H. S., McKusick, V. A., and Dronamraju, K. R., Pyruvate kinase deficient hemolytic anemia in an Amish isolate, *Am. J. Hum. Genet.* **17:**1 (1965).

34. Bowman, H. S., and Procopio, F., Hereditary non-spherocytic hemolytic anemia of the pyruvate-kinase deficient type, *Ann. Intern. Med.* **58**:567 (1963).
35. Brand, K., Arese, P., and Rivera, M., Bedeutung und Regulation des Pentosophosphateweges in menschlichen Erythrozyten I & II, *Hoppe-Seylers Z. Physiol. Chem.* **351**:501 (1970).
36. Brandt, N. J., and Hanel, H. K., Atypical pyruvate kinase in a patient with haemolytic anemia, *Scand. J. Haematol.* **8**:126 (1971).
37. Brewer, G. J., Erythrocyte metabolism and function: Hexokinase inhibition by 2,3-diphosphoglycerate and interaction with ATP and Mg^{2+}, *Biochim. Biophys. Acta* **192**:157 (1969).
38. Brock, D. J., and Singer, J. D., Red cell triosephosphate isomerase and chromosome 5, *Lancet* **2**:1136 (1970).
39. Brok, F., Ramot, B., Zwang, E., and Danon, D., Enzyme activities in human red blood cells of different age groups, *Israel J. Med. Sci.* **2**:291 (1966).
40. Brunetti, P., Puxeddu, A., Nenci, G., and Migliorini, E., Haemolytic anemia due to pyruvate kinase deficiency, *Lancet* **2**:169 (1963).
41. Bunn, H. F., Erythrocyte destruction and hemoglobin catabolism, *Semin. Hematol.* **9**:3 (1972).
42. Carbonell, J., Feliu, E. J., Marco, R., and Sels, A., Pyruvate kinase: Classes of regulatory isoenzymes in mammalian tissues, *Eur. J. Biochem.* **37**:148 (1973).
43. Cardenas, J. M., and Dyson, R. D., Bovine pyruvate kinases. II. Purification of the liver isozyme and its hybridization with skeletal muscle pyruvate kinase, *J. Biol. Chem.* **248**:6938 (1973).
44. Cardenas, J. M., Dyson, R. D., and Strandholm, J. J., Bovine and chicken pyruvate kinase isozymes: Intraspecies and interspecies hybrids, in: *Third International Isozyme Conference, Yale University, April, 1974* (C. L. Markert, ed.), Academic Press, New York (1975).
45. Carson, P. E., Flanagan, C. L., Hickes, C. E., and Alving, A. S., Enzymatic deficiency in primaquine sensitive erythrocytes, *Science* **124**:484 (1956).
46. Carter, N. D., and Yoshida, A., Purification and characterization of human phosphoglucose isomerase, *Biochim. Biophys. Acta* **181**:12 (1969).
47. Cartier, P., Labie, P., Leroux, J. P., Najman, A., and DeMaugre, F., Déficit familial en diphosphoglycerate mutase: Étude hématologique et biochimique, *Nouv. Rev. Fr. Hematol.* **12**:269 (1972).
48. Cartier, P., Habibi, B., Leroux, J. P., and Marchand, J. C., Anémie hémolytique congénitale associée à un déficit en phosphoglycérate-kinase dans les globules rouges, les polynucléaires, et les lymphocytes, *Nouv. Rev. Fr. Hematol.* **11**:565 (1971).
49. Cartier, P., Najman, A., Leroux, J. P., and Temkine, H., Les anomalies de la glycolyse au cours l'anémie hémolytique par déficit du globule rouge en pyruvate kinase, *Clin. Chim. Acta* **22**:165 (1968).
50. Cartier, P., Temkine, H., and Griscelli, C., Étude biochimique d'une anémie hémolytique avec déficit familial en phosphohexoseisomerase, *Enzym. Biol. Clin. (Basel)* **10**:439 (1969).
51. Chapman, R. G., Hennessey, M. A., Watersdorph, A. M., Huennekens, F. M., and Gabrio, B. W., Erythrocyte metabolism: Level of glycolytic enzymes and regulation of glycolysis, *J. Clin. Invest.* **41**:1249 (1962).
52. Chauffard, M. A., and Troisier, J., Anémie grave avec hémolysine dans la sérum, *Sem. Med.* **28**:904 (1908).

53. Chen, S. H., Malcom, L. A., Yoshida, A., and Giblett, E. R., Phosphoglycerate kinase: An X-linked polymorphism in man *Am. J. Hum. Genet.* **23**:87 (1971).
54. Chilcote, R. R., and Baehner, R. L., Red cell (RBC) glucose phosphate isomerase deficiency (GPI): Clinical and laboratory evidence of increased blood viscosity, *Pediat. Res.* **8**:398 (1971).
55. Cohen, G., and Hochstein, P., Generation of hydrogen peroxide in erythrocytes by hemolytic agents, *Biochemistry* **3**:895 (1964).
56. Conway, M. M., and Layzer, R. B., Blood cell phosphofructokinase in Down's syndrome, *Humangenetik* **9**:135 (1970).
57. Corash, L., and Gralnick, H. R., High yield quantitative isolation of human platelet from whole blood, *Blood* **44**:919 (1974).
58. Corash, L. M., Piomelli, S., Chen, M. C., Seaman, C., and Gross, E., Separation of erythrocytes according to age on a simplified density gradient, *J. Lab. Clin. Med.* **84**:147 (1974).
59. Dacie, J. V., Mollison, P. L., Richardson, N., Selwyn, J. C., and Shapiro, L., Atypical congenital hemolytic anemia, *Quart. J. Med.* **22**:79 (1953).
60. Davidson, W. D., and Tanaka, K. R., Continuous measurement of pentose phosphate pathway activity in erythrocytes: An ionization chamber method, *J. Lab. Clin. Med.* **73**:173 (1969).
61. deGruchy, G. C., and Grimes, A. J., The non-spherocytic congenital haemolytic anemias, *Br. J. Haematol.* **23**:Supplement 19 (1972).
62. deGruchy, G. C., Santamaria, J. N., Parson, I. C., and Crawford, M., Non-spherocytic congenital hemolytic anemia, *Blood* **16**:1371 (1960).
63. Delivoria-Papadopoulos, M., Oski, F. A., and Gottlieb, A. J., Oxygen–hemoglobin dissociation curves: Effect of inherited enzyme defects of the red cell, *Science* **165**:601 (1969).
64. Detter, J. C., Ways, P. D., Giblett, E. R., Baughan, M. A., Hopkinson, D. A., Povey, S., and Harris, M., Inherited variations in human phosphohexose isomerase, *Ann. Hum. Genet.* **31**:329 (1968).
65. Deys, B. F., Grzeschik, K. H., Grzeschik, A., Jaffé, E. R., and Siniscalco, M., Human phosphoglycerate kinase and inactivation of the X-chromosome, *Science* **175**:1002 (1972).
66. Dunham, P. B., and Gunn, R. B., Adenosine triphosphate and active cation transport in red blood cell membranes, *Arch. Intern. Med.* **129**:241 (1972).
67. Engelhardt, R., Arnold, H., and Hoffman, A., GPI-Recklinghausen: A new variant of glucosephosphate isomerase deficiency with hemolytic anemia. Erythrocytes, thrombocytes, leukocytes, in: *Recent Advances in Membrane and Metabolic Research* (E. Gerlach, K. Moser, E. Deutsch, *et al.*, eds.), pp. 180–182, Georg Thieme, Stuttgart (1973).
68. Feig, S. A., Methemoglobinemia, in: *Hematology of Infancy and Childhood* (D. G. Nathan and F. A. Oski, eds.), p. 379, Saunders, Philadelphia (1974).
69. Feig, S. A., Segel, G. B., Shohet, S., and Nathan, D. G., Energy metabolism in human erythrocytes. II. Effect of glucose depletion, *J. Clin. Invest.* **51**:1547 (1972).
70. Feig, S. A., Shohet, S. B., and Nathan, D. G., Energy metabolism in human erythrocytes. I. Effects of sodium fluoride, *J. Clin. Invest.* **50**:1731 (1971).
71. Finch, C. A., and Lenfant, C., Oxygen transport in man, *New Engl. J. Med.* **286**:407 (1972).
72. Fitch, I. I., Parr, C. W., and Welch, S. G., Phosphoglucose isomerase variation in man, *Biochem. J.* **110**:56P (1968).

73. Flory, W., Peczon, B. D., Koeppe, R. E., and Spivey, M. D., Kinetic properties of rat liver pyruvate kinase at cellular concentrations of enzyme, substrates and modifiers, *Biochem. J.* **141:**127 (1974).
74. Forget, B. G., and Kan, Y. W., Thalassemia and the genetics of hemoglobin, in: *Hematology of Infancy and Childhood* (D. G. Nathan and F. A. Oski, eds.), p. 450, Saunders, Philadelphia (1974).
75. Fritz, P. J., and White, L., 3-Phosphoglycerate kinase from rat tissues: Further characterization and developmental studies, *Biochemistry* **13:**444 (1974).
76. Fung, R. H. P., Keung, Y. K., and Chung, G. S. H.,Screening of pyruvate kinase deficiency and G6PD deficiency in Chinese newborn in Hong Kong, *Arch. Dis. Child.* **44:**373 (1969).
77. Garby, L., Anemia and hypoxia, *Clinics Haematol.* **3:**575, (1974).
78. Gardos, G., and Straub, F. B., Uber die Rolle der Adenosintriphosphorsaure (ATP) in der K-Permeabilitat der menschlichen roten Blutkorperchen, *Acta Physiol. Acad. Sci. Hung.* **12:**1 (1957).
79. Garnett, M. E., Dyson, R. D., and Dost, F. N., Pyruvate kinase isozyme changes in parenchymal cells of regenerating rat liver, *J. Biol. Chem.* **249:**5222 (1974).
80. Garreau, H., and Buc-Temkine, H., Allosteric activation of human erythrocyte pyruvate kinase by fructose-1,6-diphosphate: Kinetic and equilibrium binding studies, *Biochimie* **54:**1103 (1972).
81. Gerber, G. K., Schultze, M., and Rapoport, S. M., Occurrence and function of a high Km hexokinase in immature red blood cells, *Eur. J. Biochem.* **17:**445 (1970).
82. Giblett, E. R., Anderson, J. E., Cohen, F., Pollara, B., and Meuwissen, H. J., Adenosine-deaminase deficiency in two patients with severely impaired cellular immunity, *Lancet* **2:**1067 (1972).
83. Glatze, D., Weber, F., and Wiss, O., Enzymatic test for detection of a riboflavin deficiency: NADPH-dependent glutathione reductase of red blood cells and its activation by FAD *in vitro, Experientia* **24:**1122 (1968).
84. Grzeschik, K. M., Allerdice, P. W., Grzeschik, A., Opitz, M., Miller, O. J., and Siniscalco, M., Cytological mapping of human X-linked genes by use of somatic cell hybrids involving an X-autosome translocation, *Proc. Natl. Acad. Sci. U.S.A.* **69:**69 (1972).
85. Haidas, S., Labie, D., and Kaplan, J. C., 2,3-Diphosphoglycerate content and oxygen affinity as a function of red cell age in normal individuals, *Blood* **38:**463 (1971).
86. Harkness, D. R., A new erythrocytic enzyme defect with hemolytic anemia: Glyceraldehyde-3-phosphate dehydrogenase deficiency, *J. Lab. Clin. Med.* **68:**879 (1966).
87. Harris, H., *The Principles of Human Biochemical Genetics*, American Elsevier, New York (1970).
88. Harris, J. W., and Kellermeyer, R. W., *The Red Cell. Production, Metabolism, Destruction: Normal and Abnormal*, Harvard University Press, Cambridge, Mass. (1970).
89. Harris, S. R., Paglia, D. E., Jaffé, E. R., Valentine, W. N., and Klein, R. L., Triosephosphate isomerase deficiency in an adult, *Clin. Res.* **18:**529 (1970).
90. Heinrich, R., and Rapoport, T. A., Linear theory of enzymatic chains; its application for the analysis of the crossover theorem and of glycolysis of human erythrocytes, *Acta Biol. Med. Germ.* **31:**479 (1973).
91. Helbig, W., and Jacobasch, G., Sippenuntersuchung bei Pyruvatkinasemangel Anämie, *Folia Haematol. (Leipzig)* **91:**65 (1969).

92. Hjelm, M., and Wadam, B., Nonspherocytic hemolytic anemia with phosphoglycerate kinase deficiency, *Proc. 13th Int. Congr. Hematol., Munich,* p. 121 (1970).
93. Hoffman-Ostenhof, O., Cohen, W. E., Braunstein, A. E., Karlson, P., Keil, B., Klyne, G., Lieberg, C., Slater, E. C., Webb, E. C., and Whelan, W. J., IUPAC-IUB Commission on Biochemical Nomenclature. The nomenclature of multiple forms of enzymes: Recommendations 1971, *J. Biol. Chem.* **246:**6127 (1971).
94. Holmsen, H., and Storm, E., The adenosine triphosphate inhibition of the pyruvate kinase reaction and its dependence on total magnesium ion concentration, *Biochem. J.* **112:**303 (1969).
95. Hoyer, L., and Breckenridge, R. T., Immunologic studies of antihemophilic factor (AHF, factor VIII) crossreacting material in a genetic variant of hemophilia A., *Blood* **32:**962 (1968).
96. Huebner, R. J., Viruses in search of disease, *Ann. N.Y. Acad. Sci.* **67:**209 (1957).
97. Hultquist, D. E., and Passon, P. G., Catalysis of methemoglobin reduction by erythrocyte cytochrome b_5 and cytochrome b_5 reductase, *Nature New Biol.* **229:**252 (1971).
98. Hutton, J. J., and Chilcote, R. R., Glucose phosphate isomerase deficiency with hereditary non-spherocytic hemolytic anemia, *Pediatrics* **85:**494 (1974).
99. Ibsen, H., and Krueger, E., Distribution of pyruvate kinase isozymes among rat organs, *Arch. Biochem. Biophys.* **157:**509 (1973).
100. Ibsen, K. H., Schiller, K. W., and Haas, T. A., Interconvertible kinetic and physical forms of human erythrocyte pyruvate kinase, *J. Biol. Chem.* **246:**1233 (1971).
101. Ibsen, K., and Trippet, P., Human erythrocyte pyruvate kinase conformers obtained by electrofocusing, *Life Sci.* **10:**1021 (1971).
102. Imamura, K., and Tanaka, T., Multimolecular forms of pyruvate kinase from rat and other mammalian tissues. I. Electrophoretic studies, *J. Biochem.* **71:**1043 (1972).
103. Imamura, K., Tanaka, T., Miwa, S., Nakashima, K., and Nishina, T., Studies on pyruvate kinase (PK) deficiency. II. Electrophoretic, kinetic and immunological studies on erythrocyte and other tissue PKs, *J. Biochem.* **74:**1165 (1973).
104. Imamura, K., Tanaka, T., Nishina, T., Nakashima, K., and Miwa, S., Studies on pyruvate kinase (PK) deficiency. II. Electrophoretic, kinetic, and immunological studies on pyruvate kinase of erythrocytes and other tissues, *J. Biochem.* **74:**1165 (1973).
105. Imamura, K., Taniuchi, K., and Tanaka, T., Multimolecular forms of pyruvate kinase. II. Purification of M_2 type pyruvate kinase from Yoshida ascites hepatoma 130 cells and comparative studies on the enzymological and immunological properties of the three types of pyruvate kinase L, M, and M_2, *J. Biochem.* **72:**1001 (1972).
106. Irving, M. G., and Williams, J. F., Kinetic studies on the regulation of rabbit liver pyruvate kinase, *Biochem. J.* **131:**287 (1973).
107. Jacob, H., and Jandl, J. H., Effect of sulfhydryl inhibition on red blood cells. I. Mechanism of hemolysis, *J. Clin. Invest.* **41:**779 (1962).
108. Jacobson, K. W., and Black, J., Conformational differences in the active sites of muscle and erythrocyte pyruvate kinase, *J. Biol. Chem.* **246:**5504 (1971).
109. Jandl, J. H., and Cooper, R. A., Hereditary spherocytosis, in: *The Metabolic Basis of Inherited Disease* (J. B. Stanbury, J. B. Wyngaarden, and D. S. Fredrickson, eds.), p. 1323, McGraw-Hill, New York (1972).

110. Kahana, S. E., Lowry, O. H., Schulz, D. W., Passoneau, J. V., and Crawford, E. J., The kinetics of phosphoglucoisomerase, *J. Biol. Chem.* **235**:2178 (1960).

111. Kaplan, J. C., and Beutler, E., Hexokinase isoenzymes in human erythrocytes, *Science* **159**:215 (1968).

112. Keitt, A. S., Pyruvate kinase deficiency and related disorders of red cell glycolysis, *Am. J. Med.* **41**:762 (1966).

113. Keitt, A. S., Hemolytic anemia with impaired hexokinase activity, *J. Clin. Invest.* **48**:1997 (1969).

114. Keitt, A. S., Red cell maturation and survival factors governing red cell life span, in: *Hematology of Infancy and Childhood* (D. G. Nathan and F. A. Oski, eds.), Saunders, Philadelphia (1974).

115. Key, A. J., Studies on erythrocytes, with special reference to reticulum, polychromatophilia and mitochondria, *Arch. Intern. Med.* **28**:511 (1921).

116. Khan, P. M., Westerveld, A., Grzeschik, K. H., Deys, B. F., Garson, O. M., and Siniscalco, M., X-linkage of human phosphoglycerate kinase confirmed in man–mouse and man–Chinese hamster somatic cell hybrids, *Am. J. Hum. Genet.* **23**:614 (1971).

117. Kirkman, H, N., Glucose-6-phosphate dehydrogenase variants and drug-induced hemolysis, *Ann. N.Y. Acad. Sci.* **151**:753 (1968).

118. Kirkman, H. N., Glucose-6-phosphate dehydrogenase, *Advan. Hum. Genet.* **2**:1 (1971).

119. Kirkman, H. N., Enzyme defects, in: *Progress in Medical Genetics* (A. G. Steinberg and A. G. Bearn, eds.), Grune and Stratton, New York (1972).

120. Kleihauer, E., Kleeberg, U. R., and Besch, P., Methylene blue induced hemolytic Heinz body anemia in a newborn infant with glutathione reductase and triosephosphate isomerase deficiency, *Proc. 13th Int. Congr. Hematol., Munich,* p. 293 (1970).

121. Konrad, P. N., McCarthy, D. J., Mauer, A. M., Valentine, W. N., and Paglia, D. E., Erythrocyte and leukocyte phosphoglycerate kinase deficiency with neurologic disease, *J. Pediat.* **82**:456 (1973).

122. Kosower, N. S., Vanderholl, G. A., and London, I. M., Hexokinase activity in normal and glucose-6-phosphate dehydrogenase deficient erythrocytes, *Nature (London)* **201**:684 (1964).

123. Kraus, A. P., Langston, M. F., Jr., and Lynch, B. L., Red cell phosphoglycerate kinase deficiency; a new case of non-spherocytic hemolytic anemia, *Biochem. Biophys. Res. Commun.* **30**:173 (1968).

124. Krone, W., Schneider, G., Schulz, D., Arnold, H., and Blume, K. G., Detection of phosphohexose isomerase deficiency in human fibroblast cultures, *Humangenetik* **10**:224 (1970).

125. LaCelle, P. L., and Weed, R. I., The contribution of normal and pathologic erythrocytes to blood rheology, in: *Progress in Hematology,* Vol. VII (E. B. Brown and C. V. Moore, eds.), Grune and Stratton, New York (1971).

126. Layzer, R. B., and Conway, M. M., Multiple isoenzymes of human phosphofructokinase, *Biochem. Biophys. Res. Commun.* **40**:1259 (1970).

127. Layzer, R. B., and Epstein, C. J., Phosphofructokinase and chromosome 21, *Am. J. Hum. Genet.* **24**:533 (1972).

128. Layzer, R. B., and Rasmussen, J., Bases of muscle phosphofructokinase, *Arch. Neurol.* **31**:411 (1974).

129. Layzer, R. B., Rowland, L. P., and Ranney, H. M., Muscle phosphofructokinase deficiency, *Arch. Neurol.* **17**:512 (1967).

130. Layzer, R. B., Rowland, L. P., and Bank, W. J., Isoenzyme abnormality in human muscle phosphofructokinase deficiency, *Clin. Res.* **16**:152 (1968).
131. Layzer, R. B., Rowland, L. P., and Bank, W. J., Physical and kinetic properties of human phosphofructokinase from skeletal muscle and erythrocytes, *J. Biol. Chem.* **244**:3823 (1969).
132. Leger, J., Bost, M., Kolodie, L., Schaerer, R., and Hollard, D., Anémie hémolytique congénitale et familiale avec déficit en phospho-hexose-isomerase (PHI) et elliptocytose, *Proc. 13th Int. Congr. Hematol., Munich*, p. 293 (1970).
133. Leif, R. C., and Vinograd, J., The distribution of buoyant density of human erythrocytes in bovine albumin solutions, *Proc. Natl. Acad. Sci. U.S.A.* **51**:520 (1964).
134. Llorente, P., Marco, R., and Sols, A., Regulation of liver pyruvate kinase and the phosphoenolypyruvate crossroads, *Eur. J. Biochem.* **13**:45 (1970).
135. Löhr, G. W., Arnold, H., Blume, K. G., Engelhart, R., and Beutler, E., Hereditary deficiency of glucosephosphate isomerase as a cause of nonspherocytic hemolytic anemia, *Blut* **26**:393 (1973).
136. Löhr, G. W., and Waller, H. D., Zur Biochemie einiger angeborener hamolytischer Anamien, *Folia Haematol. (Frankfurt)* **8**:377 (1963).
137. Löhr, G. W., Waller, H. D., Anschutz, F., and Knoop, A., Biochemische Defekte in den Blutzellen bei familiarer Panmyelopathie (Typ Fanconi), *Humangenetik* **1**:383 (1965).
138. Löhr, G. W., Waller, H. D., Anschutz, F., and Knoop, A., Hexokinasemangel in Blutzellen bei einer Sippe mit familiarer Panmyelopathie (Typ Fanconi), *Klin. Wochenschr.* **43**:870 (1965).
139. Luzzatto, L., Studies of polymorphic traits for the characterization of populations: African popuiations south of the Sahara, *Israel J. Med. Sci.* **9**:1181 (1973).
140. Marks, P. A., and Gross, R. T., Erythrocyte glucose-6-phosphate dehydrogenase deficiency: Evidence of differences between Negroes and Caucasians with respect to this genetically determined trait, *J. Clin. Invest.* **38**:2253 (1959).
141. Marks, P. A., and Johnson, A. B., Relationship between the age of human erythrocytes and their osmotic resistance: A basis for separating young and old erythrocytes, *J. Clin. Invest.* **37**:1542 (1958).
142. Marks, P. A., Szeinberg, A., and Banks, J., Erythrocyte glucose-6-phosphate dehydrogenase of normal and mutant human subjects, *J. Biol. Chem.* **236**:10 (1961).
143. Matsumoto, N., Ishihara, T., Oda, E., Miwa, S., Nakashima, K., Uchino, F., and Fukumoto, Y., Fine structure of the spleen and liver in glucose-phosphate isomerase (GPI) deficiency: Hereditary nonspherocytic hemolytic anemia—selective reticulocyte destruction as a mechanism of hemolysis, *Acta Haematol. Jpn.* **36**:46 (1973).
144. McDaniel, C., Kirtley, M. F., and Tanner, M. J. A., The interaction of glyceraldehyde-3-phosphate dehydrogenase with human erythrocyte membrane, *J. Biol. Chem.* **249**:6478 (1974).
145. Mentzer, W. C., Pyruvate kinase deficiency and disorders of glycolysis, in: *Hematology of Infancy and Childhood* (D. G. Nathan and F. A. Oski, eds.), p. 315, Saunders, Philadelphia (1974).
146. Mentzer, W., and Alpers, J., Mild anemia with abnormal RBC pyruvate kinase, *Clin. Res.* **29**:209 (1971).
147. Mentzer, W. C., Jr., Baehner, R. L., Schmidt-Schonbein, H., Robinson, S. H., and Nathan, D. G., Selective reticulocyte destruction in erythrocyte pyruvate kinase deficiency, *J. Clin. Invest.* **50**:688 (1971).

148. Meuwissen, H. J., Pollara, B., Pickering, R. J., Ammann, A., Biggar, D., Brunell, P., Buckley, R., Cohen, F., Cross, V., Dissing, J., Giblett, E., Griscelli, C., Hirschhorn, R., Hong, R., Huber, J., Keightley, R., Kersey, J., de Konig, J., Lischner, H., Los, W., Meuwissen, H. J., Moore, E. C., Ochs, H. D., Pachman, L., Parks, B., Pickering, R. J., Pollara, B., Rosen, F., Singer, D., South, M. A., Wara, D., and Wolfson, J., Combined immunodeficiency disease associated with adenosine deaminase deficiency: Report of a workshop held in Albany, New York, October 1, 1973, *J. Pediat.* **86**:169 (1975).

149. Miller, D. R., The hereditary hemolytic anemias: Membrane and enzyme defects, *Pediat. Clin. N. Am.* **19**:865 (1972).

150. Mills, G. C., The physiologic regulation of erythrocyte metabolism, *Texas Rep. Biol. Med.* **27**:773 (1969).

151. Minakami, S., and Yoshikawa, H., Studies on erythrocyte glycolysis. II. Free energy changes and rate limiting steps in erythrocyte glycolysis, *J. Biochem.* **59**:139 (1966).

152. Minakami, S., and Yoshikawa, H., Studies on erythrocyte glycolysis. III. The effects of active cation transport, pH and inorganic phosphate concentration on erythrocyte glycolysis, *J. Biochem.* **59**:145 (1966).

153. Minnich, V., Smith, M. B., Brauner, M. J., and Majerus, P. W., Glutathione biosynthesis in human erythrocyte. I. Identification of the enzyme of glutathione synthesis in hemolysates, *J. Clin. Invest.* **50**:507 (1971).

154. Miwa, S., and Nagata, M., Pyruvate kinase deficiency hereditary nonspherocytic hemolytic anemia: Report of two cases in a Japanese family and review of literature, *Acta Haematol. Jpn.* **28**:1 (1965).

155. Miwa, S., Nakashima, K., Oda, S., Matsumoto, N., Ogawa, H., Kobeyashi, R., Kotoni, M., Haratta, A., Onaya, T., and Yamada, T., Glucosephosphate isomerase (GPI) deficiency. Hereditary nonspherocytic hemolytic anemia: Report of the second case found in Japanese, *Acta Haematol. Jpn.* **36**:70 (1973).

156. Miwa, S., Nakashima, K., Oda, S., Oda, E., Matsumoto, N., Ogawa, H., and Fukumoto, Y., Glucosephosphate isomerase (GPI) deficiency hereditary nonspherocytic hemolytic anemia: Report of the first case found in Japanese, *Acta Haematol. Jpn.* **36**:65 (1973).

157. Miwa, S., Nakashima, K., Oda, S., Ogawa, H., Nagafuji, H., Arima, M., Okuna, T., and Nakashima, T., Phosphoglycerate kinase deficiency hereditary nonspherocytic hemolytic anemia; report of a case found in a Japanese family, *Acta Haematol. Jpn.* **35**:57 (1972).

158. Miwa, S., Nishina, T., Kakehashi, Y., Kitamura, M., Hiratsuka, A., and Shizume, K., Studies on erythrocyte metabolism in a case with hereditary deficiency of H-subunit of lactate dehydrogenase, *Acta Haematol. Jpn.* **34**:228 (1971).

159. Miwa, S., Nishina, T., Kakehashi, Y., and Obyama, M., Studies on erythrocyte metabolism in various hemolytic anemias: With special reference to pyruvate kinase deficiency, *Acta Haematol. Jpn.* **33**:501 (1970).

160. Miwa, S., Sato, T., and Murao, H., A new type of phosphofructokinase deficiency: Hereditary non-spherocytic hemolytic anemia, *Acta Haematol. Jpn.* **35**:113 (1972).

161. Moser, K., Ciresa, M., and Schwarzmeier, J., Hexokinasemangel bei hämolytischer Anämie, *Med. Welt* **21**:1977 (1970).

162. Nakashima, K., Miwa, S., Oda, S., Oda, E., Matsumoto, N., Fukumoto, Y., and Yamada, T., Electrophoretic and kinetic studies of glucosephosphate isomerase (GPI) in two different Japanese families with GPI deficiency, *Am. J. Hum. Genet.* **25**:294 (1973).

163. Nakashima, K., Miwa, S., Oda, S., Tanaka, T., Imamura, K., and Nishina, T., Electrophoretic and kinetic studies of mutant erythrocyte pyruvate kinases, *Blood* **43**:537 (1974).

164. Nathan, D. G., Oski, F. A., Miller, D. R., and Gardner, F. H., Life-span and organ sequestration of the red cells in pyruvate kinase deficiency, *New Engl. J. Med.* **278**:73 (1968).

165. Nathan, D. G., and Shohet, S. B., Erythrocyte ion transport defects and hemolytic anemia: "Hydrocytosis" and "desicytosis," *Semin. Hematol.* **7**:381 (1970).

166. Necheles, T. F., Rai, U. S., and Cameron, D., Congenital non-spherocytic hemolytic anemia associated with an unusual erythrocyte hexokinase abnormality, *J. Lab. Clin. Med.* **76**:593 (1970).

167. Nishimura, E. T., Kobana, T. V., Takahara, S., Hamilton, H. B., and Madden, S. C., Immunologic evidence of catalase deficiency in human hereditary acatalasemia, *Lab. Invest.* **10**:333 (1961).

168. Ockel, E., Rapoport, S., Hinterberger, V., and Gerischer-Mothes, W., Die pH-Abhangigkeit der anaeroben Glykolyse und der Hexokinase, *Folia Haematol. (Leipzig)* **78**:477 (1962).

169. Oski, F. A., and Bowman, H., A low K_m phosphoenolpyruvate mutant in the Amish with red cell pyruvate kinase deficiency, *Br. J. Haematol.* **17**:289 (1969).

170. Oski, F., and Fuller, E., Glucose-phosphate isomerase (GPI) deficiency associated with abnormal osmotic fragility and spherocytes, *Clin. Res.* **19**:427 (1971).

171. Oski, F. A., and Gottlieb, A. J., The effect of deoxygenation of adult and fetal hemoglobin on the synthesis of red cell 2,3-diphosphoglycerate and its *in vivo* consequences, *J. Clin. Invest.* **49**:400 (1970).

172. Oski, F. A., Gottlieb, A. J., and Miller, L., The influences of heredity and environment on the red cells' function of oxygen transport, *Med. Clin. N. Am.* **54**:731 (1970).

173. Oski, F. A., Marshall, B. E., Cohen, P. J., Sugerman, H. J., and Miller, L. D., Exercise with anemia: The role of left shifted or right shifted oxygen hemoglobin equilibrium curve, *Am. Intern. Med.* **74**:44 (1971).

174. Oski, F. A., Miller, L. D., Delivoria-Papadopoulos, M., Manchester, S. M., and Shelburne, J. C., Oxygen affinity in red cells—Changes induced *in vivo* by propranolol, *Science* **175**:1372 (1972).

175. Oski, F. A., Nathan, D. G., Sidel, V. W., and Diamond, L. K., Extreme hemolysis and red-cell distortion in erythrocyte pyruvate kinase deficiency. I. Morphology, erythrokinetics, and family enzyme studies, *New Engl. J. Med.* **270**:1023 (1964).

176. Oski, F. A., and Stockman, J. A., III, Congenital hemolytic anemias and red cell enzyme deficiencies, *Curr. Probl. Pediat.* **3**:1 (1973).

177. Oski, F. A., and Whaun, J., Hemolytic anemia and red cell glyceraldehyde-3-phosphate dehydrogenase, *Proc. Soc. Pediat. Res. 39th Ann. Meet., Atlantic City,* p. 151 (1969).

178. Osterman, J., Fritz, P. J., and Wunteh, T., Pyruvate kinase isozymes from rat tissues: Developmental studies, *J. Biol. Chem.* **248**:1011 (1973).

179. Paetkau, V., Yoanathan, E. S., and Lordy, H. A., Phosphofructokinase: Studies on the subunit structure, *J. Mol. Biol.* **33**:721 (1968).

180. Paglia, D. E., Holland, P., Baughan, M. A., and Valentine, W. N., Occurrence of defective hexosephosphate isomerization in human erythrocytes and leukocytes, *New Engl. J. Med.* **280**:66 (1969).

181. Paglia, D. E., and Valentine, W. N., Additional kinetic distinctions between normal pyruvate kinase and a mutant isozyme from human erythrocytes: Correction of the kinetic anomaly by fructose-1,6-diphosphate, *Blood* **37**:311 (1971).
182. Paglia, D. E., and Valentine, W. D., Hereditary glucosephosphate isomerase deficiency, *Am. J. Clin. Pathol.* **62**:740 (1974).
183. Paglia, D. E., Valentine, W. N., Baughan, M. A., Miller, D. R., Reed, C. F., and McIntyre, O. R., An inherited molecular lesion of erythrocyte pyruvate kinase: Identification of a kinetically aberrant isozyme associated with premature hemolysis, *J. Clin. Invest.* **47**:1929 (1968).
184. Paglia, D. E., Valentine, W. N., and Rucknagel, D. L., Defective erythrocyte pyruvate kinase with impaired kinetics and reduced optimal activity, *Br. J. Haematol.* **22**:651 (1972).
185. Parker, J. C., and Hoffman, J. F., The role of membrane phosphoglycerate kinase in the control of glycolytic rate by active transport in human red blood cells, *J. Gen. Physiol.* **50**:893 (1967).
186. Payne, D. M., Porter, D. W., and Gracy, R. W., Evidence against the occurrence of tissue-specific variants and isoenzymes of phosphoglucose isomerase, *Arch. Biochem. Biophys.* **151**:122 (1972).
187. Pearson, P. L., Sanger, R., and Brown, J. A., Report of the commission on the genetic constitution of the X-chromosome. Human Gene Mapping 2, *Cytog. Cell Genet.* **14**:190 (1975).
188. Piomelli, S., G6PD deficiency and related disorders of the pentose pathway, in: *Hematology of Infancy and Childhood* (D. G. Nathan and F. A. Oski, eds.), p. 346, Saunders, Philadelphia (1974).
189. Piomelli, S., Corash, L. M., Davenport, D. D., Miraglia, J., and Amorosi, E. L., *In vivo* lability of glucose-6-phosphate dehydrogenase in Gd^{A-} and Gd^{Mediterranean} deficiency, *J. Clin. Invest.* **47**:940 (1968).
190. Piomelli, S., Lurinsky, G., and Wasserman, L. R., The mechanism of red cell aging. I. Relationship between cell age and specific gravity evaluated by ultracentrifugation in a discontinuous density gradient, *J. Lab. Clin. Med.* **69**:659 (1967).
191. Piomelli, S., Reindorf, A., Arzanian, L. M., and Corash, L., Clinical and biochemical interactions of glucose-6-phosphate dehydrogenase deficiency and sickle cell anemia, *New Engl. J. Med.* **287**:213 (1972).
192. Piomelli, S., Reindorf, C. A., and Corash, L., Protective effect of G6PD deficiency in sickle cell anemia, *Clin. Res.* **20**:472 (1972).
193. Piomelli, S., and Siniscalco, M., The haematological effects of glucose-6-phosphate dehydrogenase deficiency and thalassemia trait: Interaction between the two genes at the phenotype level, *Br. J. Haematol.* **16**:537 (1969).
194. Piomelli, S., and Wyss, S. R., Metabolic death of the red blood cell, *Blood* **38**:833 (1971).
195. Piomelli, S., Wyss, S. R., Rita, M., and Zondag, L., Isozymes of pyruvate kinase (PK) in human blood: Electrophoretic and kinetic properties, *Am. Soc. Hum. Genet. 24th Meet., Philadelphia,* p. 439 (1972).
196. Pirandello, L., *Six Characters in Search of an Author* (transl. by F. May), Heinemann, London (1954).
197. Rakitzis, E. T., and Mills, G. C., Relation of red cell hexokinase activity to extracellular pH, *Biochim. Biophys. Acta* **141**:439 (1967).
198. Rapoport, S., Hinterberger, V., and Hofman, E. C. G., Die begrenzende Rolle der Hexokinase-Reaktion für die anaerobe Glykolyse der roten Blutzellen, *Naturwissenschaften* **48**:501 (1961).

199. Rattazzi, M. C., Corash, L. M., von Zanen, G. E., Jaffé, E. R., and Piomelli, S., G6PD deficiency and chronic hemolysis: Four new mutants. Relationship between clinical syndrome and enzyme kinetics, *Blood* **38**:205 (1971).

200. Reynard, A. M., Hass, L. F., Jacobsen, D. D., and Boyer, P. D., The correlation of reaction kinetics and substrate binding with the mechanism of pyruvate kinase, *J. Biol. Chem.* **236**:2277 (1961).

201. Robinson, M. A., Loder, P. B., and de Gruchy, G. C., Red cell metabolism in non-spherocytic congenital haemolytic anemia, *Br. J. Haematol.* **7**:327 (1961).

202. Rose, I. A., and O'Connell, E. L., The role of glucose-6-phosphate in the regulation of glucose metabolism in human erythrocytes, *J. Biol. Chem.* **239**:12 (1964).

203. Rose, I. A., and Warms, J. V. B., Control of red cell glycolysis: The cause of triose phosphate accumulation, *J. Biol. Chem.* **245**:4009 (1970).

204. Rosenthal, A. S., Kregenow, E. M., and Moses, H. L., Some characteristics of a Ca^{2+}-dependent ATPase activity associated with a group of erythrocyte membrane proteins which form fibrils, *Biochim. Biophys. Acta* **196**:254 (1970).

205. Sanpitak, N., Supalert, Y., Chayutimonkul, L., and Flatz, G., Combined erythrocyte phosphohexose isomerase and glucose-6-phosphate dehydrogenase deficiency, *Hum. Hered.* **23**:83 (1973).

206. Sass, M. D., Caruso, C. J., and Farhangi, M., TPNH-methemoglobin reductase deficiency: A new red-cell enzyme defect, *J. Lab. Clin. Med.* **70**:760 (1967).

207. Schatzmann, H. J., ATP-dependent Ca^{2+} extrusion from human red cells, *Experientia* **22**:364 (1966).

208. Schneider, A. S., Dunn, I., Ibsen, K. H., and Weinstein, I. M., Triosephosphate isomerase deficiency. B. Inherited triosephosphate isomerase deficiency. Erythrocyte carbohydrate metabolism and preliminary studies of the erythrocyte enzyme, in: *Hereditary Disorders of Erythrocyte Metabolism* (E. Beutler, ed.), p. 273, Grune and Stratton, New York (1968).

209. Schneider, A. S., Valentine, W. N., Baughan, M. A., Paglia, D. E., Shore, N. A., and Heins, M. L., Triosephosphate isomerase deficiency. A multisystem inherited enzyme disorder. Clinical and genetic aspects, in: *Hereditary Disorders of Erythrocyte Metabolism* (E. Beutler, ed.), p. 265, Grune and Stratton, New York (1968).

210. Schneider, A. S., Valentine, W. N., Hattori, M., and Heins, H. L. J., Hereditary hemolytic anemia with triosephosphate isomerase deficiency, *New Engl. J. Med.* **272**:229 (1965).

211. Schrier, S. L., Studies of the metabolism of human erythrocyte membranes, *J. Clin. Invest.* **42**:756 (1963).

212. Schröter, W., Kongenitale nichtsphärocytäre hämolytische Anämie bei 2,3-Diphosphoglyceratemutase-Mangel der Erythrocyten im frühen Sauglingsalter, *Klin. Wochenschr.* **43**:1147 (1965).

213. Schröter, W., Brittinger, G., Zimmerschitt, E., and König, E., A new haemolytic syndrome with glucose-phosphate isomerase (GPI) and glucose-6-phosphate dehydrogenase (G6PD) deficiency of the erythrocytes: Biochemical studies, *Eur. J. Clin. Invest.* **1**:145 (1970).

214. Schröter, W., Brittinger, G., Zimmerschitt, E., and König, E., Combined glucosephosphate isomerase and glucose-6-phosphate dehydrogenase deficiency of the erythrocytes: A new haemolytic syndrome, *Br. J. Haematol.* **20**:249 (1971).

215. Schröter, W., Koch, H. H., Wonneberger, B., Kalinowsky, W., Arnold, H.,

Blume, K. G., and Hüther, W., Glucose phosphate isomerase deficiency with congenital non-spherocytic hemolytic anemia: A new variant (type Nordhorn). I. Clinical and genetic studies, *Pediat. Res.* **8**:18 (1974).

216. Scott, E. M., The relation of diaphorase of human erythrocytes to inheritance of methemoglobinemia, *J. Clin. Invest.* **39**:1176 (1960).

217. Seegmiller, J., Inherited disorders of hypoxanthine guanine phosphoribosyltransferase in X-linked uric acidemia. *Advan. Hum. Genet.* **6**: 75–163 (1976).

218. Selwyn, J. G., and Dacie, J. V., Autohemolysis and other changes resulting from the incubation *in vitro* of red cells from patients with congenital hemolytic anemia, *Blood* **9**:414 (1954).

219. Serratrice, G., Monges, A., and Roux, H., Forme myopathique du déficit en phosphofructokinase, *Rev. Neurol.* **120**:271 (1969).

220. Shohet, S. B., Hemolysis and changes in erythrocyte membrane lipids, *New Engl. J. Med.* **286**:577 (1972).

221. Shohet, S. B., Nathan, D. G., and Karnovsky, M. L., Stages in the incorporation of fatty acids into red blood cells, *J. Clin. Invest.* **47**:1096 (1968).

222. Siniscalco, M., Strategies for X-chromosome mapping with somatic cell hybrids, in: *Somatic Cell Hybridization* (R. L. Davidson and F. de la Cruz, eds.), Raven Press, New York (1974).

223. Sparkes, R. S., Carrel, R. E., and Paglia, D. E., Probable localization of a triosephosphate isomerase gene to the short arm of the number 5 human chromosome, *Nature (London)* **224**:367 (1969).

224. Srivastava, S. K., and Beutler, E., The effect of normal red cell constituents on the activities of red cell enzymes, *Arch. Biochem. Biophys.* **148**:249 (1972).

225. Staal, G. E. J., Koster, J. F., Kamp, H., Van Milligen-Boersma, L., and Veeger, C., Human erythrocyte pyruvate kinase: Its purification and some properties, *Biochim. Biophys. Acta* **227**:86 (1971).

226. Staal, G. E. J., Koster, J. F., and Nijessen, J. G., A new variant of red blood cell pyruvate kinase deficiency, *Biochim. Biophys. Acta* **258**:685 (1972).

227. Staal, G. E. J., Visser, J., and Veeger, C., Purification and properties of glutathione reductase of human erythrocytes, *Biochim. Biophys. Acta* **185**:39 (1969).

228. Stefanini, M., Chronic hemolytic anemia associated with erythrocyte enolase deficiency exacerbated by ingestion of nitrofurantoin, *Am. J. Clin. Pathol.* **58**:408 (1972).

229. Sugita, Y., and Nomura, S., Purification of reduced pyridine nucleotide dehydrogenase from human erythrocytes and methemoglobin reduction by the enzyme, *J. Biol. Chem.* **246**:6072 (1971).

230. Sutor, W. A., and Rutter, W. J., A method for detection of pyruvate kinase, aldolase and other pyridine nucleotide linked enzyme activities after electrophoresis, *Anal. Biochem.* **43**:147 (1971).

231. Tanaka, K. R., and Paglia, D. E., Pyruvate kinase deficiency, *Semin. Hematol.* **8**:367 (1971).

232. Tanaka, K. R., Valentine, W. N., and Miwa, S., Pyruvate kinase (PK) deficiency hereditary nonspherocytic hemolytic anemia, *Blood* **19**:267 (1962).

233. Tanaka, T., Marano, Y., Fumiaki, S., and Morimura, H., Crystallization, characterization and metabolic regulation of two types of pyruvate kinase isolated from rat tissues, *J. Biochem.* **62**:71 (1967).

234. Tanphaichitr, V. S., and Van Eys, J., The assay of pyruvate kinase activity in blood cells, *Clin. Chim. Acta* **41**:41 (1972).

235. Tariverdian, G., Arnold, H., Blume, K. G., Lenkeit, U., and Löhr, G. W., Zur

Formalgenetik der Phosphoglucoseisomerase (E.C. 5.3.1.9) Untersuchung einer Sippe mit PGI-Defizienz, *Humangenetik* **10**:218 (1970).

236. Tarui, S., Kono, N., Nasu, T., and Nishikawa, M., Enzymatic basis for the coexistence of myopathy and hemolytic disease in inherited muscle phosphofructokinase deficiency, *Biochem. Biophys. Res. Commun.* **34**:77 (1969).

237. Tarui, S., Okuno, G., Ikura, Y., Tanaka, T., Suda, M., and Nishikawa, M., Phosphofructokinase deficiency in skeletal muscle: A new type of glycogenesis, *Biochem. Biophys. Res. Commun.* **19**:517 (1965).

238. Tobin, W. E., Huijing, F., Porro, R. S., *et al.*, Muscle phosphofructokinase deficiency, *Arch. Neurol.* **28**:128 (1973).

239. Travis, S. F., Morrison, A. D., Clements, R. S., Winograd, A. I., and Oski, F. A., The role of the polyol pathway in methaemoglobin reduction in human red cells. *Br. J. Haematol.* **27**:597 (1974).

240. Travis, S. F., Sugarman, H. J., Ruberg, R. L., Dudrick, S. J., Delivoria-Papadopoulos, M., Miller, L. D., and Oski, F. A., Alterations of red-cell glycolytic intermediates and oxygen transport as a consequence of hypophosphatemia in patients receiving intravenous hyperalimentation, *New Engl. J. Med.* **285**:763 (1971).

241. Tsai, M. Y., and Kemp, R. G., Hybridization of rabbit muscle and liver phosphofructokinase, *Arch. Biochem. Biophys.* **150**:407 (1972).

242. Tsai, M. Y., and Kemp, R. G., Isoenzymes of rabbit phosphofructokinase: Electrophoretic and immunochemical studies, *J. Biol. Chem.* **248**:785 (1973).

243. Tsuboi, K. K., and Chervenka, C. H., Adenylate kinase of human erythrocyte: Isolation and properties of the predominant inherited form, *J. Biol. Chem.* **250**:132 (1975).

244. Tsuboi, K. K., Fukunaga, K., and Chervenka, C. H., Phosphoglucose isomerase from human erythrocyte: Preparation and properties, *J. Biol. Chem.* **246**:7586 (1971).

245. Valentine, W. N., Hereditary enzymatic deficiencies of erythrocytes, *Semin. Hematol.* **8**:307 (1971).

246. Valentine, W. N., Deficiencies associated with Embden–Meyerhof pathway and other metabolic pathways, *Semin. Hematol.* **8**:348 (1971).

247. Valentine, W. N., Hsieh, H., Paglia, D. E., Anderson, H. M., Baughan, M. A., Jaffe, E. R., and Garson, O. M., Hereditary hemolytic anemia associated with phosphoglycerate kinase deficiency in erythrocytes and leukocytes: A probable X-chromosome-linked syndrome, *New Engl. J. Med.* **280**:528 (1969).

248. Valentine, W. N., Oski, F. A., Paglia, D. E., Baughan, M. A., Schneider, A. S., and Naiman, J. L., Hereditary hemolytic anemia with hexokinase deficiency: Role of hexokinase in erythrocyte aging, *New Engl. J. Med.* **276**:1 (1967).

249. Valentine, W. N., Oski, F. A., Paglia, D. E., Baughan, M. A., Scheider, A. S., and Naiman, J. L., Erythrocyte hexokinase· and hereditary hemolytic anemia, in: *Hereditary Disorders of Erythrocyte Metabolism* (E. Beutler, ed.), p. 288, Grune and Stratton, New York (1968).

250. Valentine, W. N., Schneider, A. S., Baughan, M. A., Paglia, D. E., and Heins, H. W., Hereditary hemolytic anemia with triosephosphate isomerase deficiency: Studies in kindreds with co-existent sickle cell trait and erythrocyte glucose-6-phosphate dehydrogenase deficiency, *Am. J. Med.* **41**:27 (1966).

251. Valentine, W. N., Tanaka, K. R., and Miwa, S., A specific erythrocyte enzyme defect (pyruvate kinase) in three subjects with congenital non-spherocytic hemolytic anemia, *Trans. Assoc. Am. Physicians* **74**:100 (1961).

252. Van Berkel, J. C., Koster, J. F., and Hülsmann, W. C., Distribution of L and M-type pyruvate kinase between parenchymal and Kupffer cells of rat liver, *Biochim. Biophys. Acta* **276**:425 (1972).
253. Vico, G. B., *La Scienza Nuova* (Engl. trans. by T. C. Bergin and M. H. Fish), Cornell University Press, Ithaca, N.Y. (1968).
254. Waller, M. D., Benöhr, H. C., Heuer, B., and Nerke, O., Die Glutathionreduktion in Erythrocyten von Gesunden und Enzymdefektträgern, *Klin. Wochenschr.* **48**:79 (1970).
255. Waterbury, L., and Frenkel, E. P., Phosphofructokinase deficiency in congenital nonspherocytic hemolytic anemia, *Clin. Res.* **17**:347 (1969).
256. Waterbury, L., and Frenkel, E. P., Hereditary nonspherocytic hemolysis with erythrocyte phosphofructokinase deficiency, *Blood* **39**:445 (1972).
257. WHO Scientific Group, Standardization of Procedures for the Study of Glucose-6-phosphate Dehydrogenase, WHO Tech. Rep. Ser. No. 366, Geneva (1967).
258. Woessner, S., and Carbonell, M., Anemia hemolitica congenita no esferocitica por deficit de piruvatoquinasa: Presentation de un caso clinico, *Sangre* **13**:61 (1968).
259. Yoshida, A., Glucose-6-phosphate dehydrogenase of human erythrocytes. I. Purification and characterization of normal (B^+) enzyme, *J. Biol. Chem.* **241**:4966 (1966).
260. Yoshida, A., Hemolytic anemia and G6PD deficiency, *Science* **179**:532 (1973).
261. Yoshida, A., and Miwa, S., Characterization of a phosphoglycerate kinase variant associated with hemolytic anemia, *Am. J. Hum. Genet.* **26**:378 (1974).
262. Yoshida, A., and Watanabe, M., Human phosphoglycerate kinase. I. Crystallization and characterization of normal enzyme, *J. Biol. Chem.* **247**:440 (1972).
263. Zuelzer, W. W., Robinson, A. R., and Msu, T. H. J., Erythrocyte pyruvate kinase deficiency in non-spherocytic hemolytic anemia: A system of multiple genetic markers? *Blood* **32**:33 (1965).

Chapter 4

Population Structure of the Åland Islands, Finland

James H. Mielke,* Peter L. Workman,† Johan
Fellman, and Aldur W. Eriksson‡

Samfundet Folkhälsans Genetiska Institut
Populationsgenetiska Avdelningen
Helsinki, Finland

INTRODUCTION

The total description of population structure, as so well discussed by Harrison and Boyce,[44] requires the integration of biological, social, and demographic data set in an ecological framework. This, by itself, is understood to be an unobtainable and unapproachable goal. Moreover, we recognize that a major aim of population research is to describe and understand the complex evolution of the population structure as well as to describe it at a single point in time. Unfortunately, process as such can never be inferred from structure and thus longitudinal perspectives are obligate. The time span underlying a processual problem varies according to the focus of the research, itself partially limited by human factors and the kinds of data which can be obtained (historical, archeological, demographic, biological, etc.). The study of population structure therefore involves both studies with a short time span, such as analyses of pathological or normal biological development or recent

* Present address: Department of Sociology, Anthropology, and Social Work, Wright State University, Dayton, Ohio.
†Present Address: Department of Anthropology, University of New Mexico, Albuquerque, New Mexico.
‡Present address: Anthropogenetisch Instituut, Vrije Universiteit, Amsterdam, Holland.

sociohistoric changes, and a long-term perspective on the macroevolutionary history antecedent to the contemporary biological and social structure.

The genetic characterization of a population, for polymorphic, monomorphic, or rare traits, provides a cross-sectional component of the structure. Although contemporary biological variation in a sense carries with it the evolutionary history, one generally finds that alternative, quite dissimilar processes can be invoked to explain current patterns of variation. Studies on the mode of inheritance of traits and their expressivity in different environments provide a biological basis for viewing the contemporary social and demographic implications of genetic variability. However, for an evolutionary perspective on the forces underlying the present genetic variation, the problem of time depth becomes critical. In some studies, historical, geological, or archeological data serve to date, however crudely, the time of divergence of populations separated by large time spans or distances. For such situations, one can obtain general inference on total amounts of gene flow, estimates of genetic divergence, and some inference on the interaction between the directed (selection, gene flow) and random processes. However, for studies of the microevolutionary processes involved in variation among subgroups in a partially isolated, geographically or socially stratified population, the precision of the historical record must be much greater. Populations for which abundant archival material is available, documenting births, deaths, marriages, etc., are especially suitable for analyses of this kind.

In this chapter, we shall describe the progress, to date, which has been achieved in attempts to describe the genetic structure of the Åland Islands, containing a relatively isolated population living in the archipelago lying between Sweden and Finland. Extensive parish records dating from the late seventeenth century, selected archival material for land holdings, crop production, etc., from the fifteenth century, and a large body of archeological and ethnohistorical material provide an extraordinary time depth during which the historical processes related to contemporary variation can be specified. These studies contribute to an integrated analysis of Ålandic structure in which the genetic approaches can be seen to provide a significant tool for ethnohistorical work. Many of the genetic analyses have been made possible by developments in the analytical basis for studying genetic structure that have occurred during the past decade (see, for example,

Cannings and Cavalli-Sforza[12] and Morton[72]). Of particular utility have been the techniques for utilizing the migration data which can be obtained from the historical records.[9,12,47,64,94]

The studies which have been carried out reflect pragmatic concerns with medical problems, the availability of resources for collecting and analyzing data, and the interests of the many collaborators who have been involved in Ålandic studies. Ongoing studies in historical demography, studies on the relation between family structure and fertility, and additional genetic surveys of normal and pathological variation will add more pieces to the puzzle. Projected studies include record linkage on two of the most extremely isolated parishes for both historical and genetic analyses and a study of the influence of social and economic factors on the historical patterns of migration. Despite the enormous amount of work which remains to be done with the data available, the results obtained show clearly how much can be learned about population structure using the variety of techniques whose development has marked the recent history of human population genetics.

This chapter is not intended to be a review of the models and/or theories available for examining population structure; for this purpose there are numerous review articles which can be consulted.[12–14,69,72,73,89] Rather, we shall attempt to provide some insight into the procedures and the inference obtained in studies of the population structure of a partially isolated human population and indicate the kinds of studies which would most enhance the results thus far obtained. A brief description and history of Åland are provided first. Then the analysis is divided into two sections, the first describing the inference provided by the direct analyses of archival materials (mainly matrimonial migration data) and the second dealing with biological studies (genetics, human twinning rates, normal and pathological ophthalmological traits) and the complementary inference on population structure provided by using both data sources.

ÅLAND

Location and Description

The Åland archipelago, situated between Sweden and Finland, separates the Gulf of Bothnia to the north from the Baltic Sea to the

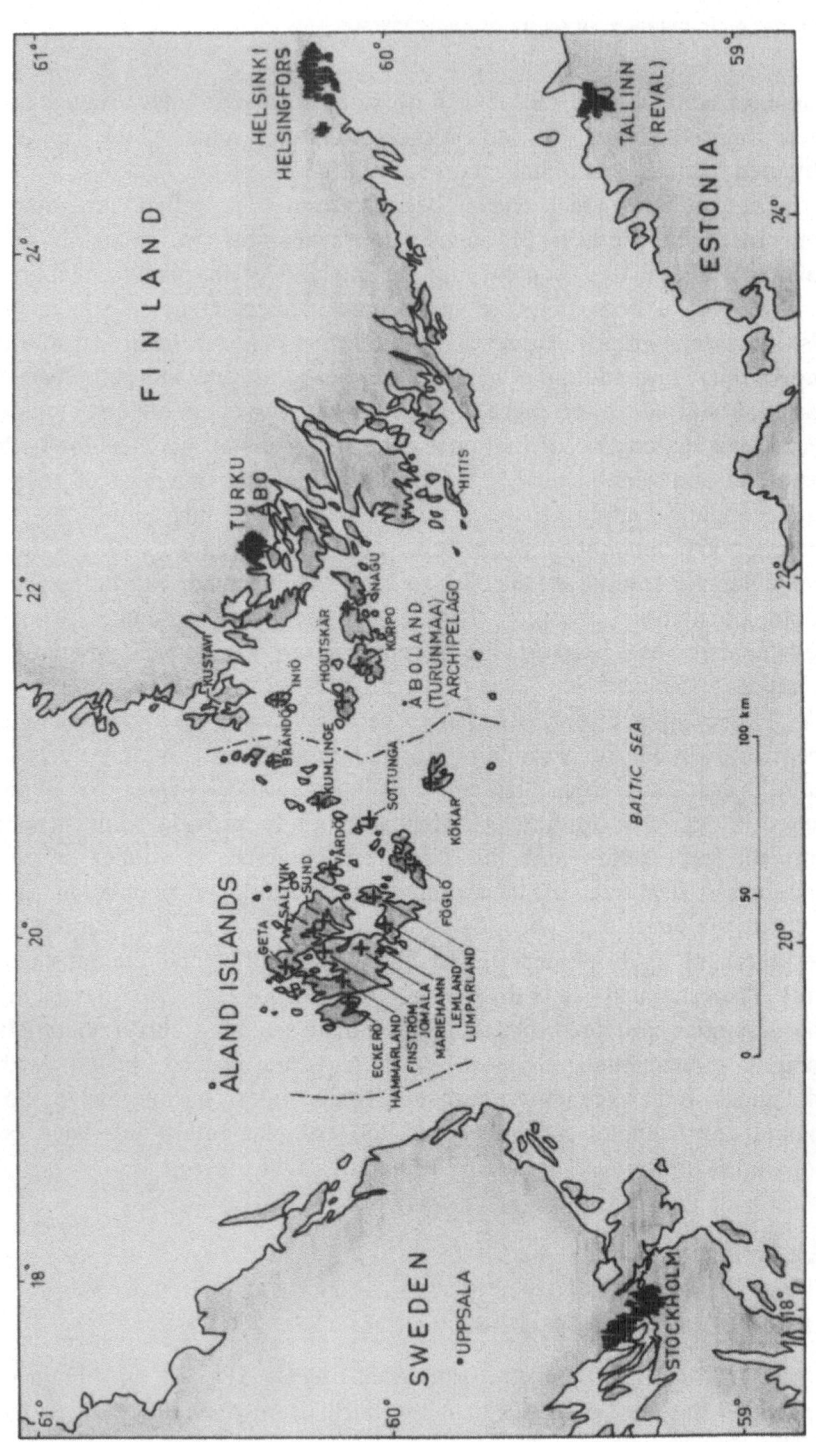

Fig. 1. Map of Scandinavia showing location of the Åland Islands and the division of Åland into 16 Lutheran parishes.

south. The Sea of Åland lies between it and Sweden on the west and
to the east is the Åboland archipelago, with more than 15,000 islands
and skerries, and Finland (Fig. 1). The land area of Åland comprises
1450 km²; however, if the sea area is also considered, the population
moves over a total area of approximately 10,000 km².[92] The archipelago
consists of roughly 6600 islands and skerries, but at the present time
fewer than 100 are inhabited.[53] The total population as of January 1971
numbered 21,211 people with 96.3% being of Swedish ancestry and the
remainder of Finnish ancestry. Almost half (41.3%) of the entire
population currently resides in the town of Mariehamn, the provincial
capital.

Since the sixteenth century, the archipelago has been divided into
Lutheran parishes or chapelries (Fig. 1). Currently there are 16
parishes: ten of these are subdivisions of the main island (Fasta
Åland), five comprised of numerous islands and skerries, and the
sixteenth parish, Mariehamn, is the only major urban center. All of the
15 county parishes were established prior to the 1650s, while Mariehamn was founded in 1905.

History

According to archeological evidence, the first inhabitants of the
Åland Islands came from the eastern coast of Finland about 5000 years
ago. However, it was not until about 600 A.D. that the population
began to increase, as a result of considerable immigration from the
west of Sweden into the main island. During the Viking era (c. 800–
1100 A.D.), the islands became one of the most densely populated areas
in Fenno-Scandia because of their location along the Viking trade
routes.[16,59] The outer islands in the archipelago are presumed to have
been populated by migrants from the main island, continuously at least
since the thirteenth century.

By the beginning of the eleventh century, Christianity was
securely established throughout the entire archipelago. From the
eleventh to the seventeenth century, there was relative political calm in
this region with few uprisings and raids, none of which seems to have
substantially affected the Åland population, primarily peasants with an
economy based on agriculture, stock raising, and fishing.[16]

In 1699, August II of Saxony united Poland, Russia, Saxony, and
Denmark-Norway in a common cause to overthrow the kingdom of

Sweden. For Åland this was a disaster, since most of its population were Swedish. The subsequent arrival of a Russian fleet prompted a mass exodus of most of the inhabitants. (approximately 7000) to Sweden. The Russians occupied Åland from 1714 to 1721, and not until the Peace of Nystad (Treaty of Uusikaupunki) in 1721 did the majority of the Ålanders return to their homes. In 1727, Åland had a population of some 6000[16] and by 1800 the population had grown to over 12,000, mostly by internal growth.

In 1808, Sweden engaged in a war with Russia which resulted in Russian control of the Åland Islands. Because of Åland's forced association with Russia, trade barriers were imposed by Sweden which affected the Åland economy rather drastically from 1838 to 1855 when they were relaxed. In 1856, the peace treaty signed at the conclusion of the Crimean War established the Åland Islands as a demilitarized zone, but under Russian supervision. After this time, freedom of trade prevailed and the economy of Åland improved. The foundation of the harbor town of Mariehamn in 1861 was both a result of and major factor in the economic improvement of the Islands. By the end of the nineteenth century, Mariehamn (population 991) was the center of culture and economic trade of the province, which by then was comprised of some 22,897 people.[16] During the nineteenth century, the rate of immigration was relatively low, possibly because of the Russian presence, and most of the increase in population was internal.

The onset of World War I once again brought Russian troops (a ground force of some 6600) to Åland, but there were no open hostilities on the islands. However, during the Russian revolution in 1917, the situation on Åland became chaotic since most of the inhabitants wanted reunion with Sweden. Åland had been part of the Grand Duchy of Finland under both Swedish and Russian sovereignty, but economically and culturally its people had always been associated with Sweden. The question of Åland was brought before the League of Nations Council in June 1920, and a year later the Council stipulated that Åland should be a semiautonomous county of Finland.

During the conflict between Finland and Russia, in the Second World War,[18,86,98] the control of Åland was again a source of dispute because of the islands' strategic importance. On April 18, 1947, a treaty signed among Finland, Russia, and Great Britain established the Åland archipelago as a nonfortified autonomous province of Finland.

Population Composition

Until the twentieth century, the Åland Islands remained relatively isolated. Immigration from Sweden and Finland, as well as interparish migration, was slight; and it was not until the end of the nineteenth century that there were major shifts in the population composition.

From 1750 to 1870, the population of Åland increased slowly. Then there was a major increase in population numbers, about the same rate in all parishes, beginning in the 1870s with a peak being reached around 1900, as shown in Table I. The population increase in the Åland archipelago (and the Åboland archipelago, also) was partially a result of the remarkable growth of the Finnish population after 1860.[40,53] In addition, developments in deep sea fishing techniques in the latter nineteenth century, as well as the introduction of dairying, increased Åland's economic opportunities. As population pressures increased in Finland, there was migration from the coastlands into the southwestern archipelago. Individuals were able to earn a livelihood almost entirely by fishing, and as a consequence unoccupied land in Åland became populated. Because of the population pressures in Åland emigration began, with the first emigrants leaving in the 1860s.[53] The highest waves of emigration were during 1901–1905 and 1949–1953. According to Jaatinen,[52] the net loss to Åland due to emigration since 1880 has been considerable, and between 1905 and 1950 the total population decreased by approximately one-eighth. During the twentieth century, much of the population loss was due to emigration to the United States. de Geer[40] estimates that the net population loss between 1905 and 1950, taking into consideration all marginal islands, totaled between 10 and 15%.

At the beginning of the twentieth century, the number of inhabited islands in Åland was 158; by 1959, this number had declined to 97.[53] There appears to have been a migration from the east to west, i.e., from Finland to Åland and then to Sweden, with migration trend power fields going in west and southwest directions.[40] The westward migration trend has been exaggerated because of the western urban center of Mariehamn.[53] However, some areas have remained rather stable or even increased in population because of their natural assets (e.g., farm economy), proximity to markets, or tourist trade and services. Examples of this are found in several of the Åland parishes:

TABLE I. Percentage of the Population in Each Parish Relative to the Total Population, 1749–1973[a]

Parish	1749[a]	1775	1800	1825	1850	1875	1900	1910	1920	1930	1940	1950	1973
Eckerö	6.2	6.3	5.5	5.8	5.8	5.7	5.4	5.1	5.5	5.3	4.8	4.3	3.4
Hammar- land	7.8	7.8	8.5	8.7	7.7	8.3	8.2	7.8	7.6	6.8	7.0	6.7	5.0
Geta	3.6	5.2	4.5	5.2	4.9	4.9	4.5	4.5	4.3	4.0	3.6	3.6	2.3
Finström	7.4	9.1	10.3	10.2	10.1	10.0	10.0	9.9	9.6	10.2	9.5	9.6	8.2
Saltvik	10.5	10.2	10.6	9.9	9.6	10.1	10.5	12.2	11.8	12.8	10.5	9.4	7.1
Sund	9.4	8.9	8.3	7.7	9.9	8.5	8.1	7.1	7.0	7.0	6.8	6.4	4.6
Vårdö	4.8	4.2	4.1	4.2	5.2	5.1	4.8	4.9	4.7	3.9	3.3	3.0	2.0
Jomala	13.3	13.7	14.0	13.7	12.5	11.9	12.8	11.3	11.6	11.0	12.9	15.7	9.9[b]
Lemland	7.7	7.0	6.9	7.1	7.9	8.4	8.0	7.6	7.1	6.8	6.9	6.2	3.3
Lumparland	2.8	2.7	2.6	2.4	2.1	2.6	2.4	2.6	2.4	2.1	2.3	2.1	1.5
Föglö	7.2	6.7	6.9	7.3	7.7	7.6	7.4	6.8	7.0	7.2	6.4	5.5	3.3
Sottunga	1.6	1.6	1.8	1.6	1.9	1.8	1.6	1.7	1.8	1.8	1.6	1.4	0.9
Kökar	5.9	5.5	3.9	3.9	3.2	2.9	3.1	4.1	4.3	4.0	3.5	3.1	1.7
Kumlinge	4.8	4.9	6.2	6.4	4.7	4.4	4.1	4.3	4.4	4.4	3.9	3.6	2.5
Brändö	6.7	6.4	5.8	5.7	6.8	5.9	5.0	5.4	5.6	5.2	4.6	4.3	3.0
Mariehamn	—	—	—	—	—	1.9	4.1	4.8	5.3	7.5	12.3	15.1	41.3
Total popu- lation	8543	11,405	12,128	12,888	15,560	18,365	24,841	21,356	20,423	19,705	21,196	21,690	21,211

[a] 1749 is an estimate.
[b] In 1961 a considerable part of Jomala was incorporated into the town of Mariehamn.

central and western Saltvik and some areas of Hammarland, Jomala, and Eckerö.[53] However, by 1971, all of the parishes except Mariehamn had experienced some depopulation since 1900.

Although there has been interisland migration and some long-range migration from Sweden and Finland into the Åland archipelago, the islands have remained, until the recent part of the twentieth century, relatively isolated. It is precisely this historical insularity of the people which offers an excellent opportunity for the study of population structure through time. Comprehensive parish records of marriages, deaths, and births, and poll-tax records, for the period 1750 to the present provide an outstanding data base for historical analysis of the population structure and its changes. Adequate documentation of the history of the Åland archipelago permits verification of the inferences drawn from parish records. Thus, by use of these data sources in conjunction with genetic studies, the Åland Islands also offer ideal conditions for the comparison and testing of models designed for the examination of partially isolated subdivided human populations.

PART I

MIGRATION ANALYSES

Kinship and Population Structure

The concept of kinship as developed by Malécot[65,66] provides a genetic model which can be used in the analysis of population structure. Kinship is the probability of genetic identity by descent; that is, it provides a measure of the genetic relationship between individuals or populations. With this model, various types of data can be used to obtain inference on the population structure; kinship can be calculated from genealogies, predicted by migration data, and, under certain assumptions, estimated from phenotypes, gene frequencies, metrics, or isonymy. Thus one is not limited to a single data base, and diverse estimates can be compared. Kinship depends on the extent of migration (gene flow), the systematic pressure (long-range migration), and the effective size of each population and thus provides a representation of many of the factors affecting population structure. It also provides a basis for examining isolation by distance and genetic topology and can be used to obtain a biological distance in terms of a measure called hybridity by Morton.[76] Thus according to Morton[76] the concept of kinship is fundamental in obtaining inference on the genetic structure of the population.

To the social anthropologist, the term "kinship" usually implies a set of social relations—a hierarchial structuring of the society, or other structural/functional aspects. However, as used in genetics, kinship is a number which measures genetic similarity and theoretically denotes the probability of genetic identity by descent.

According to Malécot,[65]

> *Nous appellerons coefficient de parehte f_{IL} de 2 individus I et L la probabilite pour que 2 loci homologues pris l'un sur I, l'autre sur L soient identiques, c'est-a-dire descendent d'un meme locus.* (pp. 7–8)

Kinship can also be defined for pairs of discrete populations. The kinship of two populations I and J is the probability that a gene drawn at random from I is identical by descent with a random gene in J. This value, ϕ_{IJ}, can be computed as the average of all individual coefficients, ϕ_{ij}, where i and j denote individuals drawn at random for I and J, respectively. Kinship is an expectation for a random gene at a random locus; so we are not concerned with all the possible values of kinship derived from different loci or alleles (caused by selection or drift) except to estimate their mean.

Suppose that the populations under consideration comprise an array of s populations. Knowledge of the population structure of this array of s populations can be provided by the symmetrical ($s \times s$) matrix (Φ) of kinship coefficients describing the genetic relationships within and between the populations. The diagonal elements of the matrix (ϕ_{ii}) describe *local kinship*, the probability that two genes drawn at random from population I are identical by descent (for the mathematics of deriving local kinship for various models of population structure, see Imaizumi et al.[51]). The predicted *mean kinship within populations* is the mean of the diagonal elements

$$\phi = \sum_i N_i \phi_{ii} / \sum_i N_i$$

and is a measure of the heterogeneity among populations. When kinship is estimated from genetic data, mean kinship is identical to Wright's F_{ST}.[110] The off diagonal elements of Φ, $\phi_{ij} = \phi_{ji}$, describe the genetic relationships between all pairs of populations.

Underlying this model is the notion of a founder or ancestral population from which the array of s populations is descended, and the kinship is defined relative to the gene pool of that founder population. For the Åland Islands, the founder population can be considered as comprised of the small population (approximately 5200) who returned to the islands after the Great Northern War in 1721.[55]

As defined, kinship coefficients depend on the evolutionary processes by which the contemporary population has descended from the founder population, and therefore any systematic or random factors would have an effect on the magnitude of the coefficient. The patterns and amount of gene flow or migration between the populations in the array and the extent of long-range migration from the outside (m) will affect the kinship coefficients. For example, if local kinship, ϕ_{ii}, is low there is probably greater than average migration into the area, or if the kinship coefficient is large we can assume less immigration. Also, the effective size of the populations in the array will have an effect on the kinship (ϕ_{ij}) since for small, relatively isolated groups there is a greater probability that two individuals are descended from some common ancestor in the not too remote past. Therefore, for any array of populations (assuming a founder population) all of the subsequent effects of genetic drift, gene flow, nonrandom mating patterns, differential fertility, etc., would be summarized in the kinship matrix Φ. Thus one approach to studying population structure is to obtain an $s \times s$ matrix whose (i,j)th element is an estimate of ϕ_{ij}. Given a genealogy, kinship can be calculated, exactly, with reference to a specific founder population. In the next section, we shall describe, briefly, how kinship in future generations may be predicted from migration data.

The Migration Matrix Model

A migration matrix, M, is a formal representation of the movement of individuals within and among a set of populations.[9] For k populations, the matrix has k rows and columns, one for each population; for Åland, M is either 15×15 or 16×16 depending on whether the urban parish of Mariehamn is excluded or included.

Ideally, the elements of M, m_{ij}, are the numbers of individuals born in the ith population (rows) whose parents are born in the jth population (columns). A matrix can be computed for both parental and maternal data, but these are usually added to obtain M. Each child is then counted twice, once for each parent. Thus the sum of the elements of M is $2N$, twice the total population size but equal to the actual number of genes. The matrix is made column stochastic. That is, by dividing each element by its column total, we get a matrix, P, with elements p_{ij} ($\sum_i p_{ji} = 1$) representing the probability that a gene in the breeding population of j goes to i by migration.

As described, such a parent–offspring matrix incorporates both migration and reproduction including differential fertility. However, for the Åland analysis we have used matrimonial migration data obtained from the marriage records. In doing so, we must assume that there is no differential fertility relative to migration. The validity of this assumption will be tested in subsequent studies, but prior experience[25,47] suggests that these data provide a good approximation to the more desirable, but more difficult to obtain, data based on parent and offspring birthplaces. Where exact parent–offspring data have been available, migration matrix models have also been used to predict changes in the relative sizes of populations due to the observed migration pattern.[64] Here, however, we must assume that each marriage produces two children, so that both reproductive variation and changes in population size cannot be considered. Our focus is on the nature of the genetic relationships which would be induced by an observed pattern of migration; thus changes in the migration patterns can be compared with respect to their genetic effect.

Suppose that for an array of populations we have determined the migration pattern within the array, and hence the matrix P, the effective sizes, N_e, of each subpopulation, and an estimate of the long-range migration or systematic pressure, m, for each subpopulation. Long-range migration can be estimated by the number of outsiders coming into the array. Then if two gametes are drawn randomly from populations I and J in the tth generation there are three possible outcomes according to Imaizumi *et al.*[51] (p. 569):

1. With probability $p_{ki}p_{kj}/2N_k$, both genes are derived from the same gene in the kth population in generation t-1.

2. With probability $p_{ki}p_{kj}[1-(1/2N_k)]$, both genes are drawn from the kth population, but from different genes in generation t-1.

3. With probability $P_{ki}P_{hj}$, the genes are drawn from different populations, k and h $(k \neq h)$, in generation t-1.

Thus, if we assume that P, N_e, and m remain constant in time, the coefficient of kinship in future generations can be approximated (predicted). The basic recurrence equation for predicting kinship between populations I and J in the tth generation was derived by Malécot[66] and slightly modified by Morton[72,74,76,77]:

$$\phi_{ij}^{(t)} = (1 - m_i)(1 - m_j)$$
$$\cdot \left\{ \sum_{k=1}^{n} \sum_{k=1}^{n} P_{ki}P_{kj}\phi_{kj}^{(t-1)} + \sum_{k=1}^{n} p_{ki}p_{kj}[1 - \phi_{kk}^{(t-1)}]/2N_k \right\}$$

Or written as a matrix recurrence equation,

$$\phi^{(t)} = \sum_{r=1}^{t} (1 - m)^{2r}(P')^r D^{(t-r)}(P)^r$$

where D is a diagonal matrix with $[1 - \phi_{kk}^{(t-1)}/2N_k]$ in the kth position. Kinship at $t^{(0)}$ will be zero; that is, we assume no initial relationships between any of the populations in the array. As t, the number of generations, increases, the kinship matrix $\phi^{(t)}$ approaches an equilibrium state, asymptotically, and independent of the initial conditions.[43] With this technique, for a given pattern of migration we can predict the kinship between populations which would result from that migration pattern and describe, generation by generation, the rate and pattern of the approach to equilibrium.

Kinship estimates can also be obtained from other sources of data. If random samples of gene frequencies are taken in the array of populations and local panmixia is assumed, kinship can be estimated from genetic data.[72,81] Methods also exist for estimating kinship from anthropometry,[3,72] isonymy (same surnames),[3,15,79] genealogies or pedigrees,[72] and phenotype pairs.[3,111] Morton[77] has also attempted to predict kinship from linguistic data; however, the assumptions and predictions may not conform to reality and the estimates are only tentative since retention and dispersion of cognates may vary greatly from subculture to subculture.[95] There are, of course, alternative algorithms and applications of the migration matrix technique,[9,47,94,101] as well as diverse models and procedures which can be used for the analysis of population structure using genetic or anthropometric data. The actual inference about structure, however, does not appear to vary among these generally equivalent models. Here the focus on the kinship model allows a consistent theoretical perspective from which the results can be interpreted and compared.

In this study, inference on kinship has thus far used data on matrimonial migration and the distribution of gene frequencies in Åland. In the following sections, we will examine the results obtained from using matrimonial migration for a 200-year time span in Åland. These results will then be compared to inference obtained from genetics.

MATRIMONIAL MIGRATION IN ÅLAND

The Swedish ecclesiastical law of 1686 prescribed that the clergy (Lutheran ministers) should keep regular records of all the marriages in each parish. Church records concerning other aspects of social life were instituted even earlier than 1686; for example, registration of births had started in the 1650s in some parishes (Table II). Since the last half of the seventeenth century, the parish records have consisted of the names and places of residence (parish, village, and often house or farm location) of the bride and groom prior to marriage. The marriage records are very complete, with only minor problems of registration occurring. For example, during certain time periods some of the clergy have registered the residence of only the bride and not the groom; so it was necessary to exclude a number of individuals from the analysis. The number of individuals of unknown origin varies from parish to parish; however, during the later years this number decreases drastically. Inconsistencies like this are due to individual clergymen's idiosyncrasy and do not follow a specific pattern throughout the archipelago.[25,26] Therefore, there is not a systematic bias operating to substantially affect the kinship coefficients. Obviously, problems of this type are unavoidable when one is working with historical documents.

In 1830, the Russian Empire began to build a fortress (Bomarsund) in the parish of Sund. As a consequence, a large number of Russian immigrants (mainly soldiers) came into Sund between 1830 and 1856.

TABLE II. Year of Commencement of Church
Registration of Births (Maternities) in Åland[a]

Parish	Year of commencement of church registration of births	
Eckerö	1669	(1672–1683, 1714–1722)
Hammerland	1653	(1710–1793)
Geta	1738	
Finström	1738	
Saltvik	1655	(1687–1698, 1715–1722)
Sund	1695	(1714–1723, 1740–1747)
Vårdö	1710	(1715–1721)
Lumparland	1684	(1697–1702, 1715–1721)
Lemland	1725	
Jomala	1741	
Mariehamn	1906	(town founded in 1861; up to 1906 part of Jomala parish)
Brändö	1739	
Kumlinge	1688	(1714–1721)
Sottunga	1722	
Föglö	1693	(1715–1722)
Kökar	1666	

[a] Years in parentheses are lacking or deficient.

Many of these Russians married local people, particularly from Sund
and Saltvik. After the peace in 1856, almost all of the couples with a
Russian marriage partner left Åland. Since these Russian immigrants
did not contribute to the local gene pool, they have been excluded from
the analysis.

Information on the place of residence before and after marriage for
each marriage partner, i.e., origin and marital residence, can be
arranged in the form of a migration matrix. An example of a
matrimonial migration matrix and the corresponding column stochastic
matrix for the period 1750–1799 are presented in Tables III and IV,
respectively. Also presented in Table III are (1) the number of
individuals coming into each parish whose origin was outside Åland,
(2) the total number of individuals used in the analysis, (i.e., the number
of individuals married during each time period), (3) the number of
individuals of unknown origin (these have been excluded from the
analysis), and (4) an estimate of the effective size, N_e, of each parish

TABLE III. Matrimonial Migration Matrix for 1750–1799 for Åland Islands

Origin	Residence														
	Ec	Ha	Ge	Fi	Sa	Su	Vå	Jo	Le	Lu	Fö	So	Kö	Ku	Br
Eckerö	397	1	1	5	2	0	0	1	0	0	0	0	0	0	0
Hammarland	16	91	10	9	6	1	0	8	0	0	0	0	0	0	0
Geta	1	0	339	16	11	3	0	4	0	0	0	0	0	0	0
Finström	4	1	21	730	16	8	2	13	0	0	0	0	0	0	1
Saltvik	0	0	13	22	738	27	1	6	1	1	0	1	0	0	0
Sund	0	0	0	6	32	517	27	6	1	5	2	0	0	0	0
Vårdö	0	0	0	0	5	20	332	3	2	5	2	2	0	1	1
Jomala	0	1	2	19	11	2	0	1061	12	1	0	0	0	0	0
Lemland	0	1	0	1	2	2	2	19	379	15	3	2	0	0	0
Lumparland	0	0	0	0	0	5	12	3	1	178	8	3	0	0	0
Föglö	0	0	0	1	0	1	1	2	6	5	656	14	3	6	0
Sottunga	0	0	0	0	0	0	2	1	0	4	16	138	3	3	1
Kökar	0	0	0	0	0	1	0	0	0	0	4	2	371	1	0
Kumlinge	0	0	0	1	4	2	3	2	1	1	5	10	1	374	7
Brändö	0	1	0	0	0	0	0	0	0	0	0	0	1	20	521
Outside of Åland	2	0	8	8	21	13	7	31	3	1	20	5	19	9	18
Total	420	96	394	818	848	602	389	1160	406	216	716	177	398	414	549
Unknown ♂	4	8	42	89	22	52	11	82	18	13	78	11	3	25	19
Unknown ♀	2	0	52	57	66	26	2	14	0	1	10	0	1	59	2
m	0.005	0	0.020	0.010	0.025	0.022	0.018	0.027	0.007	0.005	0.028	0.028	0.048	0.022	0.033
N_e	209	280	148	298	364	311	153	474	250	94	249	63	166	187	216

TABLE IV. Column Stochastic Migration Matrix per Mille for 1750–1799

Origin	Residence														
	Ec	Ha	Ge	Fi	Sa	Su	Vå	Jo	Le	Lu	Fö	So	Kö	Ku	Br
Eckerö	950	11	3	6	3	0	0	0	0	0	0	0	0	0	0
Hammarland	38	948	26	11	7	2	0	7	0	0	0	0	0	0	0
Geta	2	0	878	20	13	5	0	4	0	0	0	0	0	0	0
Finström	10	11	54	901	19	14	5	12	0	0	0	0	0	0	2
Saltvik	0	0	34	27	892	46	3	5	3	5	3	6	0	0	0
Sund	0	0	0	7	39	878	71	5	3	23	3	0	0	2	0
Vårdö	0	0	0	0	6	34	869	3	5	23	0	12	0	0	2
Jomala	0	10	5	23	13	3	0	940	30	5	4	0	0	0	0
Lemland	0	10	0	2	3	3	5	17	940	70	12	12	0	0	0
Lumparland	0	0	0	0	0	8	31	3	2	828	12	17	0	0	0
Föglö	0	0	0	2	0	2	3	3	15	23	942	81	7	15	0
Sottunga	0	0	0	0	0	0	5	2	0	19	23	802	8	8	2
Kökar	0	0	0	0	0	2	0	0	0	0	6	12	979	3	0
Kumlinge	0	0	0	1	5	3	8	2	2	5	7	58	3	923	13
Brändö	0	10	0	0	0	0	0	0	0	0	0	0	3	49	981

calculated as one-third the harmonic mean of the census sizes for the period.

In order to obtain a representation of the changes in the population structure in Åland from 1750 to 1949, it was necessary to divide the 200-year time period into a number of intervals. The time span was divided into three 50-year intervals and five 10-year periods: 1750–1799, 1800–1849, 1850–1899, 1900–1909, 1910–1919, 1920–1929, 1930–1939, and 1940–1949. For several analyses, the five 10-year periods have also been lumped into one 50-year interval for comparative purposes. The twentieth century was divided into decades because there were major population, economic, and technological changes during this time as opposed to the rather stable period from 1750 to 1900.

Parish Endogamy

Using column stochastic matrices determined from the matrimonial migration patterns, the degree of parish endogamy can be estimated assuming that individuals, but not couples, migrate. The diagonal elements, P_{ii}, of the column stochastic matrices give the probability that a random individual in population I originated in population I, and as shown by Morton[77] endogamy can be estimated by $(2P_{ii}-1)$ on the condition that $P_{ii} \geq 0.50$. The values of P_{ii} for each parish over the 200-year time period are given in Table V.

In general, the P_{ii} values decrease over the time span, indicating a decrease in the probability that an individual (and subsequently a gene) in population I originated in I. The decrease in the values corresponds to the dispersed, rather isolated characteristics of the parishes in the earlier years and to the increase in mate exchange between parishes in the later years. There is also a corresponding drop in the P_{ii} values as Mariehamn starts to influence the population structure of the archipelago. There are, however, variations in some of the parishes: for example, Sottunga has the lowest value of P_{ii} from 1750 to 1909, while Kökar and Brändö exhibit the highest values through time. Both Kökar and Brändö are the most geographically isolated parishes. The lowest values of P_{ii} are during the periods 1930–1939 and 1940–1949 for the town of Mariehamn (10.256 and 0.223, respectively), and this indicates that couples are emigrating to the urban center.

The estimated parish endogamy rates for each time period as well

TABLE V. Observed Values of p_{ii} Within Åland Parishes from 1750 to 1949

Parish	1750–1799	1800–1849	1850–1899	1900–1909	1910–1919	1920–1929	1930–1939	1940–1949
Eckerö	0.950	0.966	0.952	0.930	0.967	0.866	0.826	0.771
Hammarland	0.948	0.924	0.897	0.880	0.900	0.890	0.621	0.697
Geta	0.878	0.901	0.892	0.919	0.881	0.788	0.717	0.689
Finström	0.901	0.917	0.925	0.923	0.865	0.872	0.696	0.683
Saltvik	0.892	0.901	0.914	0.938	0.888	0.968	0.808	0.705
Sund	0.878	0.909	0.908	0.889	0.923	0.899	0.667	0.752
Vårdö	0.869	0.917	0.930	0.888	0.879	0.891	0.828	0.743
Jomala	0.940	0.933	0.927	0.907	0.848	0.859	0.689	0.587
Lemland	0.940	0.947	0.941	0.955	0.977	0.925	0.691	0.686
Lumparland	0.828	0.897	0.893	0.909	0.786	0.887	0.712	0.634
Föglö	0.943	0.952	0.950	0.912	0.935	0.970	0.835	0.829
Sottunga	0.802	0.868	0.877	0.852	0.878	0.778	0.733	0.662
Kökar	0.978	0.972	0.980	0.974	0.982	0.952	0.904	0.916
Kumlinge	0.923	0.936	0.965	0.948	0.947	0.939	0.890	0.877
Brändö	0.981	0.969	0.977	0.966	0.931	0.977	0.879	0.929
Mariehamn	—	—	—	0.865	0.855	0.833	0.256	0.223

as the average for Åland (including and excluding Mariehamn) are given in Table VI. There is a decrease in the mean endogamy for the whole of Åland from 1750 to 1949 from 84 to 31%. However, the level of endogamy is quite stable up to 1929 (81%) and then declines sharply in subsequent decades: 41% for 1930–1939 and 31% for 1940–1949. This trend is also apparent for each separate parish with the exception of Brändö, Kökar, and Kumlinge.

Sottunga exhibits the lowest values of endogamy for the periods from 1750 to 1909 and from 1920 to 1929. This trend may, in part, be due to its small effective size (less than 130). Possibly individuals were unable to obtain mates within the parish of Sottunga since it was fairly small and there was avoidance of consanguineous marriage. Then as the effective size increased the probability of finding a mate within the parish increased and parish endogamy subsequently increased.

Kökar and Brändö have the highest values of endogamy and are fairly consistent over the periods, suggesting the possibility of high values of inbreeding. Genealogical reconstruction could verify this suggestion.[34,35] Both parishes are geographically isolated from the main

TABLE VI. Percent Endogamy by Parish from 1750 to 1949 in Åland[a]

Parish	1750–1799	1800–1849	1850–1899	1900–1909	1910–1919	1920–1929	1930–1939	1940–1949
Eckerö	90	93	90	86	93	73	65	54
Hammarland	90	85	79	76	80	78	24	39
Geta	76	80	78	84	76	58	43	38
Finström	80	92	85	85	73	74	39	37
Saltvik	78	80	83	88	78	94	62	41
Sund	76	82	82	78	85	80	33	50
Vårdö	74	83	87	78	76	78	66	49
Jomala	88	87	85	81	70	71	39	17
Lemland	88	89	88	91	95	85	38	37
Lumparland	66	79	79	82	57	77	42	27
Föglö	89	90	90	82	87	94	67	. 66
Sottunga	60	74	75	70	76	56	47	32
Kökar	96	94	96	95	96	90	81	83
Kumlinge	85	87	93	90	89	88	78	75
Brändö	96	94	95	93	86	95	76	86
Mariehamn	—	—	—	73	86	88	−49	−55
Total Åland including Mariehamn	84	86	86	84	80	81	41	31
Excluding Mariehamn	—	—	—	85	83	82	52	46

[a] Endogamy estimated by $2p_{ii} - 1$.

island, and mate exchange with the other parishes appears to be slight throughout time.

During 1930–1939 and 1940–1949, Mariehamn displays negative endogamy. This result, as discussed earlier, is a consequence of the assumption that $P_{ii} \geq 0.50$ and indicates that couples are migrating to Mariehamn.

Prediction of Kinship from Matrimonial Migration Data

The division of the migration data into time periods (1750–1799, etc.) permits inference on the effect of changes in the mating patterns on the population structure over the past 200 years.

The predicted mean kinship values for each time period are given in Table VII. Since marriage records for Mariehamn start in 1906, the kinship was predicted two ways: (1) including Mariehamn and (2) excluding Mariehamn. In this way, the influence of a growing "urban" center on the migration patterns can be examined. Mean predicted kinship within populations decreases over the time period from 0.01501 to 0.00096 (0.00082 including Mariehamn), indicating an increase in mobility and mate exchange and a decrease in heterogeneity between the parishes. This decrease in parish isolation is also reflected by the drop in parish endogamy over the 200 years. The predicted mean kinship values are all consistently higher when Mariehamn is excluded from the analysis. Mariehamn has high effective size (N_e) and high mate exchange with all parishes; thus it has the effect of high long-range migration in an island model[107] and lowers the kinship values.

In order to obtain kinship values (called conditional kinship) comparable to the kinship coefficients which are estimated from gene frequencies, we first calculate estimated random kinship, i.e., kinship relative to random pairs from the finite contemporary gene pool, by

$$\phi_R = \sum_{i,j} N_i N_j \phi_{ij} / \sum_{i,j} N_i N_j$$

or by

$$\phi_R = \sum w_i w_j \phi_{ij}$$

TABLE VII. Predicted Mean Kinship Within Populations for Åland from 1750 to 1949

	Mean predicted kinship (ϕ)		Conditional kinship (r_{ij})	
	Including Mariehamn	Excluding Mariehamn	Including Mariehamn	Excluding Mariehamn
1750–1799	—	0.01501	—	0.01094
1800–1849	—	0.01302	—	0.00978
1850–1899	—	0.00841	—	0.00658
1900–1909	0.00518	0.00555	0.00413	0.00366
1910–1919	0.00535	0.00611	0.00443	0.00511
1920–1929	0.00401	0.00432	0.00333	0.00354
1930–1939	0.00103	0.00118	0.00085	0.00098
1940–1949	0.00082	0.00096	0.00067	0.00080

where $w_i = \sum N_i/N$. We then compute conditional kinship (r_{ij}), which is kinship relative to the contemporary gene pool, or as in this case relative to the finite array of populations in Åland during each time period, by

$$r_{ij} = (\phi_{ij} - \phi_R)/(1 - \phi_R)$$

The conditional kinship values, also presented in Table VII, can be used to compare to kinship coefficients estimated from the gene frequencies.

Approach to Equilibrium

According to Imaizumi *et al.*,[51] the recurrence relation, $\phi_{ij}^{(t)}$, appears to converge rather rapidly if the systematic pressure is not very small. Figure 2 plots the predicted mean kinship per generation until approximate convergence (equilibrium). If the systematic pressure is relatively small, as during the time periods 1750–1799 and 1800–1849, approximate convergence takes about 75 generations, and equilibrium, defined here as changes less than 10^{-6} per generation, is reached in 185 and 182 generations, respectively. However, if the systematic pressure is relatively large, as in 1930–1939 and 1940–1949, approximate convergence takes only five or six generations and equilibrium is reached in 23 and 21 generations, respectively. Figure 2 demonstrates that because of the increase in systematic pressure and more migration between parishes the mean predicted kinship within populations and the number of generations to convergence have decreased considerably in this population. Thus the increase in migration rates means that an equilibrium would be attained after only a few generations. Genetic variation in the contemporary population is therefore largely determined by the recent migration history and would provide little information about the historical relations among parishes.

Kinship Matrices

The predicted mean kinship within populations provides a generalized view of the relationship that exists through time in the whole of Åland. However, the kinship values within each parish (ϕ_{ii}) and between parishes (ϕ_{ij}) are also of interest. An example of a matrix of

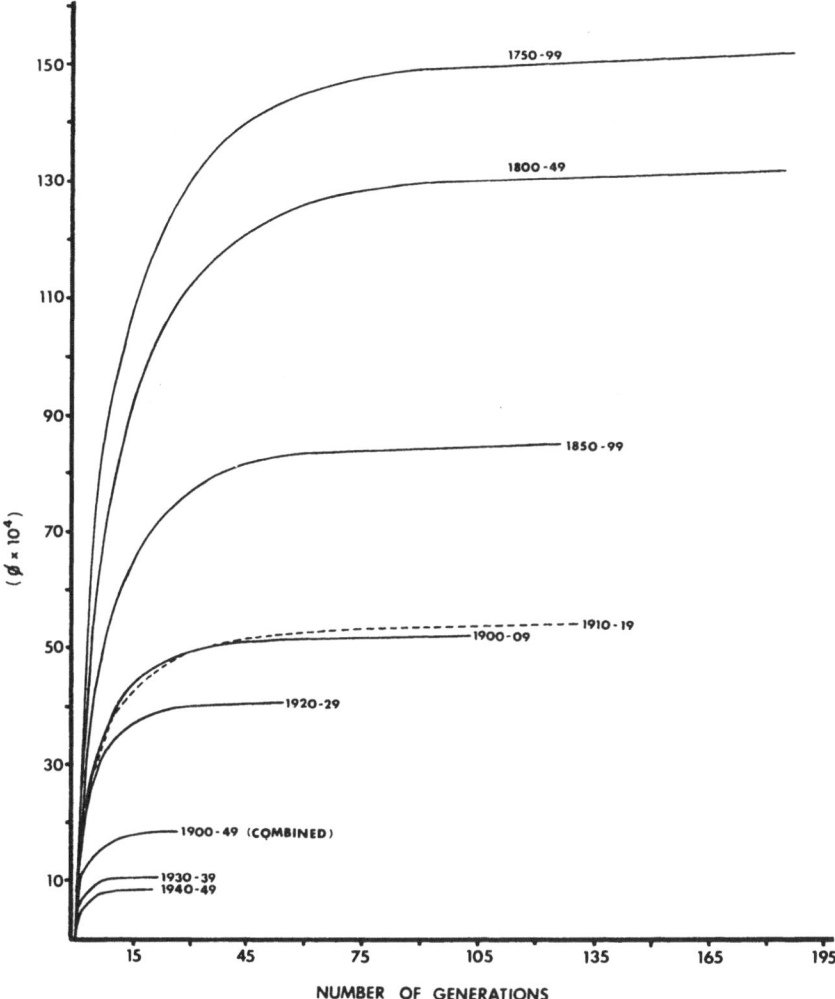

Fig. 2. Approach to equilibrium of predicted mean kinship from migration for all periods.

predicted kinship values for 1750–1799 is given in Table VIII. The diagonal elements of this matrix denote local kinship, ϕ_{ii}. Local kinship can be interpreted as the extent to which each parish in the array deviates from the mean kinship for the total array. Low values of ϕ_{ii} indicate greater than average migration, and parishes experiencing little immigration would in turn have larger values, indicating greater than

TABLE VIII. Predicted Kinship ($\phi_{ij} \times 10^4$) from Matrimonial Migration Data for 1750–1799 (above the diagonal) and Geographical Distances in Kilometers (below the diagonal) Used for Isolation by Distance and Topology[a]

Parish	Ec	Ha	Ge	Fi	Sa	Su	Vå	Jo	Le	Lu	Fö	So	Kö	Ku	Br
Eckerö	305	138	70	69	46	36	29	41	34	29	15	17	6	17	18
Hammarland	8.4	222	73	66	46	37	32	49	48	37	20	24	8	28	36
Geta	22.5	17.6	150	71	50	38	29	36	30	27	14	16	5	13	13
Finström	19.4	11.4	12.0	113	49	40	32	42	34	30	16	18	6	15	13
Saltvik	26.0	17.9	14.9	6.7	78	47	37	32	31	31	16	19	6	17	13
Sund	29.1	20.7	20.0	10.7	5.1	84	60	29	34	44	22	23	9	18	13
Vårdö	42.7	32.3	32.1	24.5	18.2	13.8	135	29	43	64	31	36	10	26	17
Jomala	20.1	12.9	24.0	12.3	14.4	13.7	24.9	82	54	38	19	20	6	14	11
Lemland	30.7	24.4	34.9	22.9	22.4	19.0	23.6	11.8	177	84	42	39	11	21	13
Lumparland	37.9	30.3	35.8	24.7	21.2	16.4	14.7	17.7	10.4	174	54	56	14	29	17
Föglö	51.1	44.3	51.3	40.0	36.7	31.7	15.8	31.4	20.4	15.5	140	77	28	41	20
Sottunga	60.0	52.1	53.1	44.2	38.6	33.7	21.3	40.1	32.5	22.7	18.1	176	31	65	35
Kökar	76.7	69.5	73.7	63.5	58.8	53.7	42.9	56.7	46.2	39.3	25.9	22.2	203	21	14
Kumlinge	64.9	56.6	51.9	46.3	39.7	35.9	22.3	46.9	43.1	32.8	34.5	17.6	36.1	181	104
Brändö	83.2	75.0	66.2	63.8	57.2	54.6	42.4	67.2	65.1	54.9	57.0	39.4	53.1	22.7	232

[a] Mean kinship within populations = 0.01501.

average isolation. The off diagonal elements, ϕ_{ij}, denote the kinship between pairs of populations. If ϕ_{ij} is larger relative to the other ϕ_{ij} values in the array, there is more similarity between these parishes; if ϕ_{ij} is small, there is less. However, the relationship between two parishes that have positive (rather high) ϕ_{ij} values can be indirect (i.e., $\phi_{ij} > 0$ means that i and j are in the same network). Since all parishes in the array are ultimately linked together to some degree, because of the mate exchange pattern, all of the ϕ_{ij} are greater than zero.

A number of features can be seen in the kinship matrix for 1750–1799. Several pairs of parishes have very large ϕ_{ij}, indicating that there are really clusters of parishes with higher rates of gene flow than with other parishes. These include Eckerö and Hammarland, Geta and Finström, Sund and Vårdö, and Lemland and Lumparland. Each of these pairs was formerly united into a single parish, but new churches were established as the population size in Åland increased. All of the outer island parishes could be viewed as being in a cluster with greater than average ϕ_{ij} within than between the outer islands and the main islands. Within the outer islands, however, Föglö and Sottunga and Brändö and Kumlinge are especially close. These special pairwise similarities can be shown to persist into the twentieth century, but the strength of the associations, at least among main island parishes, declines considerably.

For a detailed specification of the changing pattern of migration and its effect on the genetic structure, a discussion of each kinship matrix generated for the 200-year time span (i.e., 14 matrices total) would be necessary (see Mielke[69] for these details). However, both the length and the purposes of this chapter prohibit such a discussion and only a summary of the major results and trends will be presented.

Both the *predicted kinship* values between parishes, ϕ_{ij}, and the local kinship values, ϕ_{ii}, for each parish decrease in magnitude over the total time span of 200 years. Table IX summarizes the ϕ_{ii} values over each time period for each parish. In general, the values are highest during the first three 50-year periods and then there is a decrease in the values, starting in 1900–1909. Local kinship values for main island parishes decrease sooner and more rapidly than those for the outer island parishes. The outer island parishes (Sottunga, Kökar, Kumlinge, and Brändö) remain rather isolated, according to ϕ_{ii} values, until 1930, when there are major drops in the kinship values. It is also interesting to note that local kinship for Lemland in 1910–1919 is the highest it has

TABLE IX. Changes in Local Kinship ($\phi_{ii} \times 10^4$) for Each Parish from
1750 to 1949

Parish	1750–1799	1800–1849	1850–1899	1900–1909	1910–1919	1920–1929	1930–1939	1940–1949	1900–1949
Eckerö	305	307	112	54	139	30	16	10	23
Hammarland	222	90	46	32	27	43	4	6	11
Geta	150	126	69	84	51	37	14	10	22
Finström	113	88	59	38	34	30	4	4	9
Saltvik	78	90	56	38	25	30	6	4	11
Sund	84	81	57	32	31	26	5	4	11
Vårdö	135	150	95	72	35	46	17	11	23
Jomala	82	69	39	22	17	23	3	2	6
Lemland	177	133	59	69	226	43	6	4	14
Lumparland	174	203	144	108	77	87	21	12	35
Föglö	140	123	88	50	33	73	7	11	17
Sottunga	176	227	191	110	75	68	19	19	33
Kökar	203	217	344	147	152	82	60	23	60
Kumlinge	181	144	195	158	52	63	27	36	45
Brändö	232	236	85	35	60	66	31	38	42
Mariehamn	—	—	—	33	28	14	1	1	17

ever been. What this means is not clear and further research into the social and demographic changes for this specific parish during 1910–1919 is warranted.

From 1750 to 1899, Åland as a whole appears to have been rather isolated, with parish isolation and endogamy (as reflected by the kinship values) playing a major role in determining the population structure of the archipelago. The main island parishes begin to exchange mates more frequently and earlier than the outer island parishes. Local kinship values for the centrally located main island parishes are lowest for all years considered, and the outer island parishes constantly provide the highest local kinship values and the lowest ϕ_{ij} values for the area. Brändö, Kumlinge, Sottunga, and Kökar and consistently the most isolated parishes, while Kökar appears to be the most isolated of all parishes. The breakdown of isolation according to the local kinship values appears to have started in the 1900s, with the major breakdown of parish isolation becoming very apparent from 1930 to 1949 (Table IX).

GEOGRAPHICAL FACTORS AFFECTING MIGRATION PATTERNS

Isolation by Distance

In most cases, a population under consideration is not a random breeding unit because individual migration distances are usually smaller than the total distribution of the species. This phenomenon, called "isolation by distance,"[107] leads to local differentiation in gene frequencies caused by genetic drift. Wright[105-109] suggested a model in which a population is distributed uniformly over an area, with individual mobility defined by a continuous distribution. For simplicity, the normal distribution of mobility is usually used, although other distributions (e.g., leptokurtic) have been utilized.[110] The parents of an individual are assumed to be drawn at random from a small surrounding area (expressed in terms of "neighborhood size"). The neighborhood is defined as the population contained within an arbitrary circular region from which the parents of individuals born near the center may be considered as if drawn at random, or as "approximately the effective number in a circle or radius twice the standard deviation of the distribution of parent relative to offspring in one direction" (p. 332).[109] By methods of path coefficients, Wright was able to assess, using the inbreeding coefficient, the amount of differentiation of neighborhoods relative to a larger population in which they were contained. Two forms of this model, linear and two-dimensional, were analyzed; local differentiation appeared to be much stronger in the linear version.

Isolation by distance has also been incorporated into the "stepping stone model" of Kimura and Weiss.[58] In general, it has been found that the correlation coefficient of gene frequencies between colonies decreased as distance increased.[58,102]

The effects of isolation by distance have also been considered by Malécot.[67] He has shown that in infinitely large continuous populations, for particular distributions of marital distance, the coefficient of kinship, ϕ_{ij}, between two populations or individuals, I and J, decreases as the distance between I and J increases and can be approximated by

$$\phi(d) = ae^{-bd}d^{-c}$$

where a denotes local kinship or kinship at small distances [$a = \phi(0)$], *b* describes the systematic pressure, and $c = 0$, ½, or 1 for isotropic migration in one, two, or three dimensions, respectively. Observations on real populations and deterministic studies[50,68] have demonstrated that in finite populations over small distances *c* can be taken to equal zero so that

$$\phi(d) = ae^{-bd}$$

Morton[74] states that

> This limiting form has been found to hold for large distance with stepping stone, exponential, or normal migration, and evidently applies to any migration distribution with a finite variance. (p. 61)

Thus for Åland we can relate the ϕ_{ij} to the geographical distance between parishes by the above equation in an attempt to determine the effects of linear distance on local differentiation of the populations.

The effect of isolation by distance for the whole of Åland during each time period is shown in Fig. 3. It appears that linear distances between parishes had greater effects on the population structure in the

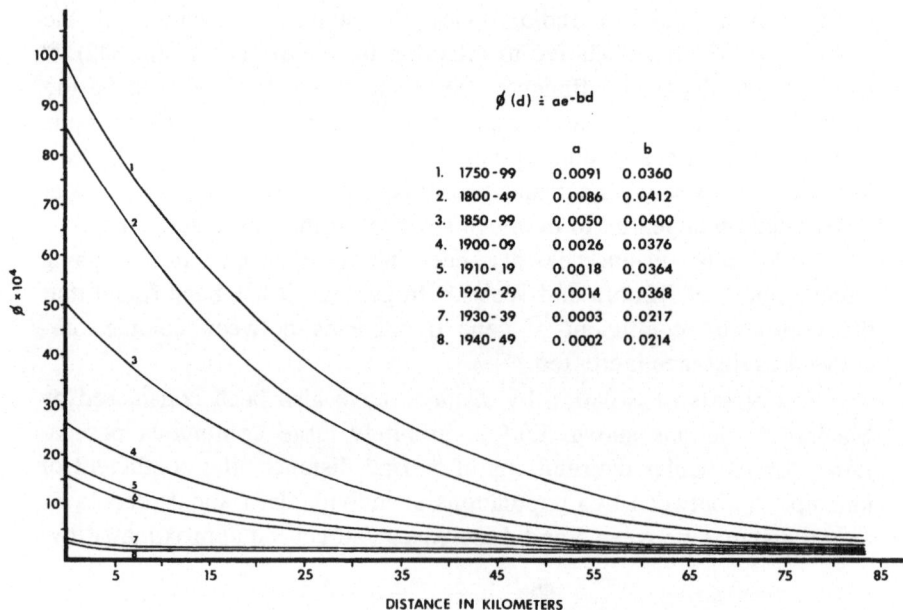

Fig. 3. Isolation by distance in the Åland Islands. Predicted from matrimonial migration data for each period.

earlier time periods, especially in the periods 1750–1799 and 1800–1849, than in the later periods, when the effects of isolation by distance seem to have been almost negligible. There appears to be a clustering of the regression lines into distinct groups: (1) 1750–1799 and 1800–1849 form one group, when isolation by distance appears to have been a major factor in parish differentiation, (2) 1850–1899 appears to have been a period when the isolation was starting to break down to some extent, (3) 1900–1909, 1910–1919, and 1920–1929 cluster together, indicating that there was further breakdown in the isolation due to distance of the parishes, and (4) 1930–1939 and 1940–1949 cluster together, exhibiting the fact that the effect of isolation by distance during these two periods was almost nonexistent.

Also presented in Fig. 3 are the a and b values for each regression. These values have been used extensively in the literature in the interpretation of the effects of isolation by distance on population structure in various areas of the world.[3,39,49,50,78,80] According to Morton et al.,[81] large values of a (>0.03) have been characteristic of primitive populations and island groups while large values of b are characteristic of continential isolates but not hunting and gathering groups or populations of oceanic islands. This simplistic classification seems wholly inappropriate given the results in Åland. Since ϕ_{ii} is dependent on the effective size and systematic pressure, the interpretation and comparison of both a and b values between different populations are now extremely limited and can generate only gross comparisons which do not add to our knowledge of population structure. Therefore, the values for both parameters (a and b) are simply reported with no interpretation attached.

By relying on $\phi(d)$ for describing the population structure for the whole area under investigation, one obtains the averaged role that linear distance has on the population structure of the area. However, this procedure obscures the role that each individual subpopulation has in contributing to, or determining, the structure of the population. Also, the interrelationships of specific subdivisions, islands, etc., and the variation in the amount of isolation are lost by this generalized approach. In order to examine the interrelationships of the individual subgroups, it is necessary to look at each population in relation to all others by plotting the ϕ_{ij} values and distance, thus not being concerned with the fitting of the data to a theoretical curve. Here we are not concerned with the exponential trend in the curve but with the peaks

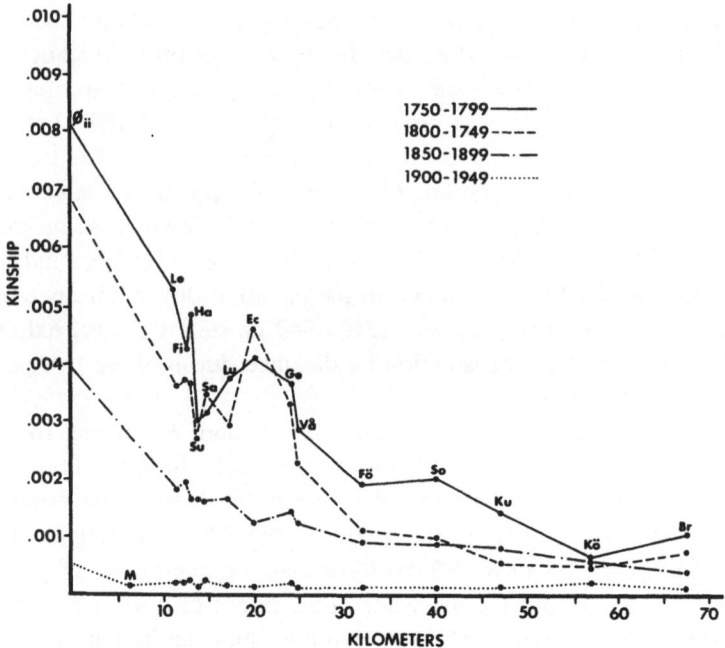

Fig. 4. Relationship of kinship and distance from Jomala.

and valleys and the change in each curve over the time periods. Figures 4, 5, and 6 show the effects of isolation by distance for selected parishes in relation to all other parishes over the 200-year time span. With this method, a more succinct description of the role that distance has on the structure of Åland, and especially specific parishes, can be examined. We do not profess to be able to explain why there are certain relationships, but hope that by describing them one may then be able to ask reasonable questions which provide a focus for future research strategies.

The 200-year time span has been broken into four 50-year periods to illustrate the changes in the isolation patterns over time. The graphs are plots of the predicted kinship values (ϕ_{ij}) between parishes relative to the distance separating them.

Jomala

Figure 4 shows the effects of isolation by distance on the parish of Jomala, which is geographically situated in the center of the main island and thus provides an example of isolation by distance for a centrally located parish. For all the time periods, the local kinship, ϕ_{ii} (Table IX), is the lowest (except for Mariehamn) in the archipelago and there is less isolation by distance for Jomala than any other parish, indicating a possible centralization in the islands.

There are few fluctuations in the lines that suggest any special relations that would not be expected due to distance alone. The

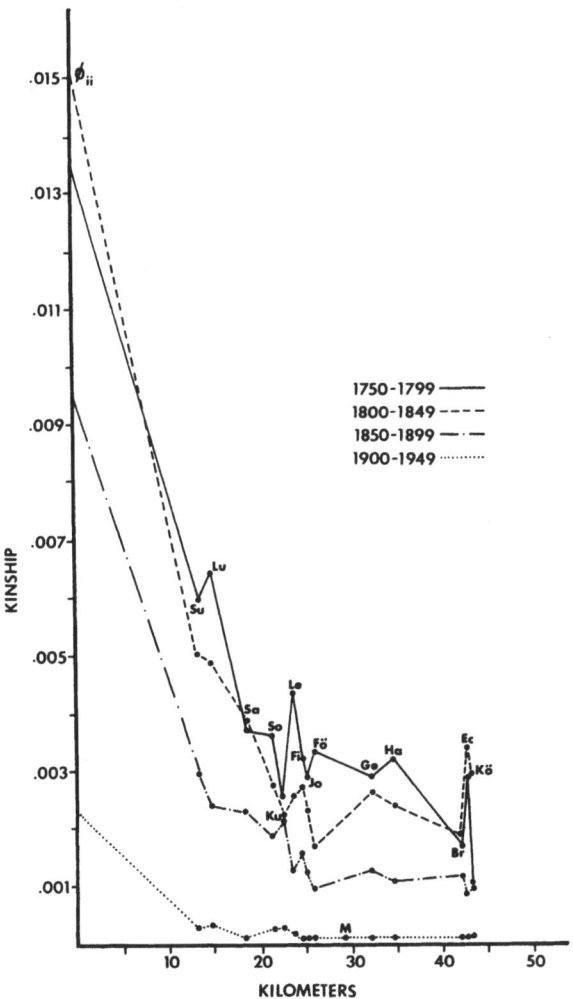

Fig. 5. Relationship of kinship and distance from Vårdö.

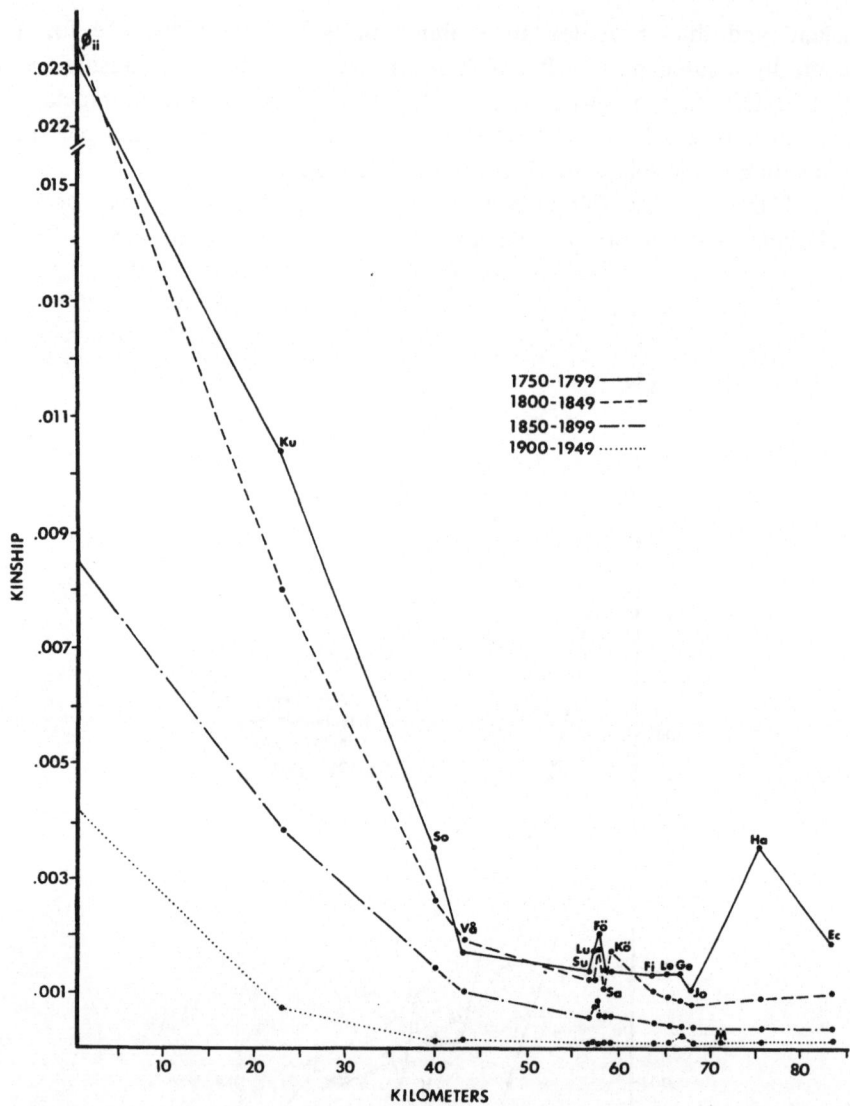

Fig. 6. Relationship of kinship and distance from Brändö.

relationship between Jomala and Sund is low when compared to the ϕ_{ij}
values for the period 1750–1799, as is Saltvik. On the other hand, the
plotted values for Eckerö and Geta are high for the periods 1750–1799
and 1800–1849. Both of these are indirect associations; that is, kinship
values are higher because of the linking of all the parishes in the

migration network. The curve for 1850–1899 is very smooth, and the isolation by distance for 1900–1949 is almost nonexistent. At least until 1900, the effect of linear distance is seen to be quite consistent. Thus, until high rates of migration opened up the isolation of this main island parish, marital frequencies showed a constant decline with linear distance throughout the Åland Islands.

Vårdö

Vårdö is situated on the northeastern side of the main island, separated by water from the rest of the main island parishes. This geographical location appears to have played a major role in determining the population structure, since the local kinship values (0.0135, 0.0150 0.0095) are rather high when compared to the values for other main island parishes such as Sund (0.0084, 0.0081, 0.0057), Saltvik (0.0078, 0.0090, 0.0056), and Jomala (0.0082, 0.0069, 0.0039) for the periods 1750–1799, 1800–1849, and 1850–1899, respectively. There appears to have been greater isolation by distance during 1800–1849 than during 1750–1799, as shown in Fig. 5. The plot is not very erratic, except the apparent relationship between Vårdö and Lemland during 1750–1799. Lemland is just south of Vårdö and is also separated from the other main island parishes by water. However, the relationship between these two parishes is indirect; that is, there is direct exchange between Lumparland and Vårdö and the exchange between Lemland and Lumparland has inflated the ϕ_{ij} values between Vårdö and Lemland (the direct exchange of mates can be seen only in the original migration matrices). Eckerö also plots high when compared to the outer island parishes, and again this relationship is indirect. The influence of isolation by distance during 1900–1949 has decreased compared to the other periods.

Brändö

The effects of isolation by distance on the parish of Brändö (Fig. 6) were apparently greater than for the other two parishes which have been discussed (i.e., Jomala and Vårdö). Local kinship values, ϕ_{ii}, are also generally greater than those for both Jomala and Vårdö, as shown in Table IX. Isolation by distance was greatest during the first two periods (1750–1799 and 1800–1849), with only a few, slightly erratic plots: Föglö plots high; however, this relationship is indirect, being linked to Brändö by way of both Sottunga and Kumlinge. Both Eckerö and Hammarland plot higher in relationship to the other values and also if one assumed that distance was the only factor operating to isolate the outer parishes. Brändö, for yet an unexplained reason, provides a large number of mates for Hammarland in 1750–1799 and subsequently the relationship between Hammarland and Eckerö in that period also raises the ϕ_{ij} between Brändö and Eckerö.

During 1850–1899 and 1900–1949, isolation by distance does not appear to have affected the population structure of Brändö as much as it did during the first 100 years; however, the isolation is much greater than that for both Vårdö and Jomala (see Figs. 4 and 5). Since Brändö actually had less mate exchange with main island parishes than with the geographically closer Åboland archipelago, this analysis may be somewhat biased. That is, Brändö may be less of an isolate within a larger population unit which would include the western part of Åboland. In future analyses, we shall attempt to distinguish the sources of long–range migration (e.g., Sweden, Finland, Åboland).

Summary

These analyses of individual parishes have demonstrated that in order to examine the effects of isolation by distance on subdivided populations it is necessary to examine each subdivision separately, not relying on the average isolation pattern for the whole area under consideration. It appears that the main island parishes have a different relation between marital frequencies and linear distance than the outer parishes. However, the main island parishes which are geographically on the fringe—Eckerö, Hammarland, Geta, Vårdö, Lemland, and Lumparland—behave differently than the centrally located ones. This fact may be related to the relatively undeveloped nature of transportation and communication systems linking the fringe main island parishes. The outer island parishes show greater isolation than the main island parishes, as might be expected due to their geographic location. The heterogeneity in the degree of local isolation (ϕ_{ij}) causes heterogeneity in the magnitudes of the corresponding ϕ_{ij}. Thus the conditions of the Malécot formulation are not satisfied and disaggregation of the parishes is essential for an interpretation of the effects of linear distance.

TOPOLOGY OF POPULATION STRUCTURE

When any pair of populations in an array has a high value of ϕ_{ij}, they have more common ancestry than pairs of populations with lower ϕ_{ij}. To the extent that geographical factors affect migration and hence kinship, the pattern of ϕ_{ij} values may reflect the geographical distances among populations. In order to analyze this possibility, kinship matrices predicted from migration and a matrix of the geographical distances separating the populations can be compared. The interdistance between each pair of parishes was calculated using the longitude and latitude of the parish church as the reference point. The distance (in kilometers) was calculated using the haversine formula for great circle arc distances.[10]

In order to investigate the topology of population structure, the kinship matrices and the matrix of geographical distances are both centroid-adjusted, producing two new matrices: A, with elements $a_{ij} = \phi_{ij} - \phi_{i.} - \phi_{.j} + \phi_{..}$, and B, with elements $b_{ij} = d_{ij} - d_{i.} - d_{.j} + d_{..}$. By using an X-Y coordinate system, the geographical distances between populations can be plotted in two-dimensional space using the first and second eigenvectors (scaled by the square root of their respective eigenvalues) of the distance matrix.[42,61] The kinship matrix and the matrix of geographical distances can be simultaneously plotted in two-dimensional space after norming and rotation to maximum congruence, so that the distance between "geography" and "kinship" locations is minimum.

The program MATFIT,[62] using the computational procedure of Schönemann and Carroll,[88] fits matrix A to matrix B by the method of least squares. The goodness of fit between the two matrices can be measured by Carroll's measure of disgreement, C_p, which expresses the distance between the two configurations relative to their norm.[61] Or the correlation between coordinates can be determined by $r_c = 1 - (C_p/2)$. Squaring r_c gives the approximate percentage of variation that is due to

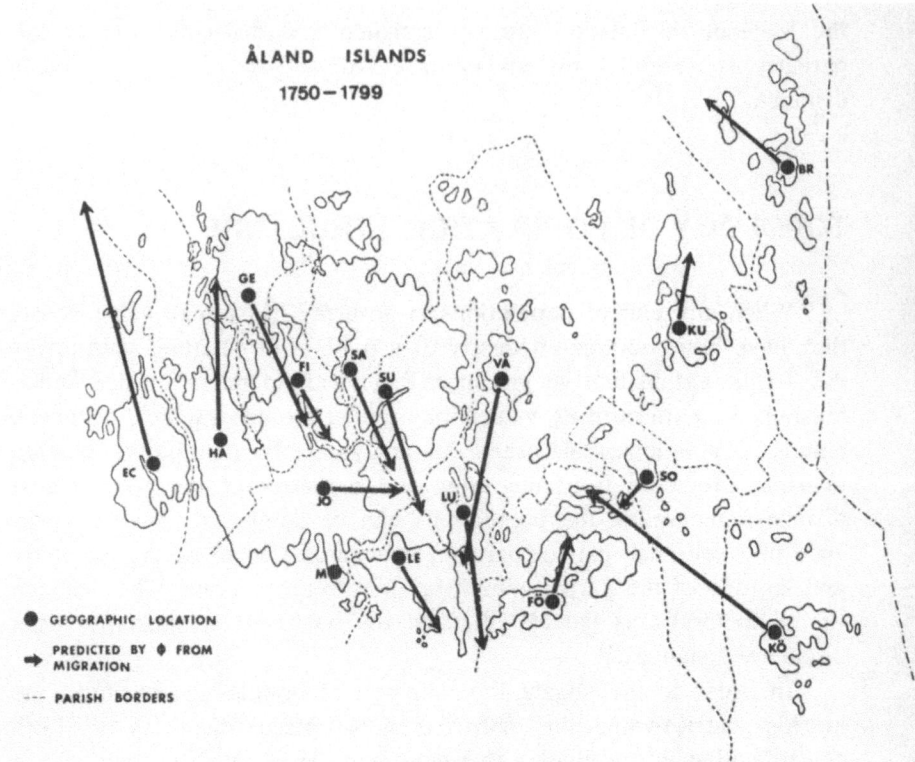

Fig. 7. Result of fitting kinship relations predicted by migration to the geographical
coordinates of the parishes for 1750–1799.

distance factors. There is a measurable amount of information loss
when this method is used because a multidimensional array is reduced
to two dimensions. However, it does provide a simple representation
from which many analytical results can be obtained.

The two-dimensional representations comparing "kinship" location
with "geographical" location are presented in Figs. 7-13. For the
period 1900–1949, the analysis was conducted twice—once with
Mariehamn included and once with it excluded—in order to examine
the influences of a single urban center on the population topology.

1750–1799

Figure 7 shows the result for 1750–1799 of fitting predicted kinship
from migration to the geographical coordinates. There is a 0.82

correlation (r_c) between the coordinates, and approximately 67% of the variation in the location predicted by ϕ_{ij} could be due to distance factors. Of the main island parishes, Eckerö is the most isolated, and both Lemland and Lumparland plot in a similar direction south and away from the main island cluster, indicating little exchange with the main island. Vårdö plots between Lemland and Lumparland, indicating greater exchange with these two parishes than the rest, or perhaps the origin of the majority of the inhabitants of Vårdö was Lemland/ Lumparland and the mating patterns have not changed drastically. The other main island parishes (Geta, Finström, Saltvik, Sund, and Jomala) all plot fairly close together, indicating mutual mate exchange among them. However, the relationship of Hammarland is not what one would

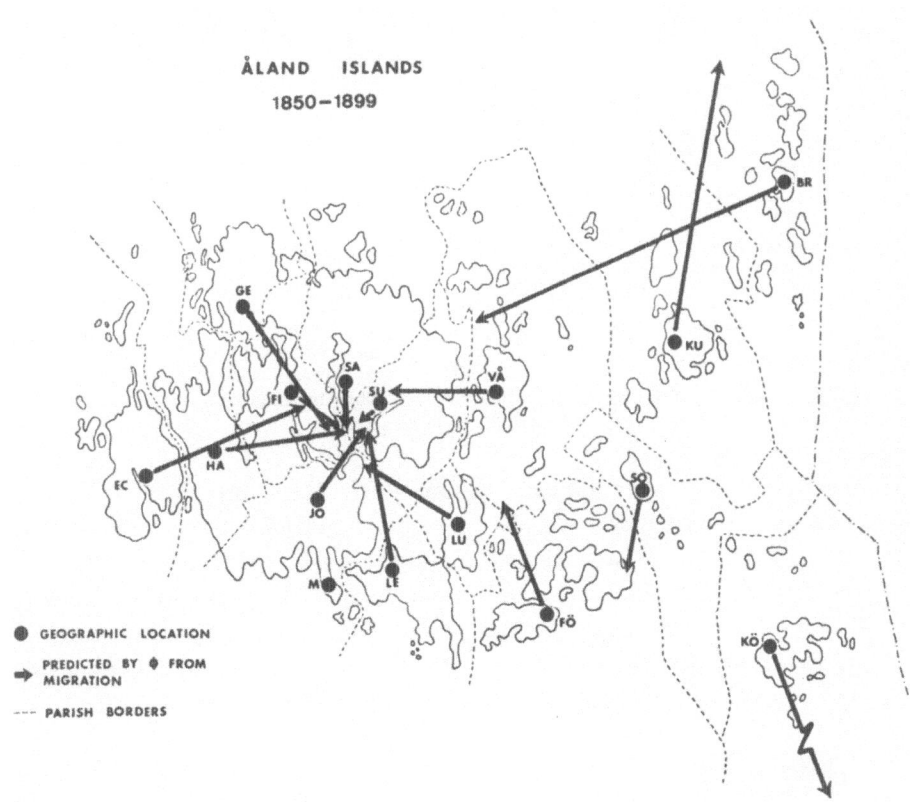

Fig. 8. Result of fitting kinship relations predicted by migration to the geographical coordinates of the parishes for 1850–1899.

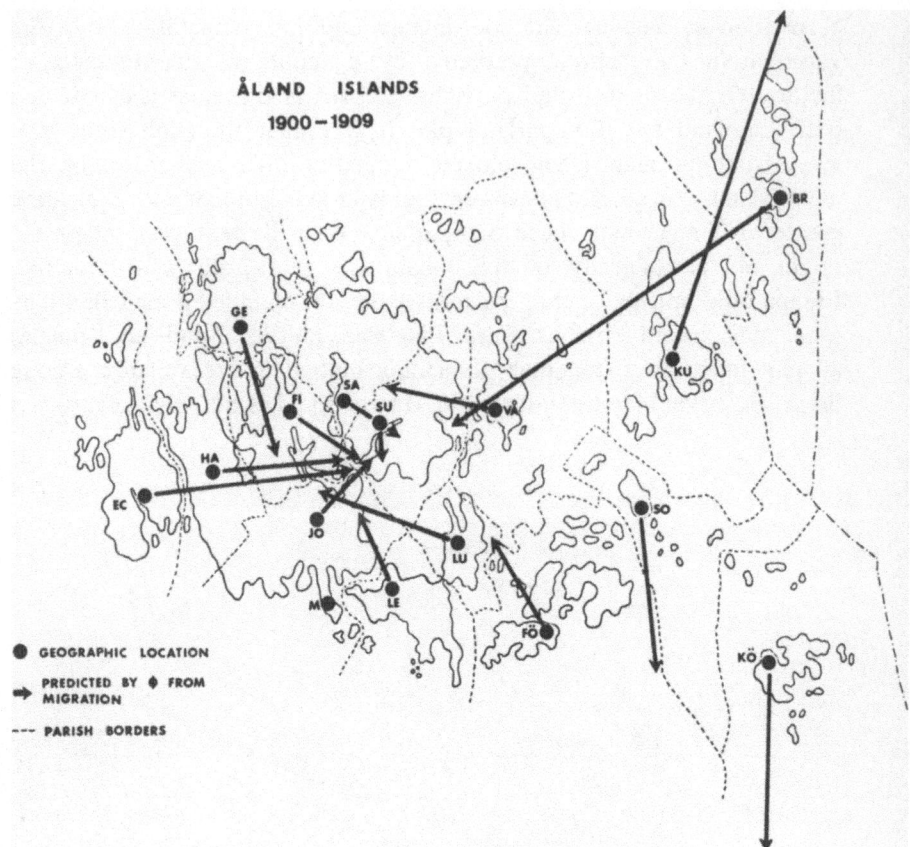

Fig. 9. Result of fitting kinship relations predicted by migration to the geographical coordinates of the parishes for 1900–1909.

expect due to geographical location alone. Hammarland plots close to Geta, suggesting considerable gene flow between these two parishes relative to the others. Föglö, Sottunga, and Kökar cluster together, suggesting possible homogeneity and similar gene frequencies among these three parishes during this period. Both Brändö and Kumlinge plot away from the rest of the archipelago, indicating greater isolation than is expected from the geographical location of these parishes.

1800–1849

The dimensional reduction for 1800–1849 is very similar to that for 1750–1799. In light of this, only a discussion of the configuration will be presented, without an accompanying figure. There is a 0.80 correlation between the coordinates of the two matrices. Most of the main island parishes tend to plot close together in the center of the island, suggesting a fair amount of gene flow between these parishes. Eckerö is still isolated, as are Lemland and Lumparland. Vårdö and Hammarland have shifted and plot toward the center of the main island grouping. As in 1750–1799, Föglö, Sottunga, and Kökar form a triad, suggesting continuation of gene flow among these three parishes and possible homogeneity in genetic structure during this period. Kumlinge and Brändö are still the most isolated of the parishes, again suggesting that there was greater isolation than would be expected due to distance.

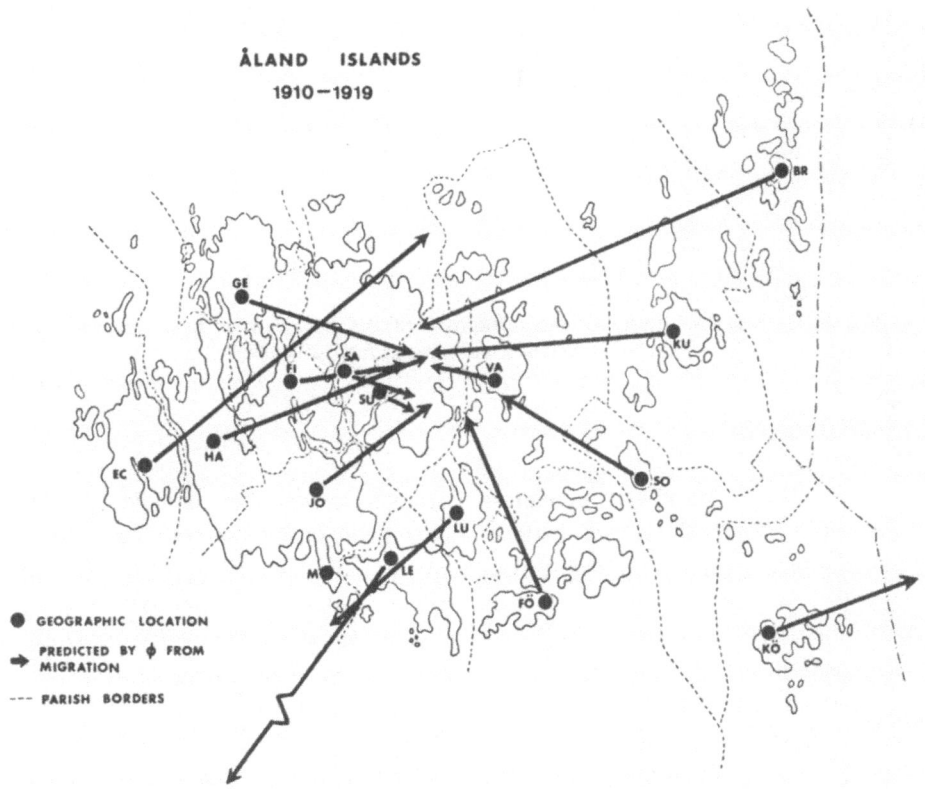

Fig. 10. Result of fitting kinship relations predicted by migration to the geographical coordinates of the parishes for 1910–1919.

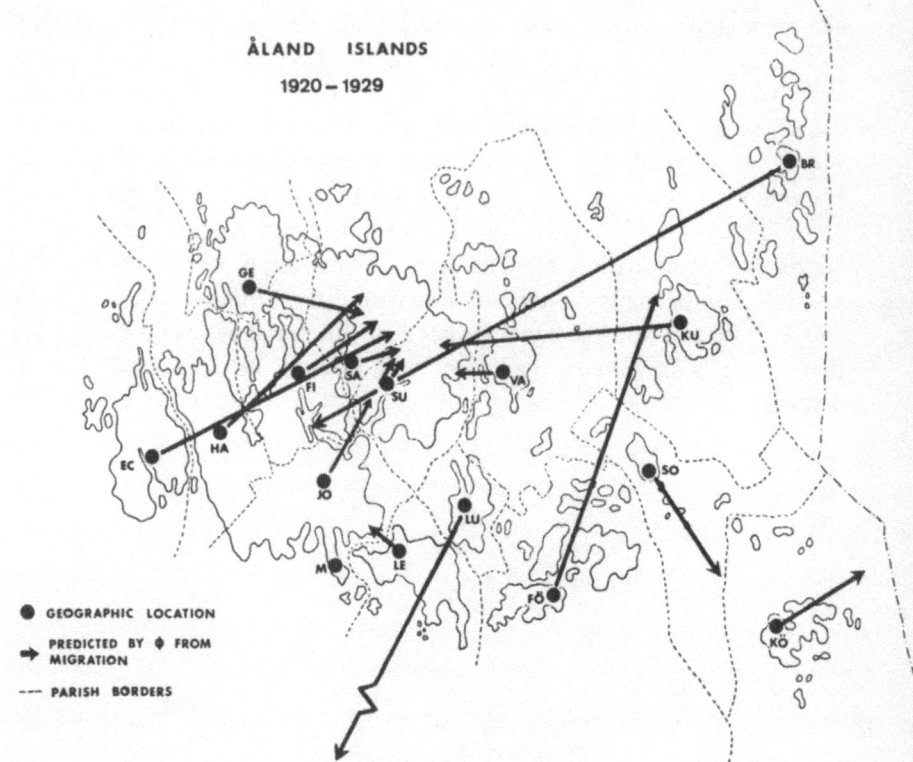

Fig. 11. Result of fitting kinship relations predicted by migration to the geographical coordinates of the parishes for 1920–1929.

1850–1899

For 1850–1899, correlation between coordinates is 0.74. During this period, all of the main island parishes plot toward the center, indicating mate exchange throughout the main island (Fig.8). Föglö and Brändö are drawn in toward the main island, in contrast to their positions during the two preceding periods, suggesting an increase in gene flow between each of these parishes and the main island cluster. Sottunga and Kökar are separated and isolated during this period, and Kumlinge is again isolated from the rest of the Åland archipelago. However, Kumlinge plots closer to Brändö than in the other periods, suggesting greater gene flow and homogeneity between these two parishes than during the earlier periods.

1900–1909

Figure 9 depicts for 1900–1909 the fit of migration and geography excluding the town parish of Mariehamn. The correlation between coordinates is 0.65. During this decade, all of the main island parishes plot close together, but they are less compact than during 1850–1899. This apparent separation may be in part due to the change in the period length (i.e., from a 50-year period to a 10-year period). The overall representation is similar to the preceding 50-year period, with the only substantial change being the predicted location of Brändö. Sottunga, Kökar, and Kumlinge again remain more isolated than would be predicted due to their geographical location. During this period,

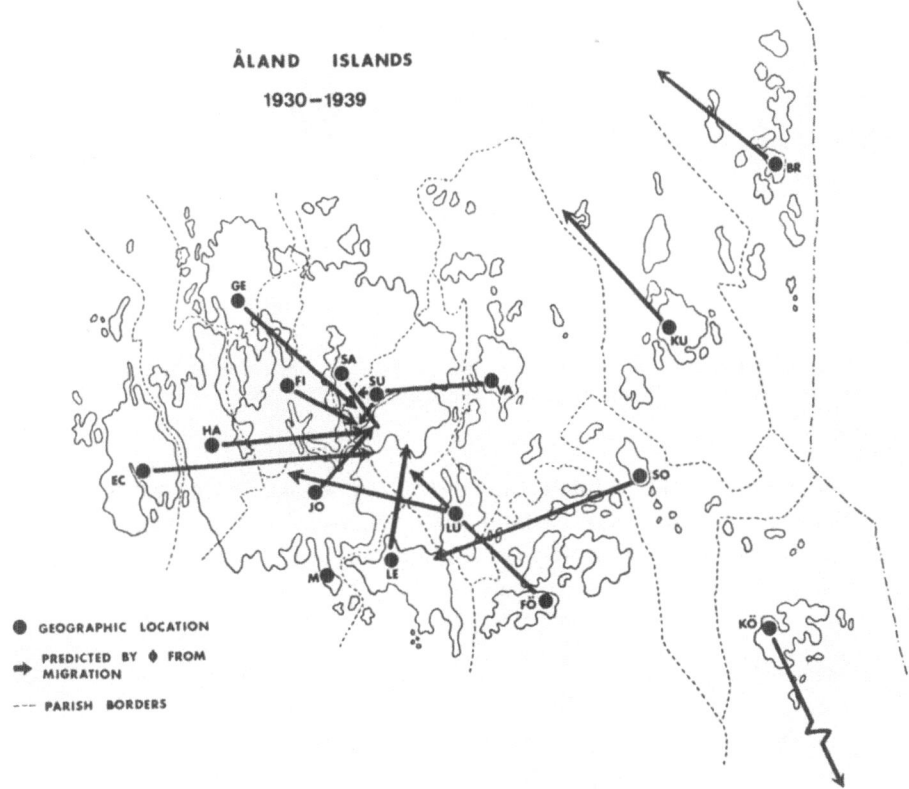

Fig. 12. Result of fitting kinship relations predicted by migration to the geographical coordinates of the parishes for 1930–1939.

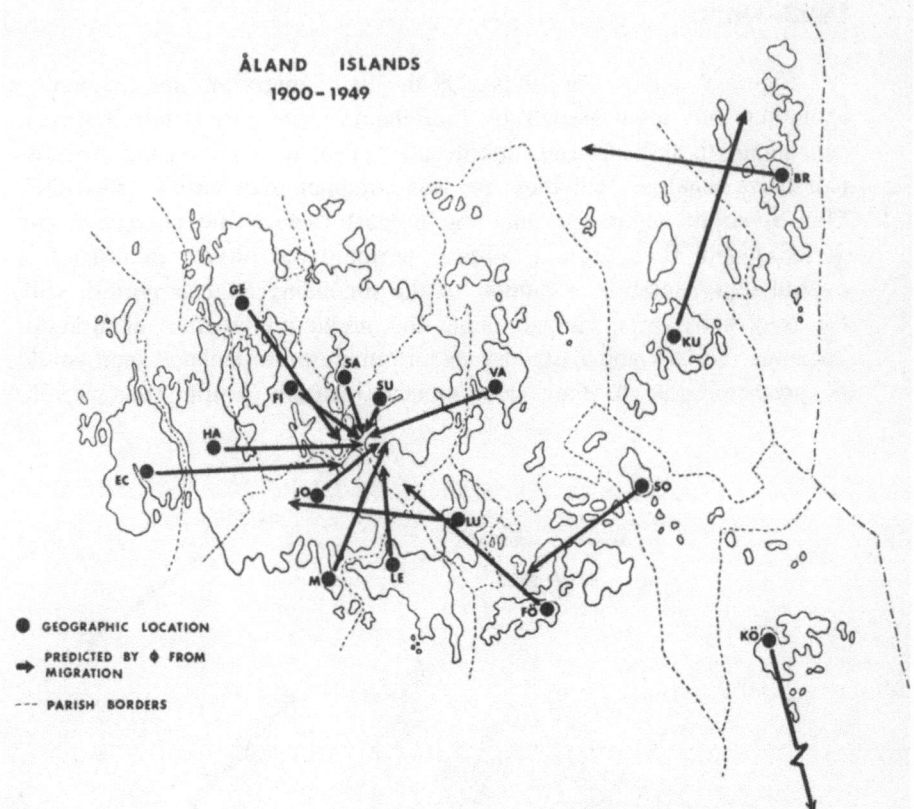

Fig. 13. Result of fitting kinship relations predicted by migration to the geographical coordinates of the parishes for 1900–1949.

emigration to the United States was at a maximum, as was the desertion of the outer islands and skerries. The change in the population composition may be partially responsible for the representation as indicated by this analysis.

1910–1919

Figure 10 represents the fit excluding Mariehamn for 1910–1919. The correlation between coordinates for this period is 0.47. During this period, the parishes become less compacted in the center of the main island than during the period 1900–1909. However, Föglö is pulled closer to the main island than before and both Kumlinge and Sottunga plot in toward the central area. This is the first period in which these two parishes seem to interact with the main island; earlier they were isolated or formed a relationship with the other outer islands. Still, both Lemland and Lumparland plot away from the rest of the grouping, indicating greater isolation than would be expected for this period. Kökar is again very isolated, plotting away from all of the rest of the archipelago.

1920-1929

For 1920–1929, the correlation between coordinates is 0.46. During this decade, there is a northeast shift of the plotted values for the main island parishes, tending to separate them from the other parishes except for Brändö (Fig. 11). Lemland plots back toward the main island, but Lumparland plots even farther away than in 1910–1919. Föglö appears to be exchanging with both Kumlinge and Brändö more than with the main island. Both Sottunga and Kökar are isolated, plotting away from the archipelago, with Sottunga plotting toward Kökar.

1930-1939

For 1930–1939, the correlation between coordinates is 0.73. All of the ten main island parishes plot closer together near the center of the island, indicating extensive gene flow among all of the subdivisions (Fig. 12). Sottunga and Föglö appear to be exchanging with the main island more than with the other outer island groups. The outer island parishes of Brändö, Kumlinge, and Kökar exhibit more isolation than during the preceding decade than would be expected due to the increased mate exchange.

1940-1949

Since the period 1940–1949 is similar to 1930–1939, no illustration will be provided. The correlation between coordinates is 0.51. Isolation by distance is not the major factor in determining the population topology of the Åland Islands during this decade. However, both Brändö and Kumlinge are again isolated (even more than during the preceding decade). Kökar is exchanging more with the main island grouping than ever before, suggesting a breakdown of its long-term isolation from the rest of the archipelago.

1900-1949

In order to obtain an overall view of the population topology during the first half of the twentieth century, the five 10-year periods were pooled together into one 50-year period. Figure 13 shows the result of fitting the predicted kinship from migration to the geographical location of the parishes for the 50-year period from 1900 to 1949. During this period, all of the main island parishes plot close to the center of the island, suggesting extensive breakdown of isolation by distance and increased gene flow as compared to the other 50-year periods. Of the outer island parishes, only Föglö and Sottunga appear to plot near the main island cluster, while Kökar, Kumlinge, and Brändö are isolated. The resultant configuration between Kumlinge and Brändö suggests that there is more gene flow between these two parishes than with the rest of the archipelago. In speculating, we suggest that the main island parishes plus Föglö and Sottunga are becoming genetically more homogeneous while Kumlinge and Brändö are becoming one unit but are drifting away from the main island. Kökar is the most isolated of all of the parishes, and this fact suggests that extensive genetic drift is likely.

The Inclusion of Mariehamn

If the urban parish of Mariehamn is included in these analyses of the population topology, there is little change in the resultant configurations. Mariehamn has less effect on the interrelationships of the other parishes early in time (i.e., 1900–1920), however, from 1920 to 1949 Mariehamn appears to act like long-range migration in an island model. The magnitude of the local kinship per parish drops slightly and all the plots are drawn closer together in the center of the main island.

TABLE X. Correlation between Coordinates, r_c, for All Time Periods and Geography

| Time period | Geography | Time period | | | | | | | |
		1750–1799	1800–1849	1850–1899	1900–1909	1910–1919	1920–1929	1930–1939	1940–1949
1750–1799	0.82	—							
1800–1849	0.80	0.95	—						
1850–1899	0.74	0.57	0.60	—					
1900–1909	0.65	0.51	0.54	0.96	—				
1910–1919	0.47	0.46	0.53	0.56	0.48	—			
1920–1929	0.46	0.44	0.57	0.61	0.60	0.67	—		
1930–1939	0.73	0.54	0.59	0.87	0.76	0.60	0.57	—	
1940–1949	0.51	0.53	0.49	0.53	0.57	0.19	0.22	0.49	—

Correlation between Coordinates

Table X summarizes the correlation between coordinates, r_c, for each time period and geography and between each period. There is a general decrease in the coefficients relating geography and kinship through time. This trend corresponds to the rather isolated parishes during the late eighteenth and early nineteenth centuries, and then the breakdown of isolation during the twentieth century. Table X also provides a summary of the relationship of each time period to all other periods. The periods 1750–1799 and 1800–1849 form one group (r_c = 0.95) and both of these time periods are different in their topology when compared to all the others. The periods 1850–1899 and 1900–1909 appear to be similar when judged according to the correlation between coordinates (r_c = 0.96), and it is also interesting to note that 1900–1909 and 1930–1939 are topologically similar; both of these time periods correspond to major emigration times in Åland's history. In general, there is more correspondence between time periods which are temporally close together than those temporally separated, indicating a gradual shift in the total population topology over the 200-year time span.

Summary of Topology

The two-dimensional representations comparing predicted kinship to the geographical location of the parishes provide a clear visual representation of population topology. In general, in the two earlier periods (1750–1850) the parishes were quite isolated, the general geographical location (main island, east or west; outer islands, north and south) having an important role in the differentiation of the subpopulation units. After 1850, it appears as though there was more exchange within the main island parishes, whereas the outer island parishes remained rather isolated even through 1949. Both Kökar and Brändö were almost always quite separated from the other parishes over the entire 200-year time span, indicating long-term isolation.

DISCUSSION OF MIGRATION ANALYSES

As shown by these analyses, the historic isolation of the Åland Islands continued into the latter half of the nineteenth century. Up to that time, parish endogamy remained high (greater than 80%) and long-range migrants contributed no more than 2.5% of the marriage partners. The actual isolation, however, may have been even higher than indicated. Åland was a stratified society with a small upper class of landowners, clergy, professionals, and sea captains. Preliminary studies indicate that this class was relatively endogamous, but its small size made it necessary to obtain marriage partners from other parishes or from outside of Åland. A large number of landless tenant farmers, servants, artisans, and their families made up the relatively more isolated lower classes. For these individuals, marriages were almost always with mates from the same parish; in fact, special dispensation from the church was required for interparish migration. Although the present analysis has focused on the parish, subdivision of each parish into a larger number of villages or community groupings showed that there was also very high local endogamy within parishes and that interparish matings were quite often between communities at short distances but separated by parish boundaries.

Technological changes in fishing techniques may have contributed much to the increase in migration which occurred between the middle nineteenth century and the first decades of the twentieth century. The farm owners also owned the fishing rights for areas adjacent to their land, and up to the middle nineteenth century most of the fishing was in these immediate offshore waters. Beginning in the 1840s new techniques permitted fishing in open, uncontrolled waters, and in the late 1880s deep sea fishing nets were introduced. This permitted formerly landless tenant farmers to earn their living solely by fishing, and new settlements both on the main island and on formerly uninhabited islands were established. An investigation of the migration patterns among social and economic classes should contribute to our understanding of the effects of this change on the isolation. The influence of urbanization and its impact on commerce, and hence the opportunity for social and geographical mobility, must be explored. Genealogical analyses are also necessary. The extent to which marriages between partners from different parishes actually represent gene flow, and not the continued interaction of already related but dispersed groups, must be established.

The striking changes which occurred from 1930 on can be seen in Table XI, which shows both the proportion of mates from outside Åland and the proportion of marriage partners in a parish coming from other parishes. Prior to the 1930s, these proportions had risen slowly; for all of Åland, the increase in long-range marriage partners was only 0.037 from 1750 to 1929. The subsequent rise to 0.225 as well as the increase in exchange among parishes meant that within one decade the average percentage of all mates from outside the parish of residence rose from 0.208 in 1920–1929 to 0.687 in 1930–1939. A number of factors may be involved in this change. The first motorized sea transport among parishes was introduced in 1930 and this must have led to a great increase in the mobility of all of the Ålanders. At the same time, increase in the Baltic fishing industry and in diversified commercial enterprises in the main island must also have led to greater movement. During the depression years, many Ålanders who had previously emigrated to Sweden or the United States returned, at least temporarily, to Åland; there, the essentially agricultural base of the economy appears to have minimized the effects of the primarily commercial disaster. This may also account, in part, for an increased immigration from outside of Åland. An analysis of the socioeconomic factors which may have been involved in this increase in movement is clearly required.

TABLE XI. Proportion of Mates from Outside (O) the Åland Islands and from Parishes Within (I) Åland Which Differ from the Parish (or Parishes) of Marital Residence

Time period	Total population[a]		Mariehamn		Jomala		Geta		Kökar		Brändö		Brändö and Kumlinge		Outer island parishes	
	O	I	O	I	O	I	O	I	O	I	O	I	O	I	O	M[b]
1750–1799	0.022	0.103	—	—	0.027	0.059	0.020	0.119	0.048	0.020	0.033	0.018	0.028	0.015	0.027	0.012
1800–1849	0.017	0.086	—	—	0.022	0.065	0.016	0.097	0.041	0.026	0.013	0.031	0.016	0.022	0.025	0.009
1850–1899	0.024	0.172	—	—	0.030	0.071	0.027	0.106	0.018	0.021	0.055	0.022	0.039	0.011	0.031	0.011
1900–1909	0.036	0.107	0.075	0.125	0.047	0.089	0.010	0.080	0.034	0.025	0.120	0.030	0.076	0.029	0.051	0.023
1910–1919	0.053	0.144	0.084	0.133	0.069	0.142	0.050	0.100	0.035	0.018	0.040	0.066	0.059	0.028	0.051	0.016
1920–1929	0.059	0.149	0.184	0.095	0.033	0.139	0.029	0.206	0.055	0.046	0.071	0.021	0.070	0.025	0.056	0.024
1930–1939	0.225	0.462	0.410	0.439	0.218	0.244	0.131	0.246	0.066	0.090	0.085	0.104	0.112	0.069	0.162	0.061
1940–1949	0.251	0.484	0.394	0.471	0.259	0.306	0.187	0.253	0.211	0.067	0.102	0.058	0.095	0.060	0.163	0.074

[a] Including Mariehamn.
[b] Main island parishes.

One feature which emerges from all the analyses is the marked heterogeneity between main island and outer island parishes. Prior to the middle of the eighteenth century, the effects of migration were much the same throughout the Åland Islands. However, as can be seen in Table XI for the entire period from 1750 to the present, there is more long-range migration to the outer islands than migration from the main island parishes. The data show that much of this is due to mate exchange with the Swedish-speaking inhabitants in the geographically closer Åboland archipelago. This pattern is especially true for Brändö and Kumlinge, which form a subgroup still quite isolated within Åland. There are also special parish associations, such as between Lemland and Lumparland, or Föglö/Sottunga/Kökar, which have existed for centuries. Presumably, this reflects their geographical proximity, but it also suggests that migration among parishes within such clusters may not have much effect on reducing genetic isolation. Research using genealogies and exact individual mating distances may provide more insight into these questions.

Originally, the focus on Åland suggested a unique opportunity to examine the structure of an extremely isolated population, itself composed of isolated subpopulations. The present results suggest that studies in Åland will also tell us as much about the process of a rapid breakup of isolation and its genetic consequences. Since the changes occurred so recently, the present population contains both individuals whose inbreeding coefficient must be relatively high due to long periods of isolation and consanguinity and those whose parents were relatively unrelated Ålanders or included one mate from outside of Åland. The marked heterogeneity among parishes should also be reflected in the distributions of individuals homozygous for rare recessive disorders. Thus the contemporary population, although numerically small, contains both a genetically heterogeneous urban population and subgroups with widely varying degrees of genetic homogeneity. In the design of future research programs, this stratification can be utilized in many ways. For example, genetic analyses can stratify samples by age, by place of birth vs. place of residence, or by the birthplaces of parents, grandparents, or more remote ancestors, in order to demonstrate the changing patterns of genetic heterogeneity which must have occurred in the past century. Such data can then be compared with migration matrices from different periods. Given the high rate of migration since 1930, and the demonstrated rapid approach to equilibrium under such migration pressure, structure revealed by these data sources should become more congruent as the time period under study becomes more contemporary. These results also show that for historical inference from genetic structure present-day distributions of gene frequencies would not be of much use without the information supplied by the historical material.

PART II

BIOLOGICAL STUDIES

Research in Åland has been concerned with diverse aspects of human biological variation including twinning,[19-22,24] anthropometry,[2,56,57] epidemiology,[87] hematology,[54,63] normal and pathological ophthalmological traits,[17,23,32,33,35-38,99,100] and population genetics.[23,25,26,29-31] In the following sections, we shall review some of the major results of this work, show how it relates to our understanding of Åland population structure, and discuss the present and proposed contributions which are facilitated by the use of the parish records.

Genetic Analyses

Analyses of the genetic structure of the Åland Islands, using contemporary gene frequencies, were designed to give insight into the relative roles of gene flow and genetic drift among Åland parishes as well as to compare the gene pool in Åland with that in surrounding regions. Without ancillary historical or archival (genealogical) material, however, interpretations of patterns of genetic variation are subject to considerable uncertainty. The process underlying contemporary genetic variation can never be inferred directly from a structural analysis since the time depth of the process is unknown and diverse processual models can be shown to fit the data equally well. However, with the use of genealogical records, the contemporary genetic sample can be partitioned into subgroups reflecting different amounts of short- or long-range gene flow and the historical factors affecting current variation can be better understood.

Field studies were carried out in the Åland Islands in 1958–1962,[23] on the main island in 1968,[56] and in the outer island parishes in 1970.[29-31] For all of the main island parishes, we have thus far obtained gene frequencies for only the ABO, Rhesus, MN, P, and PTC (taste test) systems. For some of the smaller main island parishes, very small samples were obtained, and in order to study genetic differentiation among these groups it has been necessary to combine certain parishes so that adequate sample sizes could be used.[26] Those parishes which were historically united in a single parish and, as already discussed, show high similarity throughout the eighteenth and nineteenth centuries were combined in the analyses as follows: Eckerö and Hammarland; Geta and Finström; Sund and Vårdö; and Lemland and Lumparland. For each of these pairs, a high degree of genetic similarity between parishes was observed in the migration analyses for 1750–1900. The outer island parishes, especially Kökar, have been studied much more extensively, and in these groups there are also observations on the Kell, Kidd, Duffy, and Lewis blood group systems, and on serum protein types (haptoglobin, transferrin, group specific) and red cell enzymes (phosphoglucomutase, adenylate kinase, adenosine deaminase, acid phosphatase). In addition, smaller samples of the γ-globulin allotypes[96] and pseudocholinesterase[91] have been examined.

Genealogical information was collected for each individual in the sample, both by direct interview and by examination of the parish records, regarding at least four generations of ancestors. Subjects with ancestors born outside of matrimony, or of unknown origin, or with ancestors not coming from the province of Åland were excluded from the analyses. In this way it was hoped that we could obtain a relatively "pure" Ålandic sample not affected by long-range migration during the past century or two, and for which recent historical gene flow, among Åland parishes, could be specified. In the analysis discussed here, the sample was further restricted to individuals with at least three of the four grandparents from the same parish. Their phenotypes were assigned to a parish on the basis of grandparental origin, regardless of the present residence. In this sample, such stratification provides an approximation to the pattern of genetic variation which may have

TABLE XII. Gene Frequencies in Åland, Sweden, and Finland

	Åland[26,29-31,96]			Sweden			Finland		
	Sample size	Weighted mean frequency	Range among parishes	Sample size	Gene frequency	Reference	Sample size	Gene frequency	Reference
A_1		0.202	0.096–0.280		0.222			0.213	
A_2	1818	0.079	0.018–0.133	10,457	0.086	(4)	5,536	0.096	(82)
B		0.070	0.019–0.136		0.077			0.132	
O		0.649	0.548–0.819		0.616			0.559	
R^0		0.014	0.000–0.116		0.018			0.037	
R^1		0.437	0.327–0.556		0.415			0.429	
R^2	1702	0.137	0.074–0.245	8,488	0.170	(4)	5,536	0.184	(82)
R^z		0.006	0.000–0.035		—			—	
r		0.402	0.246–0.516		0.381			0.338	
r'		0.005	0.000–0.016		0.013			0.011	

M	1153	0.545	0.409–0.661	10,457	0.570	(4)	5,536	0.643	(82)
k	857	0.950	0.939–0.981	4,527	0.964	(45)	5,536	0.980	(82)
Jk^a	376	0.412	0.279–0.486	—	—		—	—	
Fy^a	381	0.560	0.451–0.614	344	0.422	(46)	5,536	0.471	(82)
Le	453	0.582	0.501–0.787	—	—		—	—	
Hp^1	828	0.339	0.312–0.383	1,003	0.375	(6, 97)	5,536	0.381	(82)
Gc^1	666	0.668	0.643–0.690	1,744	0.743	(48, 70)	5,536	0.795	(82)
PGM_1^1	379	0.839	0.789–0.909	412	0.772	(5)	406	0.761	(29)
AK^1	379	0.960	0.906–0.991	505	0.965	(93)	406	0.967	(30)
ADA^1	383	0.914	0.826–0.971	342	0.936	(1)	1,404	0.903	(31)
P^A	378	0.271	0.150–0.342	517	0.372	(11)	264	0.375	(31)
P^B		0.656	0.579–0.733		0.558			0.494	
P^C		0.073	0.039–0.117		0.070			0.131	
Tf^C	557	0.980	0.951–1.000	2,395	0.995	(7)	5,536	0.978	(82)
Tf^B		0.012	0.000–0.016		0.005			0.013	
$Tf^D Chi$		0.008	0.000–0.034		0.001			0.009	

characterized the Åland Islands during the middle and latter nineteenth century, prior to the subsequent increase in local and long-range migration already demonstrated by migration analyses of data in the archival records.

Genetic Variation in Åland, Sweden, and Finland

The gene frequencies in this Åland sample and in Sweden and Finland are presented in Table XII, for loci where comparable data are available. The Swedish frequencies are based on samples from throughout the contemporary population. The Finnish gene frequencies are primarily from the study of Nevanlinna,[82] in which the sample, drawn randomly from the entire country, was restricted to individuals born in the same rural village from which their parents came. These data correspond to a genetic characterization of rural Finland at the end of the nineteenth century. In general, gene frequencies throughout Finland and Scandinavia are similar,[8,20] and the mean parish frequencies in Åland clearly resemble those in the surrounding countries. The largest Finnish–Swedish differences are at the M allele (MNSs system) and the B allele (ABO system). For both of these alleles, as would be expected, the frequencies in Åland correspond to those in Sweden.

Research in progress may add much to our present understanding of the larger patterns of regional differentiation in Fenno-Scandia. The Ålanders are believed to be primarily derived from the Swedish population in the region around Uppsala, and later gene flow from this group may have taken place when the Ålanders moved, temporarily, back to Sweden during the Great Northern War at the start of the eighteenth century. There is sufficient regional differentiation within Sweden[4] that a partition of the Swedish population itself may make more suitable comparisons with Ålandic frequencies. In addition, in Finland, there are two separate regions of Swedish-speaking Finns, only partly intermixed with the native Finnish population. Historical records indicate migration fields from Sweden to Finland, as well as from Finland to Sweden, which cross the Åboland and Åland archipelagos. Genetic and genealogical studies in these areas are now being completed,[82] and a partition of Finland into regions with differing likelihoods of affinities with Åland will also be possible. Given the large numbers of polymorphisms which can be utilized, and the existence of archival material of great time depth in both Finland and

Sweden, the prospects for more detailed and informative regional studies appear promising.

Genetic Differentiation among Åland Island Parishes

The general similarity of the average Ålandic frequencies to those in Sweden suggests that differentiation among Åland parishes would be due more to isolation and drift or interparish patterns of gene flow than to differential gene flow from the non-Swedish outside world. Inference on the possible occurrence of long-range gene flow was presented by Steinberg et al.,[96] who found the Gm haplotype[1,5,13,14] in two distantly related individuals born in the same parish. Since this haplotype is common in Negroids and Melanesians, one could speculate on the possibility that the ancient Viking travels may have resulted in the incorporation of genes of quite distant origin. Nevertheless, excepting a small historical contribution from the Finns, the Ålanders are likely to be almost entirely descended from an eastern Swedish founder population. The marital migration matrices show that the contribution from Sweden during 1750–1900 was generally quite low; and according to histories of earlier centuries the effect of Sweden on Ålandic frequencies is likely to have been small for several centuries.

As can be seen in Table XII, the ranges of gene frequencies among parishes are often quite large, suggesting a rather striking degree of isolation and drift and/or extensive differences in founder populations. The outer islands are known to have been settled by migrants from the main island several centuries earlier and these original founders may have represented small groups of related individuals. The observed genetic variation is also accompanied by substantial morphological differentiation. For example, the parishes of Sottunga and Kökar formerly shared a single parish church, and, today, their respective churches are only 25 km apart. Yet, individuals in these parishes differ rather substantially in both gene frequencies and physical appearance. Eriksson and Forsius[23] note differences in hair pigmentation, and their observations on the distribution of eye color types are shown in Table XIII. The percentages of brown eyes among males and females are 8.1 and 5.9 in Sottunga and 20.3 and 23.4 in Kökar. Genealogical studies also have confirmed the extreme marital isolation of these parishes over the past ten to 12 generations.

TABLE XIII. Percent Frequencies of Eye Color Types on the Åland
Islands According to the Martin–Saller Classification[a]

Region	Eye color types								Number tested
	1	2	3	4	5	6	7	8	
Main island									
Males	18.2	25.0	17.1	33.2	2.4	2.4	1.7	—	292
Females	9.7	29.0	18.8	30.4	4.8	3.2	3.2	0.8	372
Sottunga									
Males	24.3	27.0	18.9	21.6	8.1	—	—	—	37
Females	9.8	43.1	19.6	21.6	3.9	—	2.0	—	51
Kökar									
Males	42.6	25.0	6.8	5.4	10.8	4.7	4.1	0.7	148
Females	20.8	33.5	17.0	5.3	13.8	5.3	3.2	1.1	188

[a] Columns 5–8 represent brown iris types. On the main island, Sottunga, and
Kökar, the respective frequency figures for the total numbers of brown eyes
are 6.5, 8.1, and 20.3% among males and 12.1, 5.9, and 23.4% among
females. The differences between the three regions are highly significant. The
neighboring island parishes of Kökar and Sottunga differ markedly in regard
to iris pigmentation.

The effect of isolation and inbreeding, as well as the impact of
gene flow, is also apparent in the studies on Kökar. Seppälä *et al*[90]
examined the distribution of the transferrin phenotypes in a large
sample of Kökar Islanders. The distribution observed was CC, 315;
B_2C, eight; CD_{Chi}, two. The two CD_{Chi} individuals were a father and
child, the father having emigrated to Åland from Finland. The eight
B_2C individuals were found to be members of three different families,
two of which were closely related. Further genealogical analysis
showed that all three families had a common female ancestor born in
1787 whose ancestors were all from Kökar, at least back to the middle
seventeenth century. This woman was married twice and in both of her
descendencies there are B_2C subjects.

Genetic differentiation among parishes can also be examined by
calculation of matrices of similarity or dissimilarity (e.g., distance)
coefficients.[41,42] For the Åland data, we have used the BIOKIN
computer program developed by Morton and his associates.[113] This
program utilizes phenotype data and yields a symmetrical matrix of

coefficients, r_{ij}, analogous to those derived from a straightforward variance/covariance matrix over gene frequencies in an array of populations. The diagonal elements of this matrix, r_{ii}, denote what has been called "local kinship." That is, r_{ii} denotes the net genetic divergence of the frequencies in the ith population from the mean frequencies in the array. The off diagonal elements, r_{ij}, describe the extent of covariation among corresponding gene frequencies for a pair of populations. Under Morton's model these frequencies are taken to represent a sample from an idealized and unknown founder population in the same region, and the coefficients are taken as estimates of "conditional kinship."[73] True kinship relative to a founder population, denoted by ϕ_{ij}, which is predicted directly from a migration matrix analysis, is assumed to be related to the r_{ij} by the relation $\phi_{ij} = r_{ij} + (1-r_{ij})\phi_R$, where ϕ_R is the kinship of random individuals from the region. Since alternative models using no assumptions about kinship and treating the data solely in terms of contemporary genetic correlations have been shown to provide the same inference on population structure,[104] the importance of the kinship interpretation need not be of concern here.

The matrix of conditional kinship coefficients is given in Table XIV. For some analyses, a squared genetic distance,[26] θ, was derived from these coefficients. Another squared distance measure for populations i and j can be computed directly by $d^2_{ij} = r_{ii} + r_{jj} - 2r_{ij}$. In this model of genetic structure, the coefficients are all scaled relative to the mean gene frequencies in the total array. This procedure assumes a phylogenetic derivation from a common population, likely in the present case. However, BIOKIN uses sample sizes as weights assuming that these figures represent equivalent proportions of the total census population, or of the purported founder populations. However, with unequal sample sizes there can be a bias of the array means toward the values of the larger samples. In that case, the diagonal values would reflect both real divergence and the degree to which the local sample contributed to the grand mean. The diagonal values in Table XIV are probably subject to such a bias. Although Kökar is known to be very isolated, the intensive studies in that parish resulted in a sample size providing a much larger proportion of the total sample than its census size would otherwise warrant. Thus Kökar does not appear to be one of the most isolated populations. Despite this bias,

TABLE XIV. Estimates of Conditional Kinship ($r_{ij} \times 10^4$) for the Åland Islands Obtained from BIOKIN[a] (above the diagonal) and Geographical Distances in Kilometers (below the diagonal[b])

Parish		1, 2	3, 4	5	6, 7	8	9, 10	11	12	13	14	15
Eckerö/ Hammarland	1, 2	163	49	−135	34	54	−8	7	6	43	57	−31
Geta/Finström	3, 4	16.8	59	15	51	24	−52	13	−102	−21	38	−97
Saltvik	5	22.6	12.1	131	−3	101	−103	43	49	−48	−17	23
Sund/Vårdö	6, 7	30.5	21.7	9.6	50	−40	−45	43	−134	−2	13	−49
Jomala	8	14.5	18.8	15.3	19.3	71	−62	−10	−9	−30	21	10
Lemland/ Lumparland	9, 10	30.6	31.1	21.4	16.9	16.2	175	−111	39	−13	25	125
Föglö	11	44.3	43.2	32.1	24.4	29.8	13.7	138	28	−38	−7	−78
Scottunga	12	54.0	48.6	36.6	27.1	39.9	25.3	14.7	346	−101	−17	38
Kökar	13	74.2	72.0	60.1	51.0	59.8	43.6	29.9	24.9	85	−69	−79
Kumlinge	14	56.5	46.2	34.9	26.1	44.3	34.1	29.0	17.1	38.7	107	23
Brändö	15	76.4	62.9	53.8	46.9	66.2	58.2	53.6	40.4	56.0	24.7	160

[a] Omitting P and Lewis systems.
[b] Based on longitude/latitude of parish church; pooled parishes-midpoint between churches taken for location.

the coefficients in this table do indicate general features of the genetic structure of Åland.

The most divergent or isolated parish appears to be Sottunga, which has, among Åland parishes, the highest frequencies of P^A (acid phosphatase locus), R^0 (Rh system), P (P blood group locus), O (ABO locus), and Gc^2, and PGM_1^2, as well as the lowest frequencies of B (ABO locus) and r (Rh system). The least divergent parishes are those central in the main island: Geta/Finström, Sund/Vårodö, and Jomala. Among the main island parishes, numbered 1 to 8, seven of the ten r_{ij} are positive, which indicates a common pattern of covariation. For genetic data, the average degree of covariation would have $r_{ij} = 0$; positive r_{ij} indicate a greater than average similarity in the pattern of gene frequencies, negative values a less than average degree of similarity. The outer island parishes are relatively less similar to each other; only three of the ten r_{ij} are positive. Between the main island (1–8) and outer island parishes there is also a low degree of similarity, with 13 of 30 r_{ij} being positive. Thus, excepting the geographically more isolated main island parishes of Lemland and Lumparland, the main island seems to comprise a relatively homogeneous subgroup within Åland. Among the outer island parishes, Brändö and Kumlinge to the north show positive covariation with each other but much less so with the three southeastern parishes, Föglö, Sottunga, and Kökar. This pattern is also apparent in the migration analyses.

Geography and Genetic Structure

The Influence of Linear Distance

Using the matrix of coefficients and geographical distances in Table XIV, one can also explore the possibility of a relation between genetic divergence and either linear geographical distances among parishes or the general two-dimensional geographical location of the parishes. As discussed previously, for particular distributions of marital distances, in infinitely large populations, the coefficient of kinship, ϕ, decreases with increasing distance according to the relation $\phi(d) = ae^{-bd}d^{-c}$. Morton[75-77] has shown that for genetic estimates $r_{ij} = (1 - L)\,ae^{-bd} + L$, where $L = \phi_R(1 - r)$, provides the appropriate

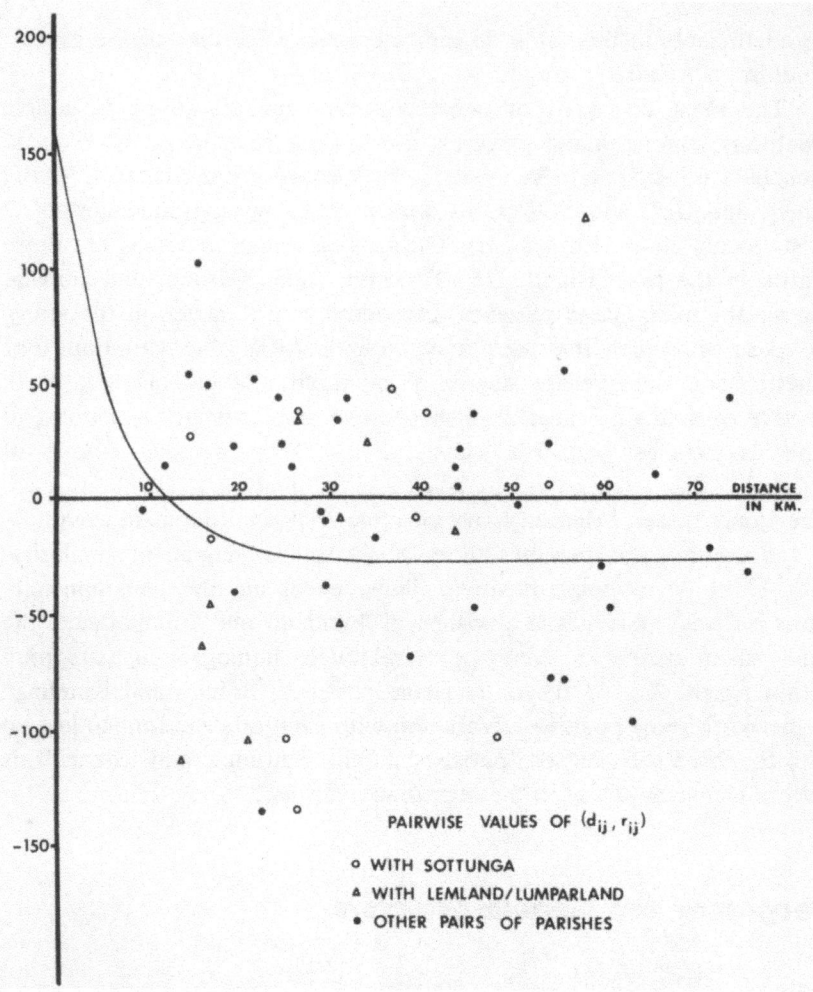

Fig. 14. Genetic covariation and linear distance in Åland. Theoretical curve
$[r(d) = (1 - L)ae^{-bd} + L]$ fitted to seven distance classes.

basis for the estimation of the Malécot parameters. In Fig. 14, each of
the 55 values of (d_{ij}, r_{ij}) is plotted together with the curve resulting from
a fit of the theoretical curve to a seven-class partition. The estimates of
the parameters are $a = 0.0156 \pm 0.0008$, $b = 0.539 \pm 0.0439$, $L =$
-0.0029. The published studies on other populations show that only
Alpine isolates have an equivalently high b value. The actual data as

seen in the scattered points and Table XIV are more informative than a simple analytical reduction. There are generally shorter distances among the parishes on the main island (18.1 km among groups 1–8 and 19.8 km among groups 1–10) than among the outer islands (32.9 km among groups 11–15). The greater covariation (and shorter genetic distances) among the main island parishes presumably reflects increasing mate exchange facilitated by land passages over shorter distances. However, if all pairs of parishes are considered within this region there is no apparent relation between distance and the value of r_{ij} in the points. Nor is there any apparent association within the outer islands or between the main and outer islands. Thus any decline noted in the grouped curve would seem to reflect a pattern of regional heterogeneity in the intensity of mate exchange and not a relation between distance and "kinship" *per se*.

Underlying the attempt to understand the effect of linear distance by fitting a theoretical curve is the concept of systematic effect of distance which is homogeneous throughout the population. Such an assumption is directly incorporated into Malécot's theoretical results. On the other hand, disaggregation of the data on the supposition that there may be heterogeneous distance relations proves to be a more meaningful approach to the study of Åland population structure.

The parishes of Sottunga and Lemland/Lumparland appear to be isolates whose patterns of covariation with other parishes do not reflect any systematic relation between the r_{ij} and linear distance. Lemland and Lumparland show positive covariation only with Sottunga, Brändö, and Kumlinge, all outer island parishes. This may reflect the water passages which link these parishes and the geographical structure of the main island, in which the road distance to Lemland and Lumparland greatly exceeds the straight-line distance. Examination of the relation between the r_{ij} and distance with and without these parishes reveals an otherwise obscured role of geographical distance on genetic covariation. In Fig. 15, the cumulative (unweighted) average of the r_{ij} over increasing pairwise distances is plotted together with the same function omitting the isolates. For the curve averaged over all parishes there appears to be a decline of the average r_{ij} only within a radius of 25 km and this curve closely resembles the results of fitting the modified Malécot function to the grouped data. However, when the two isolated groups are excluded there is a marked peak around 20 km followed by a consistent decline which reflects a generally decreasing

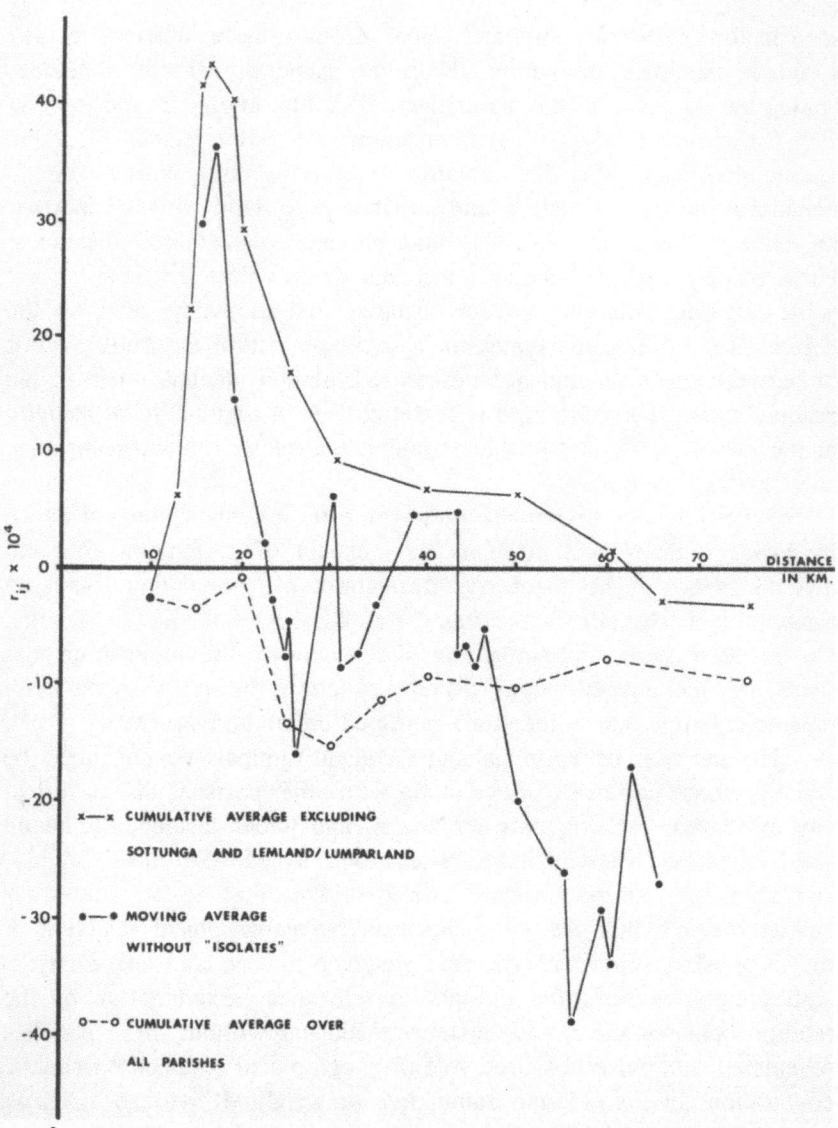

Fig. 15. Cumulative average of r_{ij} with increasing geographical distance among Åland Island parishes and moving average of the r_{ij} over every seven consecutive distances.

r_{ij} with increasing distance. In Fig. 15 a moving average of the r_{ij}, taken over every seven consecutively increasing pairwise distances, is also shown. In this curve there are seen to be two peaks, one just under 20 km and one about 40 km. Closer inspection of the data of Table XIV shows that the first peak and decline relate to relations among main island parishes, for which all distances are less than 31 km. The second peak and subsequent decline reflect primarily relations between main island and outer island parishes, whose distances range from 24.4 to 76.4 km. Up to 50 km, seven of the ten r_{ij} are positive; beyond 50 kilometers, only four of ten are positive. Among the outer island parishes, Brändö and Kumlinge, about 25 km apart, have a positive covariation; all other pairs show a negative relation. Thus there appear to be different functional relations between distance and genetic similarity relating to large regional considerations, i.e., a difference for exchanges among main island parishes and between the main and outer island parishes. In addition, isolation of some parishes and, probably, special ancestral or marital exchange relations must be involved. Overall, the effect of linear distance can be inferred to have a major role on a portion of the pattern of covariation. This result supports the point discussed with respect to migration analyses; within finite subdivided populations, pooled data and analyses do not accurately reflect the effects of isolation by distance.

Two-Dimensional Space and Genetic Distance

By procedures already discussed, a two-dimensional reduction of the genetic structure can be rotated to optimal congruence with the geographical structure of the Åland Islands. Using the genetic distance derived by the BIOKIN program, Θ, and "conditional" kinship computed without using the P and Le systems, the configuration shown in Fig. 16 was obtained. The Le and P systems are especially subject to typing errors, and, as discussed by Eriksson et al.,[26] their exclusion from this analyses seemed warranted. The actual correlation between coordinates, approximately 0.5, suggests that perhaps 25% of the total variation might be related to geographical structure. However, the effect of the isolation of Lemland and Lumparland and the anomalous position of Sottunga on the total correlation is misleading. The general geographical locations of the parishes are reflected in their genetic location. The main island parishes form a western cluster within which differentiation seems to be quite random. Brändö and Kumlinge are positioned to the northeast and Kökar and Föglö to the southeast. Despite the evident random genetic differentiation not related to geographical structure, there is clearly an influence of the regional geography on the pattern of genetic variation.

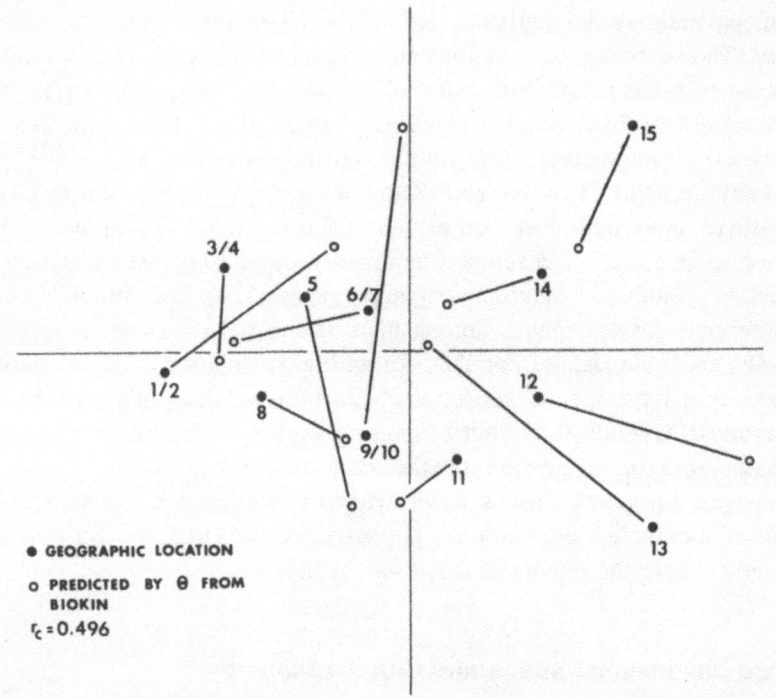

Fig. 16. Two-dimensional representation of θ estimated by BIOKIN from 14 genetic systems rotated to best fit with the geographic location of Åland Island parishes (without P and Lewis systems).

Comparison of Genetic and Migration Inference

Comparisons of the structure suggested by migration and genetic analyses should provide some understanding of the time depth of the genetic inference and of the relative influences of genetic drift and recent gene flow on population structure. Predicted kinship from migration describes covariation relative to the "founder" population in which the marital migration was actually observed. Genetic variation, however, reflects the effects of gene flow and drift with respect to some unknown ancestral population, possible, at least to a certain degree, of considerable antiquity. Extreme isolation of some but not all subpopulations, unknown relations among groups derived from common ancestors, and differential patterns of gene flow over space and time, as well as drift and sampling effects, may all be factors in the origin of contemporary genetic covariation. Thus differences between genetic and migration configurations are not only expected, they may also be used to gain inference on the migration which occurred prior to the periods for which observations are available.

The matrimonial exchanges for the period 1750–1799 show direct exchange among Sottunga, Lemland, and Lumparland, and the predicted coefficients among these parishes are relatively large. Lumparland and Sottunga also appear somewhat isolated within the array and show no effect of linear distance in their affinities with the other parishes. The genetic data show much greater divergence of these parishes from the rest of Åland, as well as a positive association between these parishes. Since the migration studies showed that both Lumparland and Sottunga were generally divergent up to 1900, it is clear that migration from 1750 to 1900 had only a moderate effect on reducing the divergence of these parishes from the rest of the parishes. Relations present in the migration results are not uniformly seen in the genetic patterns. It seems likely that historical relations among these parishes (founder or gene flow) preceded the eighteenth century but that the earlier patterns of gene flow and isolation were sufficiently strong, or of sufficient duration, that the degree and precise pattern of genetic variation reflect forces operative in those earlier periods.

There are numerous specific points of agreement and disagreement which can be shown to distinguish the genetic and migration analyses. Between Jomala and Sund/Vårdö the migration data show a low rate of exchange and the genetic data show a negative covariation ($r_{ij} = -0.004$). Brändö and Kumlinge show high mate exchange and a positive genetic covariation. On the other hand, Eckerö/Hammarland have a relatively higher rate of mate exchange from 1750 but an extremely different pattern of gene frequencies ($r_{ij} = -0.0135$). Föglö and Sottunga have frequent exchanges between 1750 and 1900 and a positive genetic covariation; however, Föglö is very dissimilar, genetically, to Lemland and Lumparland ($r_{ij} = -0.0111$), which do resemble Sottunga. Where agreement is noted, one may postulate that eighteenth- and nineteenth-century marital migration was a continuation of exchange practices common in earlier times. The low rate of migration, as already discussed, is insufficiently strong to have had much effect on prior kinship relations. Assuming that sampling effects have not distorted the genetic structure, or that isolation in recent times has not resulted in substantial new variation due to drift, genetic patterns may be assumed to reflect factors acting prior to the eighteenth century.

The genetic data are in general agreement with the migration data in terms of the broader patterns of association. Interchange among main island parishes is likely to have been greater than among the outer islands for a long period of time. Isolation prior to the eighteenth century was probably greater, and small population sizes would have enhanced the opportunity for genetic drift, so the noticeable random differentiation among main island parishes is not surprising. The extent to which particular associations reflect real historical events may be better understood following additional archival research, especially on the earlier historical periods. However, data for that period are scanty and much of the observable variation may never be explained. Isolation and variation among the outer island parishes appear more marked in the genetic studies, again suggesting a much greater time depth of the processes affecting genetic variation.

One line of historical research has been suggested by these studies. The data as a whole suggest that prior to the eighteenth century there was probably much greater local isolation in Åland than is observed for the period from 1750. The social consequences of being refugees from a common region, during the temporary emigration to Sweden during the Great Northern War (1714–1720), as well as increased intermarriage with Swedes during that period, may have contributed to a breakdown of social barriers to interparish exchange. For a study of this possibility, future research into both the Swedish archives and those in Åland for the years prior to 1714 is projected. Similarly, genealogical studies on the outer island parishes, in progress, will provide a description of a sample of marriage patterns dating back to the sixteenth century. These studies, in conjunction with other genetic portions of the Åland data, may provide a more precise assignment of the roles of drift and gene flow on the population structure in Åland.

Twinning in and around Åland

As reviewed by Eriksson,[20] there are considerable ethnogeographical variations in human twinning rates, and numerous studies indicate that genetic, ecological, and demographic factors are probably all involved. In Europe there appears to be a cline showing a progressive decrease in the frequency of twins from north to south. The highest rates, ranging between 13 and 17 per 1000 births, occur in the Nordic countries, and, in isolated populations in Finland and Scandinavia, rates exceeding 20 per 1000 have been reported. There are also many studies which show that the twinning rate, especially with regard to dizygotic twins, has been declining during the past century. The availability of extensive archival records suggested that analysis of twinning rates in the Åland Islands would add considerably to our understanding of the factors influencing twinning rates and to an analysis of secular variations since the latter seventeenth century.[24]

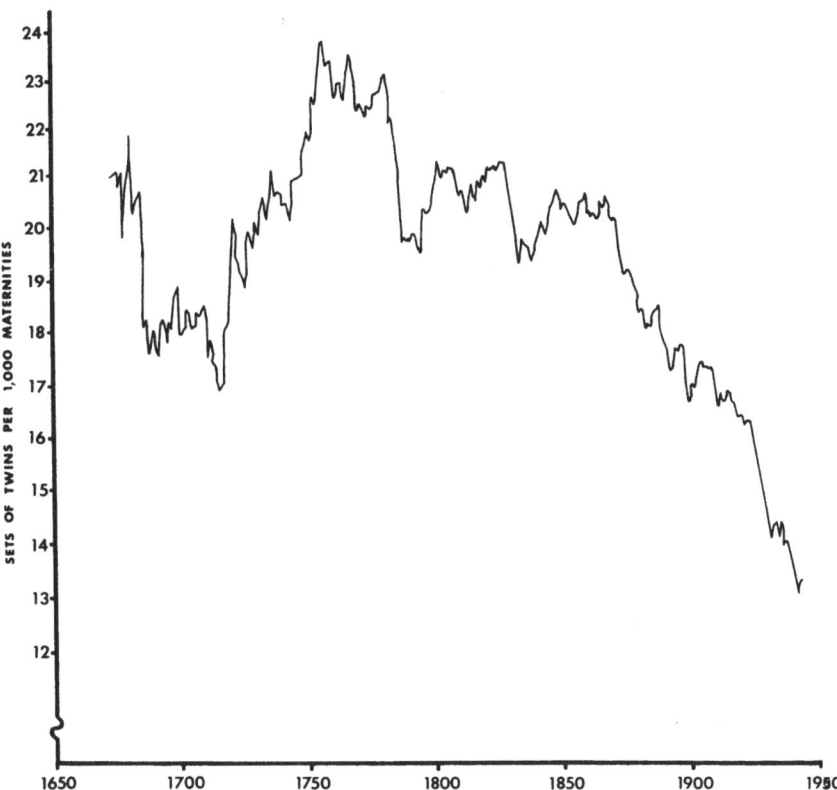

Fig. 17. Moving average of the frequencies of twin maternities in Åland, 1653–1959. The value given for each year is the twinning rate for 33 consecutive years, of which the year in question is the seventeenth.

TABLE XV. Areal and Temporal Fluctuations in the Twinning Rate in Åland, 1653-1949

Region	1653-1749		1750-1849		1850-1949		1653-1949	Temporal differences	
	Total maternities (number)	Twinning rate (‰)	Total maternities (number)	Twinning rate (‰)	Total maternities (number)	Twinning rate (‰)	Twinning rate (‰)	$\chi^2(2)$	P
1. Hammarland and Eckerö	2,216	19.9	3,896	16.2	6,540	18.2	17.9	1.2	>0.05
2. Finström and Geta	589	13.6	6,664	21.2	7,607	16.6	18.5	5.0	>0.05
3. Saltvik	2,262	17.7	4,330	21.2	5,685	17.9	19.1	1.7	>0.05
4. Sund and Vårdö	1,634	25.7	6,027	20.6	6,653	16.2	19.1	7.4	<0.025
5. Jomala (and Mariehamn)	406	19.7	6,058	19.6	8,703	19.4		0.0	>0.05
6. Lemland and Lumparland	1,024	19.5	4,565	19.9	5,066	18.6	19.2	0.2	>0.05
7. Kumlinge and Brändö	1,070	18.7	4,931	23.7	4,976	20.9	22.0	1.5	>0.05
8. Föglö and Sottunga	1,423	19.0	4,176	22.0	4,629	12.5	17.3	11.9	<0.005
9. Kökar	1,368	19.0	2,035	28.0	2,091	17.7	21.8	5.8	<0.05
Total	11,992	19.6	42,682	21.0	51,950	17.7	19.2	14.0	<0.0005
Differences $\chi^2(8)$ between regions P		4.8 >0.05		12.2 >0.05		13.3 >0.05	10.1 >0.05		

The earliest records which could be used for this purpose date from 1653 for the parish of Hammarland, and records for all parishes are available from 1741. The overall twinning rates, per parish, are shown in Table XV for the years 1653–1949. The total rate of 19.2 per 1000 births shows that Åland has experienced one of the highest twinning rates among all Caucasian populations. There has been some variation among parishes. The highest rates occurred in Brändö and Kumlinge (22 per 1000) and the lowest in the related parishes of Föglö and Sottunga (17.3 per 1000). Although such variation may reflect the genetic affinities of the parishes and differences in founder populations, overall, there was no statistically significant heterogeneity among parishes in any of three 100-year periods, 1653–1749, 1750–1849, and 1850–1949 (Table XV). However, secular variation over the whole of Åland was considerable and statistically very significantly different over time. Figure 17 shows a moving average, over 33-year periods, of the twinning rate for all of the combined parishes.

Analyses of the data considered a variety of factors which might be involved, including maternal age, parity, legitimacy, occurrence of twinning in parents of twins, multiple recurrent twinning within sibships, and local endogamy.[20–22,24] In addition, there are also extensive records for the neighboring Åboland archipelago and both Sweden and Finland which have permitted regional comparisons.

Maternal age was found to be of considerable importance. Twinning rates according to maternal age in Åland, Finland, and Sweden in this century are shown in Fig. 18. A considerable portion of the decrease in twinning seems to be related to the general decline in maternal age over the last two centuries, which is shown in Fig. 19. Using estimates of the proportion of monozygotic and dizygotic twins, it was clear that both regional and secular variation in Åland were largely due to variations in the dizygotic rates. Similar striking declines in the incidence of DZ twins occurred in Sweden and Åboland, where maternal ages also declined at about the same time. The pattern in Finland, for twentieth-century data, was not parallel to these results. However, the demographic structure in Finland has been approaching that of Sweden more rapidly since the beginning of the 1950s and, in recent years, Finland has also shown a decline in twinning rates.

Eriksson concluded that changes in the matrimonial migration patterns also have had an effect on the twinning rate. The increase in rate during the eighteenth century presumably reflects, in part, the

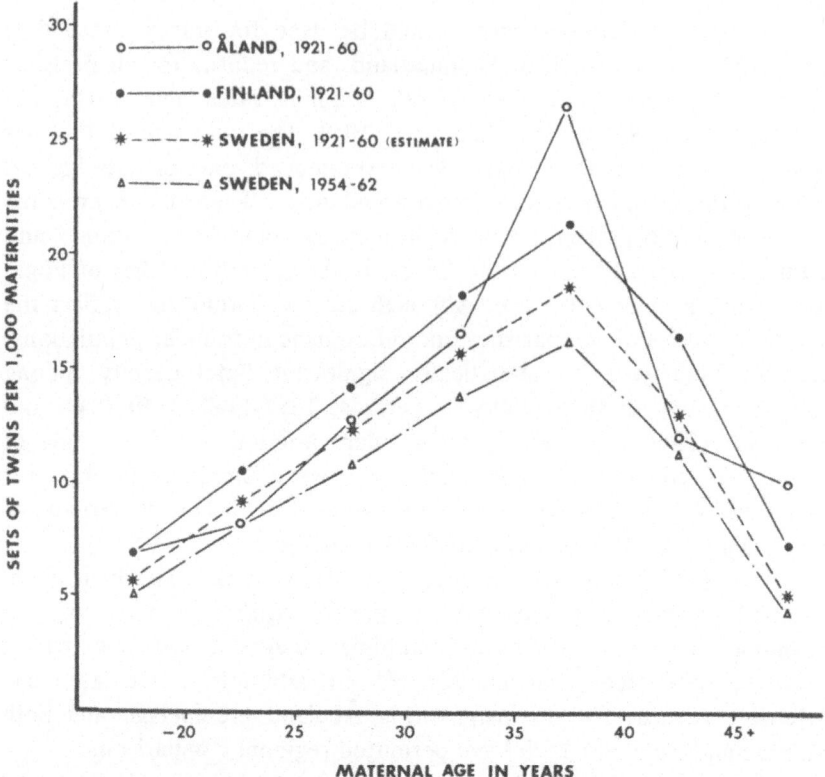

Fig. 18. Twinning rates according to maternal age in Åland, 1921–1960; Finland, 1921–
1960; and Sweden, 1921–1960 (estimated) and 1954–1962.

increasing endogamy made possible by demographic increase. The drop
in the twinning rate in the latter nineteenth century and the accelerated
decline following World War I are also matched by the changing
pattern of parish and regional endogamy in the Åland Islands. The
extremely low rate in the urban, highly intermixed town Mariehamn, of
7.9 per 1000 births, also is consistent with this hypothesis. Analysis of
the trends in Sweden relative to maternal age, local isolation, and
urbanization showed that the twinning rates in rural and urban Sweden,
and their changes, were likely due to the same factors which operated
in Åland. The higher overall rate in Åland and in Åboland may well

reflect the effect of inbreeding in these isolated groups descended from a relatively small founder group.

Studies in progress on the genealogical linking of Ålanders in particular parishes will be used to provide inference on the possible genetic basis for twinning. Prior studies have indicated a genetic factor in dizygotic twinning, but the maternal genotype and phenotype seem to be more important than are paternal factors. Using genealogical material, one can compute the coefficient of kinship among mothers or fathers of twins relative to the random kinship in the population, and it is hoped that this procedure will answer questions not suitably treated by contemporary cross-sectional samples.

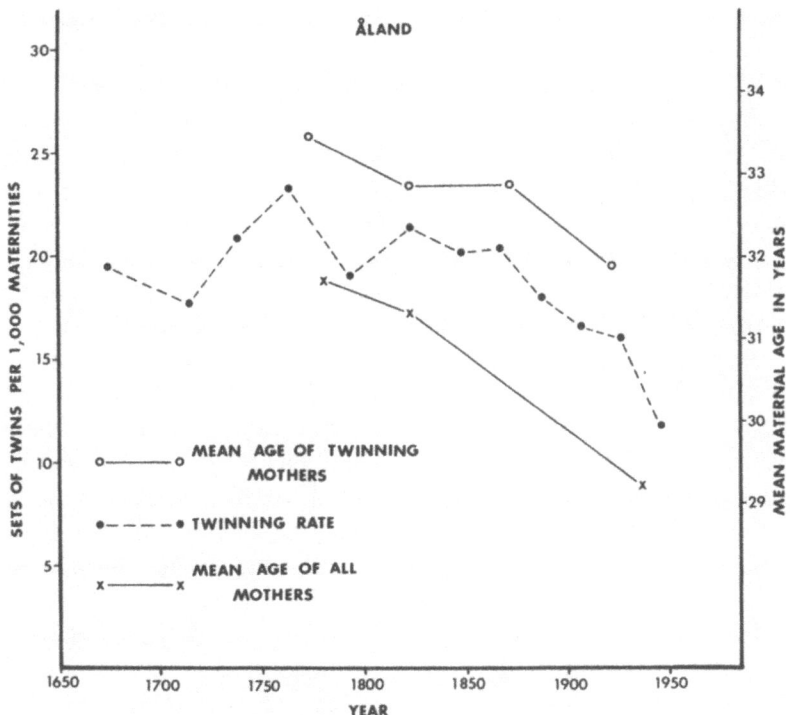

Fig. 19. Mean ages of twinning mothers with recorded ages in Åland, 1653–1949. The mean ages of all mothers were estimated from 6676 maternities, 1774–1790; from a sample of 4840 maternities in Finström, Lemland, and Kumlinge, 1800–1849; and from the 15,374 maternities for which maternal age is known in Åland, 1920–1959 (compiled from sources at the Central Statistics Office, Finland).

Ophthalmological Studies

Studies in the Kökar Isolate

The parish of Kökar has a census population of almost 600 individuals, but only about 400 of these are resident throughout the year. Kökar was selected for intensive study because of its extreme isolation and because there is especially useful ethnohistorical research on this parish which supplements the archival material. Thus far, field studies have provided data on anthropometrics, physiological variables such as serum vitamin B_{12} levels,[84] quantitative haptoglobin levels,[28] and plasma creatinine[60]; and observations on genetic polymorphisms in the blood groups and serum proteins and enzymes have been made in a sample of over 450 individuals. In addition, studies on a sample of almost 500 individuals have provided a detailed characterization of normal and pathological variation in ophthalmological characters.

Eye examinations included refraction, dark adaptation, dazzling test, color vision tests, and measurements of ocular pressure. In addition, the radius and width of the cornea,[27] the degree of arcus senilis and of iris atrophy, opacities of the lens, changes of the fundus, etc., were noted. A hypothesis of a major hereditary factor in horizontal corneal refraction was supported by the observation of highly significant parent–offspring correlations for the trait.[36]

A series of color photographs of the iris (146 men, 180 women) was studied with respect to the breadth of the pupillary zone (the interior of the iris), color, resorption, and degree of atrophy of the iris and the occurrence of Wolfflin's nodules. Family studies showed high parent–offspring correlations for the width of the pupillary zone and weak (but significant) correlations between midparent and offspring for the denseness of the ciliary zone of the iris and for the denseness of the total surface of the iris (pupillary and ciliary zones).[38]

Pterygium, a patch of thickened, usually fan-shaped conjunctiva extending over a part of the cornea, was observed in 19 of 479 (4.0%) subjects.[32] For those over 40 years of age (no case of pterygium was observed in younger subjects), there were 7.8% affected. Given the observed high rate of consanguinity in the parents of the probands, one might simply assume a recessive mode of inheritance. However, a genealogy spanning 12 generations could be constructed in which all 19 probands were included. Many could be shown to have common ancestors within this genealogy. In addition, despite the difficulty of obtaining two-generation data in a trait with such late age at onset there were two parents of the probands still alive; one of these had pterygium. Of the 21 siblings of 11 probands, however, none had pterygium. These observations support a hypothesis of a dominant mode of inheritance with, probably, reduced penetrance. This would be in agreement with the literature on the anomaly.[32]

The amount of definite color blindness, determined with the aid of Stilling's pseudoisochromatic tables, was low, about 1%. The occurrence of severe astigmatism, both with and against the rule, was relatively high. The frequency of embryotoxon corneae posterius was also relatively high.[37] Myopia of high degree was quite rare.

A genealogy of this population tracing as many ancestral ties as possible, and linking Kökar Islanders to related individuals in other Åland parishes, is expected to be completed within the next few years. The founders which have been thus far traced are generally from the middly sixteenth century. When this record is combined with the biological observations, more precise studies on the modes of inheritance of the traits, inheritability of quantitative variables, and the effects of inbreeding on developmental variation will be possible. Recent developments in the theory and computer methodology needed for studies of segregation analysis and the role of major genes in quantitative traits greatly enhance the utility of such genealogical reconstruction.

Tapetoretinal Degeneration

Investigations of Åland families afflicted with blindness revealed various types of tapetoretinal degeneration: Leber's congenital amaurosis, degeneration retinal pigmentosa juvenalis, and retinitis punctata albescens.[35] Both severe and mild forms, as well as marked variation in the age at onset, occurred within families. Observations over a period of 10 years have permitted studies of the progression of this disorder; several patients have been studied by electroretinography (ERG), electrooculography (EOG), electronystagmography (ENG), anomaloscopy, the Farnsworth 100 Hue test, fluorescein angiography, etc.[35] A major concern has been to determine whether these clinically different retinal abiotrophies of the autosomal recessive type could be due to the same mutant gene, with varying symptoms related to pleiotropy and the progression of the disorder.

In Kökar, where 565 subjects were examined, afflicted individuals belonging to five families were found; all showed clinical patterns manifesting as retinitis punctata albescens or as a central atrophic degeneration of the fundus. A search of the church records showed that these individuals could be related in different ways and that many ancestors in the Kökar pedigree had a record of night blindness, poor vision, or blindness. Similarly, four families in a Föglö/Sottunga pedigree with analogous fundal degeneration were also identified. Further studies revealed subjects in four families in a main island pedigree and in two families in a Kumlinge pedigree in which the clinical diagnosis was Leber's congenital amaurosis. There were a variety of connections among all of these groups of families, but no single common ancestor could be located for all of the probands. Thus, while the data are consistent with a hypothesis of a single mutant, it may be the case that more than one locus is involved. Analytical inference on this could be effected if the entire Åland Islands were linked in a genealogical reconstruction. Such a record would allow comparison with the degree of relatedness among randomly selected families within and between Åland parishes.

The Åland Eye Disease (Forsius–Eriksson Syndrome)

In 1963, a family was identified in which there was an X chromosomal eye syndrome characterized by a combination of poor sight, axial myopia, regular astigmatism after the rule, and defective night vision.[49,83] In all cases, there was a pigment deficiency of the eyeground, not unlike that seen in classical ocular albinism. In all but one case, spontaneous nystagmus, mainly horizontal oscillating, was observed. ERG revealed defective function of both scotopic and photopic retinal mechanisms.[17] An electronystagmographical examination was made of 25 members of this kindred.[99] Of nine investigated females, only two showed a slight latent nystagmus; in seven males with the Åland eye syndrome, there were five with classical latent nystagmus and two with only slight manifestations of latent nystagmus.

Pleiotropic gene action with varying expressivity of the nystagmus appears the most likely explanation thus far. The genealogy of this family, obtained through the church records, revealed a common ancestor for all probands (born 1836), who was noted to have had "poor sight and restless eyes."

The Åland Bleeder Syndrome (von Willebrand–Jürgens)

In 1926, von Willebrand[103] reported a large family of bleeders living in the Åland Islands. The family contained 66 members, 23 of whom were bleeders. Numerous studies since that time[63] have contributed to our present understanding of this disorder, which involves a lengthening of the bleeding time, a deficiency of factor VIII, and, possibly, a platelet disturbance.[54] This disease, which has an autosomal dominant mode of transmission, occurs in extraordinarily high frequencies (up to 10–20%) in the population in the southeastern part of the Åland archipelago. Archival studies have revealed numerous links among the many kindreds with affected individuals. The high gene frequency suggests that selection, if any, must be very weak against this trait and that the original introduction of the gene (assuming a single introduction) must have occurred very early in the history of the population. Construction of all the genealogies would not be likely to demonstrate a single common ancestor. However, the locations of the earliest locatable ancestors might reveal a clustering which would reflect the pattern of gene flow following the initial origin (by mutation or gene flow). In addition, a more precise characterization of the present distribution of this gene would provide considerable inference on historical patterns of gene flow (and drift) within the Åland Islands. A genetic distance based on the frequency of the allele would provide a basis for estimating the net gene flow among parishes over a period of many centuries. The distributions of genes whose frequencies may be very rare or absent in some groups, but at high frequencies in others, are among the most informative genetic markers for inference over long periods of time.[83] Projected field studies on the bleeder syndrome, including archival studies of the pattern of mortality in ancestors of affected individuals relative to the rest of the population, promise to have considerable ethnohistorical utility.

ACKNOWLEDGMENT

This research was supported in part by a grant from the Sigrid Juselius Foundation, Helsinki-Helsingfors, Suomi Finland.

BIBLIOGRAPHY

1. Ageheim, H., and Bergström, M., Adenosine deaminase polymorphism in a Swedish population, *Acta Genet. Med. Gemellol.* **21**:135. (1972).
2. Arho, A. O., Anthropologische untersuchungen in den Land shaften Åland und Varsinais-Suomi, *Ann. Acad. Sci. Fenn. A* **40**:2. (1934).
3. Azevedo, E., Morton, N. E., Miki, C., and Yee, S., Distance and kinship in northeastern Brazil, *Am. J. Hum. Genet.* **21**:1–22. (1969).
4. Beckman, L., A contribution to the physical anthropology and population genetics of Sweden: Variation of the ABO, Rh, MN and P blood groups, *Hereditas* **45**:1. (1959).
5. Beckman G., Beckman L., and Cedergren B., Population studies in Northern Sweden. II. Red cell enzyme polymorphism in the Swedish Lapps. *Hereditas* **69**:243. (1971).
6. Beckman, L., and Mellbin, T., Haptoglobin types in the Swedish Lapps, *Acta Genet. (Basel)* **9**:306. (1959).
7. Beckman, L., Holmgren, G., and Mårtensson, E. H., Transferrin variants in the Swedish population, *Proc. 2nd Int. Congr. Hum. Genet., Rome*, p. 737.(1961).
8. Berg, K., Studies of polymorphic traits for the characterization of populations: The populations of Scandinavia. *Israel J. Med. Sci.* **9**:1147. (1973).
9. Bodmer, W. F., and Cavalli-Sforza, L. L., A migration matrix model for the study of random genetic drift, *Genetics* **59**:565–592. (1968).
10. Bradley, A. D., *Mathematics of Air and Marine Navigation*, American Book Company, New York. (1942).
11. Broman, P., Grundin, R., and Lins, P. E., The red cell acid phosphatase polymorphism in Sweden: Gene frequencies and application to disputed paternity, *Acta Genet. Med. Gemellol.* **20**:77. (1971).
12. Cannings, C., and Cavalli-Sforza, L., Human population structure, *in: Advances in Human Genetics*, Vol. 4 (H. Harris and K. Hirschhorn, eds.), pp. 105–171, Plenum Press, New York. (1973).
13. Cavalli-Sforza, L. L., Some data on the genetic structure of human populations. *Proc. X Int. Congr. Genet.* **1**:389–407. (1959).
14. Cavalli-Sforza, L. L., Some current problems of human population genetics, *Am. J. Hum. Genet.* **25**:82–104. (1973).
15. Crow, J. F., and Mange, A. P., Measurement of inbreeding from the frequency of marriages between persons of the same surname, *Eugen. Quart.* **12**:199–203. (1965).
16. Dreijer, M., *Glimpses of Åland History*, Ålands Museum, Mariehamn, Åland Islands. (1968).
17. Elenius, V., Eriksson, A., and Forsius, H., ERG in a case of X-chromosomal

pigment deficiency of fundus in combination with myopia, dyschromatopsia and defective dark-adaptation, *in: The Clinical Value of Electroretinography*, ISCERG Symposium on Genetics, pp. 369–377, Karger, Basel. (1968).

18. Engle, E., and Paananen, L., *The Winter War: The Russo-Finnish Conflict 1939–1940*, Charles Scribner's Sons, New York. (1973).

19. Eriksson, A. W., Variations in the human twinning rate, *Acta Genet. (Basel)* **12**:242. (1962).

20. Eriksson, A. W., Human twinning in and around the Åland Islands, *Comment. Biol. Suppl.* **64**:1–159. (1973).

21. Eriksson, A. W., and Fellman, J., Twinning and legitimacy, *Hereditas* **57**:395. (1967).

22. Eriksson, A. W., and Fellman, J., Twinning in relation to the marital status of the mother, *Acta Genet. (Basel)* **17**:385. (1967).

23. Eriksson, A. W., and Forsius, H., Studies on human population genetics and anthropology in isolates on the Åland Islands, *J. Genet. Hum.* **13**:60. (1964).

24. Eriksson, A. W., Eskola, M.-R., Fellman, J., and Forsius, H., The value of genealogical data in population studies in Sweden and Finland, *in: Genetic Structure of Populations* (N. E. Morton, ed.), pp. 102–118. University of Hawaii Press, Honolulu, (1973).

25. Eriksson, A. W., Fellman, J., Workman, P. L., and Lalouel, J. M., Population studies on the Åland Islands. I. Prediction of kinship from migration and isolation by distance, *Hum. Hered.* **23**:422–433. (1973).

26. Eriksson, A. W., Eskola, M.-R., Workman, P. L., and Morton, N. E., Population studies on the Åland Islands. II. Historical population structure: Inference from bioassay of kinship and migration, *Hum. Hered.* **23**:511. (1973).

27. Eriksson, A. W., Fellman, J., Nieminen, H., and Forsius, H., Influence of age on the position and size of the iris frill and the pupil, *Acta Ophthalmol.* **43**:629 (1965).

28. Eriksson, A. W., Kirjarinta, M., Fellman, J., and Forsius, H., Quantitative haptoglobin studies, *Scan. J. Clin. Lab. Invest.* **21**:59, Suppl. 101 (1968).

29. Eriksson, A. W., Kirjarinta, M., Lehtosalo, T., Kajanoja, P., Lehmann, W., Mourant, A. E., Tills, D., Singh, S., Benkmann, H. G., Hirth, L., and Goedde, H. W., Red cell phosphoglucomutase polymorphism in Finland Swedes, Finns, Finnish Lapps, Maris (Cheremisses) and Greenland Eskimos, and segregation studies of PGM₁ types in Lapp families, *Hum. Hered.* **21**:140. (1971).

30. Eriksson, A. W., Fellman, J., Kirjarinta, M., Eskola, M.-R., Singh, S., Benkmann, H. G., Goedde, H. W., Mourant, A. E., Tills, D., and Lehmann, W., Adenylate kinase polymorphism in populations in Finland (Swedes, Finns, Lapps), in Maris, and in Greenland Eskimos, *Humangenetik* **12**:123. (1971).

31. Eriksson, A. W., Kirjarinta, M., Fellman, J., Eskola, M.-R., and Lehmann, W., Adenosine deaminase polymorphism in Finland (Swedes, Finns, and Lapps), the Mari Republic (Cheremisses), and Greenland (Eskimos), *Am. J. Hum. Genet.* **23**:568. (1971).

32. Forsius, H., and Eriksson, A. W., Pterygium in an isolated population, *Acta Genet. Med. Gemellol.* **11**:397. (1962).

33. Forsius, H., and Eriksson, A., Ein neues Augensyndrom mit X-chromosomaler Transmission: Eine Sippemit Fundusalbinismus, Foveahypoplasie, Nystagmus, Myopie, Astigmatismus und Dyschromatopsie, *Klin. Mbl. Augenheilk.* **144**:447 (1964).

34. Forsius, H., and Eriksson, A., Ett nytt ögonsyndrom med X-kromosomal överföring. *Finska Läk.-Sällsk. Handl.* **108**:245–246. (1964).

35. Forsius, H., and Eriksson, A. W., Tapeto-retinal degenerations with varying clinical features in Åland Islanders, *J. Med. Genet.* **7**:200. (1970).
36. Forsius, H., Eriksson, A. W., and Fellman, F., Corneal refraction according to age and sex in an isolated population and the heredity of the trait, *Acta Ophthalmol.* **42**:224. (1964).
37. Forsius, H., Eriksson, A., and Fellman, J., Embryotoxon corneae posterius in an isolated population, *Acta Ophthalmol.* **42**:42. (1964).
38. Forsius, H., Fellman, J., and Eriksson, A. W., On the heredity of the iris configuration, *Acta Fac. Med. Univ. Brun.* **25**:251. (1966).
39. Friedlaender, J. S., Isolation by distance in Bougainville, *Proc. Natl. Acad. Sci. U.S.A.* **68**:704–707. (1971).
40. de Geer, E., Migration in the archipelago of southwestern Finland during the last hundred years, *Fennia* **84**:67–90. (1960).
41. Goodman, M. M., Genetic distances: Measuring dissimilarity among populations, *in: Yearbook of Physical Anthropology*, Vol. 17, pp. 1–38., American Association of Physical Anthropology, Washington, D.C. (1973).
42. Gower, J. C., Some distance properties of latent root and vector methods used in multivariate analysis, *Biometrika* **53**:325–338. (1966).
43. Harris, D. E., OBELIX, *in: Genetic Structure of Populations* (N. E. Morton, ed.), pp. 308–310, University of Hawaii Press, Honolulu, (1973).
44. Harrison, G. A., and Boyce, A. J., The framework of population studies, *in: The Structure of Human Population*, (E. A. Harrison and A. J., Boyce, eds.), pp. 1–16, Clarendon Press, Oxford. (1972).
45. Heiken, A., Distribution of the Kell blood group factor K in the Swedish population, *Acta Genet. (Basel)* **12**:352. (1962).
46. Heiken, A., The frequency of the Duffy blood group factor Fy^a in Sweden, *Acta Pathol. Microbiol. Scand.* **55**:84. (1962).
47. Hiorns, R. W., Harrison, G. A., Boyce, A. J., and Kuchemann, C. F., A mathematical analysis of the effects of movement on the relatedness between populations, *Ann. Hum. Genet. (London)* **32**:237–250. (1969).
48. Hirschfeld, J., The Gc-system—Immunoelectrophoretic studies of normal serum system, *Progr. Allergy* **6**:155–186. (1962).
49. Imaizumi, Y., and Morton, N. E., Isolation by distance in Japan and Sweden compared with other countries, *Hum. Hered.* **19**:433–443.(1969).
50. Imaizumi, Y., and Morton, N. E., Isolation by distance in New Guinea and Micronesia, *Archaeol. Phys. Anthropol. Oceania* **5**:218–227. (1970).
51. Imaizumi, Y., Morton, N. E., and Harris, D. E., Isolation by distance in artificial populations, *Genetics* **66**:569–582. (1970).
52. Jaatinen, S., Regionala drag i belfolkningsutvecklingen på Åland 1900–1950, *Fennia* **76**:Nó. 4. (1953).
53. Jaatinen, S., Expansion and retreat of settlement in the southwestern archipelago of Finland, *Fennia* **84**:39–65. (1960).
54. Jürgens, J., Lehmann, W., and Eriksson, A. W., The platelet aggregation defect in the von Willebrand–Jürgens-syndrome on the Åland Islands: The possible existence of an "anti-Willebrand-factor," *Hemostase* **6**:225. (1966).
55. Jutikkala, E., Die Bevölkerung Finnlands in den Jahren 1721–1749 (dissertation.), *Ann. Acad. Sci. Fenn. B* **55/4**:1–130. (1945).
56. Kajanoja, P., A study in the morphology of the Finns and its relation to the settlement of Finland, *Ann. Acad. Sci. Fenn. (A)* **146**:1–61. (1971).
57. Kajanoja, P., A contribution to the physical anthropology of the Finns: Variations

of the ABO, Rhesus, MN, P and Lewis blood group frequencies, PTC taste ability and colour blindness, *Ann. Acad. Sci. Fenn. (Med.)* **153**:1–12. (1972).

58. Kimura, M., and Weiss, G. H., The stepping stone model of population structure and the decrease of genetic correlation with distance, *Genetics* **49**:561–576. (1964).

59. Kivikoski, E., *Kvarnbacken, ein Gräberfeld der jüngeren Eisenzeit auf Åland*, Finnische Altertumsgesellschaft, Helsinki. (1963).

60. Kuhlbäck, B., Eriksson, A. W., and Forsius, H., Plasma creatinine in different sex and age groups of a healthy isolated island population, *Acta Med. Scand. Suppl.* **412**:83. (1964).

61. Lalouel, J. M., Topology of population structure, in: *Genetic Structure of Populations*, Vol. III of *Population Genetics Monographs* (N. E. Morton, ed.), pp. 139–149. University of Hawaii Press, Honolulu, (1973).

62. Lalouel, J. M., MATFIT, in: *Genetic Structure of Populations*, Vol. III of *Population Genetics Monographs* (N. E. Morton, ed.), pp. 303–304, University of Hawaii Press, Honolulu, (1973).

63. Lehmann, W., Jürgens, J., and Eriksson, A. W., The platelet function of the thrombopathy on the Åland Islands, *Thrombos. Diathes. Haemorrh. (Stuttgart)* **12**:148. (1964).

64. Malcolm, L. A., Booth, P. B., and Cavalli-Sforza, L. L., Intermarriage patterns and blood group gene frequencies of the Bundi people of the New Guinea Highlands, *Hum. Biol.* **43**:187–199. (1971).

65. Malécot, G., *Les Mathématiques de l'Hérédite*, Masson, Paris. (1948).

66. Malécot, G., Quelques schemas probabilistes sur la variabilité des populations naturelles, *Ann. Univ. Lyon Sci. Sec.* A **13**:37–60. (1950).

67. Malécot, G., Les modèles stochastiques en genetique de population, *Publ. Inst. Statis. Univ. Paris* **8**:173–210. (1959).

68. Malécot, G., Structure géographique et variabilité d'une grande population, *Excerpta Med.* **3**:18. (1972).

69. Mielke, J. H., Population structure of the Åland Islands, Finland, from 1750 to 1949, Unpublished dissertation, University of Massachusetts, Amherst. (1974).

70. Monn, E., Berg, K., Reinskou, T., and Teisberg, P., Serum protein polymorphisms among Norwegian Lapps: Studies on the Lp, Ag, Gc and transferrin systems, *Hum. Hered.* **21**:134 (1971).

71. Morton, N. E., Models and evidence in human population genetics: Genetics today, in: *Proceedings of the Ninth International Congress of Genetics, The Hague,* Pergamon Press, London (1963).

72. Morton, N. E., Human population structure, *Ann. Rev. Genet.* **3**:53–74. (1969).

73. Morton, N. E., ed., *Genetic Structure of Populations*, Vol. III of *Population Genetics Monographs*, University of Hawaii Press, Honolulu. (1973).

74. Morton, N. E., Population structure, in: *Computer Applications in Genetics* (N. E. Morton, ed.), pp. 61–71, University of Hawaii Press, Honolulu, (1969).

75. Morton, N. E., Kinship and population structure, in: *Genetic Structure of Populations*, Vol. III of *Population Genetics Monographs* (N. E. Morton, ed.), pp. 66–70, University of Hawaii Press, Honolulu, (1973).

76. Morton, N. E., Prediction of kinship from a migration matrix, in: *Genetic Structure of Populations*, Vol. III of *Population Genetics Monographs* (N. E. Morton, ed.), pp. 119–123, University of Hawaii Press, Honolulu, (1973).

77. Morton, N. E., Population structure of Micronesia, in: *Methods and Theories of Anthropological Genetics* (M. Crawford and P. Workman, eds.), pp. 333–356, University of New Mexico Press, Albuquerque, (1973).

78. Morton, N. E. and Hussels, I., Demography of inbreeding in Switzerland, *Hum. Biol.* **42**:65–78. (1970).
79. Morton, N. E., Harris, D. E., Yee, S., and Lew, R., Pingelap and Mokil Atolls: Migration, genealogy, *Am. J. Hum. Genet.* **23**:339–360. (1971).
80. Morton, N. E., Yasuda, N., Miki, C., and Yee, S., Population structure of the ABO blood groups in Switzerland, *Am. J. Hum. Genet.* **20**:420–429. (1968).
81. Morton, N. E., Yee, S., Harris, D. E., and Lew, R., Bioassay of kinship, *Theoret. Pop. Biol.* **2**:507–524. (1971).
82. Nevanlinna, H. R., The Finnish population structure, a genetic and genealogical study, *Hereditas* **71**:195. (1972).
83. Norio, R., Nevanlinna, H. R., and Perheentupa, J., Hereditary diseases in Finland; rare flora in rare soil, *Ann. Clin. Res.* **5**:109–141. (1973).
84. Nyberg, W., Eriksson, A., Forsius, H., and Fellman, J., Serum vitamin B_{12} levels in an isolated island population, *Acta Med. Scand. Suppl.* **412**:79 (1964).
85. Pipping, K., Settlement in the outer archipelago of Kumlinge and Brändö, in: *Atlas of the Archipelago of Southwestern Finland.* (1960).
86. Platt, R., ed., *Finland and Its Geography,* Dull, Sloan, and Pearce, New York. (1955).
87. Salminen, A., Eriksson, A. W., and Oker-Blom, N., Hemagglutination-inhibiting antibodies in the human population of an endemic area of diphasic tick-borne meningoencephalitis, *Arch. Ges. Virusforsch.* **11**:215. (1961).
88. Schönemann, P. H., and Carroll, R. M., Fitting one matrix to another under choice of a central dilatation and rigid motion, *Psychometrika* **35**:245–255. (1970).
89. Schull, W. J., and McCluer, J. W., Human genetics: Structure of populations, in: *Annual Review of Genetics,* Vol. 2 (H. L. Roman, L. D. Sandler, and G. S. Stent, eds.), pp. 279–304, Johns Hopkins Press, Baltimore. (1968).
90. Seppälä, M., Eriksson, A. W., and Forsius, H., Distribution of transferrin variants in Kökar, Finland, *Ann. Med. Exp. Fenn.* **42**:50. (1964).
91. Singh, S., Saternus, K., Münsch, H., Altland, K., Goedde, H. W., and Eriksson, A. W., Pseudocholinesterase polymorphism among Ålanders (Finno-Swedes), Maris (Cheremisses, USSR) and Greenland Eskimos, and the segregation of some E_1 and E_2 locus types in Finnish Lapp families, *Hum. Hered.* **24**:352. (1974).
92. Sjöund, F., *Åland-Mariehamn Guide,* Kuultokuva, Helsinki, Finland. (1972).
93. Skude, G., and Jakobsson, A., Determination of adenylate kinase phenotypes employing agar gel, *Hum. Hered.* **20**:319. (1970).
94. Smith, C. A. B., Local fluctuations in gene frequencies, *Ann. Hum. Genet. (London)* **32**:251–260. (1969).
95. Spielman, R. S., Migliazza, E. C., and Neel, J. V., Regional linguistic and genetic differences among Yanomama Indians, *Science* **184**:637–644. (1974).
96. Steinberg, A. G., Tiilikainen, A., Eskola, M.-R., and Eriksson, A. W., Gammaglobulin allotypes in Finnish Lapps, Finns, Åland Islanders, Maris (Cheremis), and Greenland Eskimos, *Am. J. Hum. Genet.* **26**:223. (1974).
97. Tarukoski, P. H., Gene frequencies of haptoglobin types in a Swedish population, *Nord. Med.* **62**:1425–1426. (1959).
98. Upton, A. F., *Finland in Crises 1940–41: A Study in Small-Power Politics,* Cornell University Press, Ithaca, N. Y. (1964).
99. van Vliet, A. G. M., Waardengurg, P. J., Forsius, H., and Eriksson, A. W., Nystagmographical studies in Åland eye disease, *Acta Ophthalmol.* **51**:782. (1973).
100. Waardenburg, P. J., Eriksson, A. W., and Forsius, H., Åland eye disease (syndroma Forsius–Eriksson), in: *Proceedings of the Second International Con-*

gress of Neuro-genet. Neuro-Genetics and Neuro-ophthalmology: Progress in Neuro-Ophthalmology, pp. 336–339, Excerpta Medica International Congress Series No. 176, Amsterdam (1969).

101. Wagener, D. K., An extension of migration matrix analysis to account for differential immigration from the outside world, *Am. J. Hum. Genet.* **25**:47–56. (1973).

102. Weiss, G. H., and Kimura, M., A mathematical analysis of the stepping stone model of genetic correlation, *J. Appl. Prob.* **2**:129–149. (1965).

103. von Willebrand, E. A., Hereditär pseudohemofili, *Finska Läk-Sällsk Handl.* **68**:87. (1926).

104. Workman, P. L., Harpending, H., Lalouel, J. M., Lynch, C., Niswander, J. D., and Singleton, R., Population studies on southwestern Indian tribes. VI, in: *Genetic Structure of Populations*, Vol. III of *Population Genetics Monographs* (N. E. Morton, ed), pp. 166–194, University of Hawaii Press, Honolulu, (1973).

105. Wright, S., Size of population and breeding structure in relation to evolution, *Science* **87**:430–431. (1938).

106. Wright, S., Breeding structure of populations in relation to speciation *Am. Naturalist* :232–248. (1940).

107. Wright, S., Isolation by distance, *Genetics* **28**:114–138. (1943).

108. Wright, S., Isolation by distance under diverse systems of mating, *Genetics* **31**:39–59. (1946).

109. Wright, S., The genetical structure of populations. *Ann. Eugen.* **15**:323–354. (1951).

110. Wright, S., *Evolution and the Genetics of Populations*, Vol. 2: *The Theory of Gene Frequencies*, University of Chicago Press, Chicago, (1969).

111. Yasuda, N., An extension of Wahlund's principle to evaluate mating type frequency, *Am. J. Hum. Genet.* **22**:24–49. (1968).

112. Yasuda, N., and Morton, N. E., Studies on human population structure, in: *Proceedings of the Third International Congress on Human Genetics* (J. F. Crow and J. V. Neel, eds.), Johns Hopkins Press, Baltimore, (1967).

113. Yee, S., BIOKIN, in: *Genetic Structure of Populations*, (N. E. Morton, ed.), pp. 293–297, University of Hawaii Press, Honolulu, (1973).

Chapter 5

Population Genetics and Health Care Delivery: The Quebec Experience

Claude Laberge

Department of Medicine
Laval University Medical Center
Quebec City, Canada

INTRODUCTION

The main objective of this chapter is to define the potentialities for genetic studies in the French Canadians. Different levels of approach to the problem have been tried in the last 6 years and are presented herein in sequence. It is hoped that as we go from population genetics to medical genetics the reader will understand the paths that led us from the definition of the genetic structure of a population to daily involvement in genetic care delivery for specific genetic conditions.

The consequences and limitations of each project will be discussed. A logical sequence of decisions will be described: from a consanguinity study, to an isolate study, to an inbreeding survey, to a study of a regional genetic disease, and finally to development of a genetic care delivery system.

Each project constituted a step in the direction of applied genetic knowledge to a population, and in this regard the projects were not undertaken for the purpose of comparative studies with other populations. The methodologies were not sophisticated but were used only to understand problems that led eventually to an operational approach to the genetic problems of a population. This whole approach may in itself be criticized, but each level of research could be approached again, now that mechanisms have been established to use rapidly the results of such researches in the population.

A SHORT HISTORY OF FRENCH CANADA

The term "French Canada" as used in this chapter refers to the Province of Quebec, where in 1971 there were 4.8 million people. There are French-speaking persons in other parts of Canada, notably in New Brunswick and the Prairies Provinces, but these will not be considered.

Although there was a settlement at Port Royal on the Bay of Fundy in 1605, the ancestors of the present French Canadians are descendants of the settlement of Quebec in 1608. Thirty men came with Champlain at that time. The first family settled in 1617, but it was not until after 1638 that the number of births exceeded the number of deaths in the colony, thus starting an amazing population growth.

In 1651, New France numbered 680 inhabitants. The first phase of immigration ended in 1663, when the Charter of the Company of the Hundred Associates, which had favored fur trading but had neglected colonization, was revoked.

In 1666, the first official census showed 3215 inhabitants in 537 families. In 1668, only 2 years later, the population was 5870.

When New France came under British rule in 1763, the population was 65,000–70,000 persons, most of them descendants of about 10,000 immigrants who came over during the French regime. They were Roman Catholics as the colony had been closed to Huguenots.

Of the immigrants, about 3900 were brought over by companies of seigneurs, 3500 were soldiers who had stayed in Canada, 1100 were *filles du roi* (orphan wards of the king) or widows, 1000 were prisoners, and 500 were free colonists who came on their own. Most of immigrants came from northwestern and western France.

The population growth during the French regime was the result of an unusually high birth rate. This was encouraged by the king, who gave allowances for young brides and grooms and for large families. Essentially all girls and widows had to marry, and the birth rate was at times as high as 50–60 per 1000 per year. This was high enough to counteract a death rate of over 20 per 1000 and still allow for population increase.

At the Conquest (1763), about 66,000 inhabitants decided to remain in Canada. They were French speaking, Roman Catholics, and farmers, the majority having been born in Canada of Canadian parents and considering themselves "Canadians." At this point, all immigration stopped completely and thereafter growth of the population had to depend on an excess of births over deaths.

The English immigrated to Canada and settled in the Maritimes and in Upper Canada (Ontario). This was more significant in that it blocked the West to French Canadian expansion. Coassimilation of the two groups did not occur and the French Canadians were confined in a limited even if vast territory. The population had settled near the St. Lawrence River for convenience of travel and other reasons. Even today, the population is spread around waterways, occupying only a small proportion of the geographical area of the province. In 1830, the narrow land strip around the St. Lawrence River was overpopulated, the population was very reluctant to move to parts of the province away from it, and industries in New England were attractive. Thus started a migration to the United States that is estimated at 1 million emigrants from 1830 to 1932.

The birth rate was maintained very high until 10 years ago. It has been the main factor in a hundredfold increase of the French Canadian population from 1763 to 1971, since there was no immigration until recent years.

At first glance, a population which in 300 years, or 12 generations for the average French Canadian, has increased from 6000–8000 founding ancestors to 4 million must have a suitable homogeneity to permit studies of genetic traits.

The present-day population is thus large in terms of an isolate, but some characteristics are important and help us to understand how to attack the problem.

For record purposes, the population is Roman Catholic and until recently all births, deaths, and marriages were kept in parish records. Even if the population is spread over a large geographical area, the history of the province, at least for rural areas, is that of small separate isolates from few founding fathers, so there is regional homogeneity as depicted by regional genetic diseases. The province has a modern standard of living and has high standards of medical care with universal hospitalization insurance and Medicare systems.

These characteristics and history prompted the first study of consanguinity. Such a study seemed to utilize the best source of data available in the population with genetic content, the Roman Catholic Church records of marriages and special dispensations for consanguinity. The oldest diocese in the Province was chosen for this study.

A CONSANGUINITY STUDY

Objectives

The immediate objective of the consanguinity study was to ascertain the coefficient of inbreeding in the Archdiocese of Quebec, to measure its variations, and to delineate areas where consanguinity had remained high and where detailed genetic studies might be useful.

A more remote objective was to evaluate the utility of inbreeding coefficients as real measures of homogeneity of a population and their correlation with real inbreeding.

Introduction

The Roman Catholic Church requires dispensations for marriages between cousins. All requests for dispensation to marry in the Archdiocese of Quebec have been registered with the chancellor of the archdiocese.

Although the founding of the archdiocese dates back more than two centuries, reports on total number of marriages per parish are centralized only since 1885. As this total number of marriages is necessary to calculate the inbreeding coefficient, we started our study with the year 1885.

We chose four decades for study, 1885–1895, 1915–1925, 1945–1955, and 1955–1965.

Demographic Aspect

At the time of the study, the latest available figure for the archdiocese came from the federal census of 1961. The population was 731,843. Urban areas—Quebec City and suburbs and the City of

Levis—numbered 357,568 inhabitants and the remaining rural areas had 374,275.

The population is 96% of French Canadian descent, and their ancestors are the original settlers of Canada. The geography of the archdiocese corresponds closely to the land originally settled by these ancestors and is a factor of homogeneity greater than in other parts of the province. Even the cities are not of a cosmopolitan nature but have remained rather provincial both in character and in tradition.

Sources and Material

The records of the Chancellor of the Archdiocese of Quebec were used for this study. In addition to the requests for dispensation, they contained the total number of marriages per parish per year and the list of parishes constituting the archdiocese for each period studied.

Each request for dispensation contains a genealogy giving the names of all the ancestors contributing to the consanguinity for which dispensation is asked. The importance of family and religion in this population helps prevent falsification of reports. False declarations at the prenuptial inquest could invalidate the subsequent marriage as far as canonical law is concerned. Any deviation in the inbreeding coefficient due to errors in genealogies, voluntary or otherwise, is likely to be in only one direction, i.e., an underestimation of consanguinity.

Canonical law requires dispensation for consanguineous unions up to second cousins. Before 1917, dispensation was necessary up to third cousins. In order to compare results between periods, only those marriages requiring dispensation up to second cousins have been analyzed. It might be suggested that the periods are then not necessarily comparable, since sociological conditions might not be the same under a system that requires dispensation for a third cousin marriage as compared to one that does not. However, sociological pressure on marriages of second and third cousins would probably not be great, the tendency being that the more remote the consanguinity the more readily the dispensation be granted.

The mean coefficient of inbreeding for autosomal loci (F_w) was calculated according to Sewall Wright's method,[49] which corresponds to the α value of Bernstein for a population. F_w is then the probability

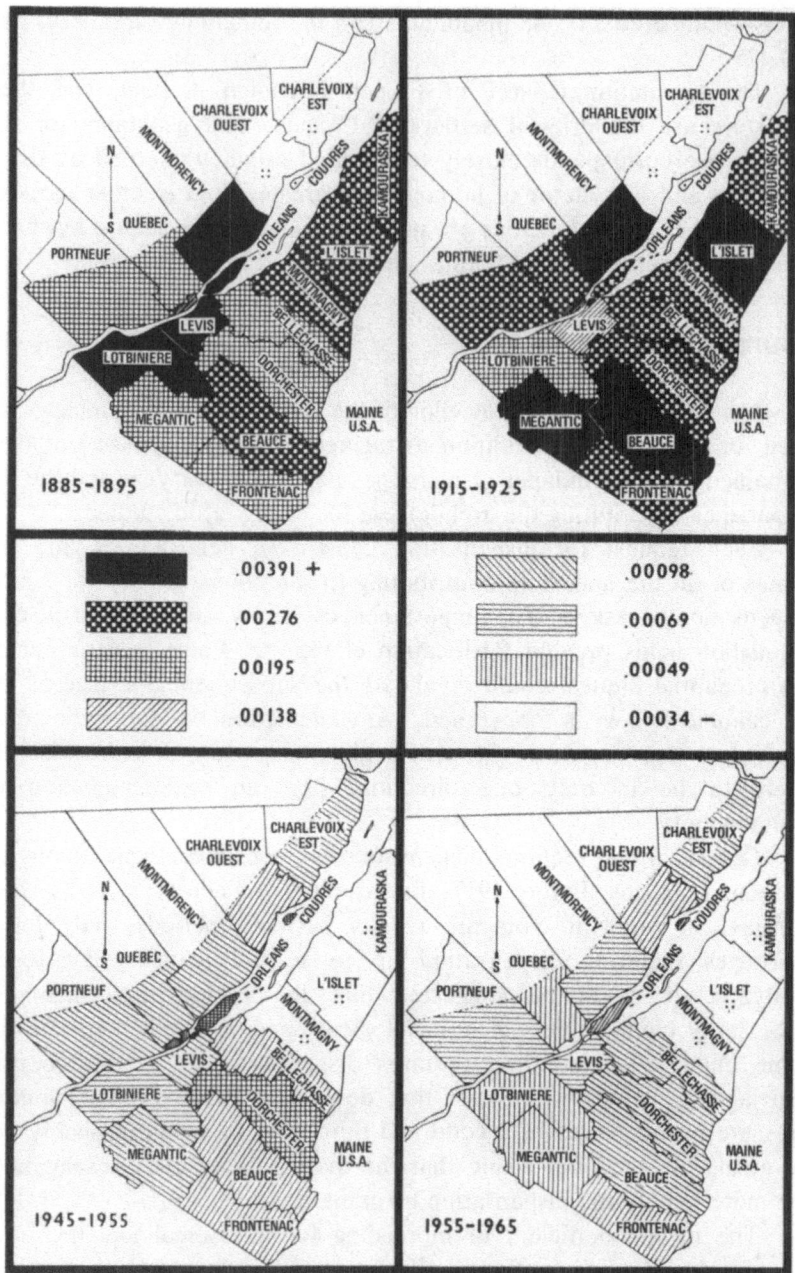

Fig. 1. Variation of coefficient of inbreeding at county level for four periods studied.

of homozygosity through a common ancestor in a child of a consanguineous mating. At the population level, the value F_w represents the decrease of heterozygosity (or heterosis) for autosomal loci as compared to a panmictic population. It represents also the average probability that two homologous loci on autosomes of one individual chosen at random in the population studied carry alleles identical by descent. This probability of identity of autosomal loci characterizes a population better than the simple frequency of consanguineous marriages (consanguinity), as it represents the direct effect of inbreeding in this population.

Results

Of the complex array of results obtained during that study, only the most important ones will be given.

In Table I, variations in the inbreeding coefficient for the archdiocese are given according to periods and areas. Taking 1920 as the highest period, variations in percentage are given for each period and finally the decrease in consanguinity since 1920 is given for each period.

Figure 1 represents the variations at each county level for the mean county coefficient of inbreeding for the four periods.

TABLE I. Variations in F_w over the Periods Studied

Period	Total	Urban	Rural
1885–1895	0.002855	0.001904	0.003027
1915–1925	0.003156	0.001902	0.003384
1945–1955	0.001342	0.000722	0.001455
1955–1965	0.000860	0.000406	0.000942
Percent (1915–1925 taken as maximum)			
1885–1895	90.45	100.14	89.47
1915–1925	100.00	100.00	100.00
1945–1955	45.23	37.98	43.00
1955–1965	27.24	21.36	27.84
Decrease in consanguinity (percent)			
1920–1950	57.47	62.02	57.00
1950–1960	35.95	43.76	35.24

TABLE II. Variations of the Different Types of Consanguineous Marriages in the Archdiocese of Quebec

Period	Type[a]				Other	Consanguinity
	I	II	III	IV		
1885–1895	0.055	2.033	1.098	3.597	0.414	7.197
1915–1925	0.123	2.159	1.271	3.873	0.507	7.933
1945–1955	0.017	0.550	0.550	1.969	0.258	3.344
1955–1965	0.008	0.371	0.361	1.362	0.126	2.228
Percent (1915–1925 taken as maximum)						
1885–1895	44.71	94.16	86.39	92.87	81.66	90.79
1915–1925	100.00	100.00	100.00	100.00	100.00	100.00
1945–1955	13.82	25.47	43.27	50.84	50.89	42.12
1955–1965	6.50	17.18	28.40	35.17	24.85	28.12
Decrease in consanguinity (percent)						
1920–1950	86.18	74.53	56.73	49.16	49.11	57.88
1950–1960	52.94	32.55	34.36	30.83	51.16	33.23

[a] Type I, uncle–niece; II, first cousin; III, first-and-a-half cousin; IV, second cousin.

TABLE III. Contributions of Types of Consanguineous Marriages to F_w and to Total Consanguineous Marriages

Period	Type of consanguinity (%)[a]				Other
	I	II	III	IV	
1885–1895					
F_w	2.80	51.31	13.85	22.69	9.35
TCM[b]	0.77	28.25	15.25	49.97	5.76
1915–1925					
F_w	5.46	47.74	14.06	21.41	11.33
TCM	1.56	27.21	16.03	48.81	6.39
1945–1955					
F_w	2.17	35.32	17.66	31.62	13.23
TCM	0.51	16.44	16.44	58.89	7.72
1955–1965					
F_w	1.58	36.70	17.86	33.69	10.17
TCM	0.36	16.65	16.20	61.14	5.65

[a] Types as in Table II.
[b] Total consanguineous marriages.

Table II presents the variations of the different types of consanguineous marriages as their percentage relative to all mariages of that period. Consanguinity is defined as the percent of marriages that are consanguineous. Again, 1920 is taken as the maximum and variations of the different types are compared to it in percentage. Finally, the decrease in type of consanguineous marriages is given for periods after 1920.

Table III gives for each period the contribution of each type of consanguineous marriage to the coefficient of inbreeding and to the consanguinity.

Discussion: Consanguinity and the Mean Coefficient F_w

The mean coefficient of inbreeding F_w represents the probability of identity by descent of two homologous autosomal loci in the child born to the average mating in a given population. Many sociocultural factors will influence this probability, and this fact requires that a segmentary study of the population first be done to minimize these influences. This segmentary study will allow the determination of geographical zones where consanguinity is high, reflecting cultural and ancestral isolates within the total population. This information would be lost in a global study of the population. It seems logical to think of a population as composed of subpopulations each having its social characteristics such as particular consanguinity rate, migration patterns, population density, and ancestral genetic pool. The parish is recognized as a social and cultural unit in the French Canadian population by many sociologists,[38] and by definition the study of consanguinity from Church dispensation records in such parishes is necessarily easy.

A list of all the parishes and their coefficient of inbreeding would, on the other hand, be too long and too detailed to permit an analysis of regional and diocesan variations and tendencies. Thus coefficients have been calculated per county, taking into account also, however, the individual parish values.

Figure 1 shows the evolution of inbreeding (F_w) in the Archdiocese of Quebec from 1885 to 1965. The counties are hatched to indicate the value of F_w for a given period, the darker the hatching the greater the value of F_w. The range is from 0.00391 and over (third cousins or closer) to 0.00034 and under (less than fourth-and-a-half cousins). It can be seen from the figure that the period of highest consanguinity was 1915–1925 and that since then there has been a sharp decline in inbreeding over the whole archdiocese.

The variances of the coefficients F_w for the average parish of each county were calculated and also showed a tendency to decrease over the years, a fact which suggests that at the county level not only is the consanquinity rate decreasing but also the variations in inbreeding from one parish to another have decreased as the isolates have broken up. The F_w coefficients have become more uniform, suggesting that the isolate is now more at the county level than at the parish level as it was in the 1880s and 1920s. The decrease in variances for a given county over the years suggests also that the population of the county is becoming more homogeneous and that it now constitutes the geographical location of the isolate. If this were not true, we would expect the variances to increase, not decrease, as the number of consanguineous marriages per parish decreases. The subpopulations have become larger and this phenomenon has been general in the rural as well as in the urban regions. Parochial subisolates most useful for genetic studies should be found in the county that shows the greatest inbreeding coefficient and variance.

A better idea of the drop in F_w in rural and urban counties can be derived from Table I, where the coefficients for comparable counties from one period to another are analyzed. The 1915–1925 period is taken as maximum (100%), and the drop in inbreeding is expressed as percent of the maximum. It can be seen that the decrease in inbreeding is more marked and rapid in the cities than in the rural regions, a fact which reflects the important migration to cities from the rural areas after 1920.

Table II also shows a decrease in the percentage of consanguineous marriages and in the different types of such marriages. The drop in the percentage of consanguineous marriages is almost identical to that of F_w and suggests a close association between these two measures. However, in theory, this association is not obligatory. When the percentage of consanguineous marriages remains identical but the frequencies of the different types change, F_w will drop without a concomitant decline of the percentage. Four marriages between second cousins give the same F_w value as a single first cousin marriage and a modification of the latter in favor of the former would give a decrease in F_w by a factor of 75% for each marriage.

This concomitant drop of F_w and consanguinity is thus a coincidence and resides only in the equilibrium that has taken place between the different types of consanguineous marriages at the archdiocese level. Table II shows that third (uncle–niece type) and fourth degree (first cousin) types decreased and that this decline took place between 1920 and 1950. This phenomenon means that the sociocultural factors that influence consanguinity affect more the marriages of close consanguinity and that, by reaction, a tolerance is manifested toward less consanguineous unions.

The contribution of the different types of consanguineous marriages is not the same for the F_w coefficient as for the percentage of consanguinity which cannot measure the contribution of the average individual to the genetic pool and cannot give an idea of the mean coefficient of inbreeding in a population. Even the percentage of first cousin marriages cannot give by itself an exact idea of the genetic constitution of a population, because, depending on the population, this percentage will represent a more or less important fraction of the totality of consanguineous marriages, being very sensitive, for example, to the influence of particular sociocultural factors. The principle that only the first cousin marriages are of importance is doubtful since for the 1955–1965 period they represent 16.65% of the consanguineous marriages and contribute only 36.70% to F_w. For the same period, the second cousin marriages contributed to F_w almost as much, 33.69%.

The mean coefficient of inbreeding for autosomal loci is thus better for determining changes in consanguinity for a population than is the percentage of consanguineous marriages or of those between first cousins. The coefficient represents a probability and thus measures much more accurately the participation of the average child of consanguineous matings in the ancestral genetic pool of the population. The sociocultural patterns and their influences on consanguinity are better analyzed against F_w than against any other measure of consanguinity because any conclusions derived will directly correlate with the genetic pool.

The principal cultural factor influencing consanguinity in Catholic populations is the need to obtain a dispensation for consanguineous marriages. Even when such dispensations are easily obtained, a certain cultural pressure against such marriages exists, a pressure which is greater the more consanguineous the union. Other factors which could influence consanguineous marriages are folklore and regional or parochial experiences arising from such marriages. If by folklore or experience consanguineous marriages are considered dangerous to the life or health of children of such marriages, the cultural pressure against such matings will increase up to a point where consanguineous matings are considered ''taboo.''

Among social factors that could influence consanguinity are migration, mean number of children per family, and genetic drift. Migration is the most important factor acting to decrease consanguinity, being the major force that breaks up the isolates. The number of marriages in the cities increases much more rapidly than in rural regions and reflects an important urban migration between 1920 and 1950. Urban marriages were 8400 for 1915–1925 and 21,450 for 1955–1965 as compared to 20,770 in 1915–1925 and 28,680 in 1955–1965 for rural areas. While an analysis of all the marriages over all the years since 1920 would have measured accurately the nature and duration of this migration, this study does show the importance of such a migration, even though done at both ends of this period. In general, this period corresponds to the years of economic depression and of rapid industrialization in the Province of Quebec. This migration had as a consequence the effect of decreasing or at least maintaining the rural population density at the same level, thus reducing the number of available partners for marriage in the immediate region of the future spouse. Marriage between cousins became more difficult because of the extraordinary conditions necessary to its realization, such as distance.

The peasant and sedentary character of the rural regions will always keep them more consanguineous than the urban ones unless massive population movements take place to mix the regional genetic pools. Migration, however, does not have an unlimited effect on consanguinity. The restricted number of common ancestors in a given region will always maintain a certain level of consanguinity by simple random genetic drift and by participation of the average individual of such a region in the ancestral patrimony. In many counties, the population density has remained the same for many years, one descendant only staying on the familial farm, the others having to migrate to cities where they work in industry or commerce. Geographical location has a given maximum occupancy for an adequate living environment and colonizing virgin territories has less appeal than life in cities. This constant population density works together with random genetic drift to keep the rural regions more consanguineous because the same family population will always be represented in a given region.

Another factor, which will influence consanguinity in the future more than it has in the past, is the mean number of children per family. As other factors affecting consanguinity decline in importance as a result of the breaking up of isolates, this factor will have a major effect. Stern[45] and Sutter and Goux[46] have shown that the number of partners available for cousin marriages depends directly on this factor. If the mean number of children per family is 7, an individual can marry 42 first cousins, 130 first-and-a-half cousins, and 500 second cousins as compared to 6, 14, and 36 if this mean number per family is 3. The mean number of children per family is at the present time at its lowest level in the Province of Quebec mainly because of the introduction of contraceptive methods for young couples, resulting from the increasing socioeconomic hardships that numerous children bring in a modern society where industrialization and education are of prime importance. A further decrease in consanguinity may thus be expected in the future, at least in the French Canadian population, as measured by the method of Church dispensation records. This does not, however, mean complete disappearance of isolates, because genetic drift and the founder effect will continue tò contribute to the inbreeding coefficient. Isolates will still be found for some time but will depend on existing local conditions, such as geographical or social isolation. French Canadians will always have a higher mean coefficient of inbreeding that their fellow North Americans of Anglo-Saxon extraction because of common descent from only about 6000 or 8000 ancestors. The value of F_w calculated from Church dispensation records will probably fall to a very low level in the near future because of mounting pressure in the society against close consanguinity.

Conclusions and Decisions

The study of request for dispensations for consanguinity done in the Archdiocese of Quebec showed that inbreeding coefficients had followed the known trend of rapid decrease accompanying the breakup of isolates.

Detailed analysis, however, showed that there were still rural isolates where consanguinity was elevated and that, although pressure was felt against close consanguinity, they would remain genetically isolated for some time.

Such studies did not allow analysis of sociocultural, regional, and family reasons for maintaining consanguinity or calculation of the real inbreeding of the population containing all ancestral information. The feeling was that real consanguinity was probably about fourfold higher than that calculated from Catholic Church records.

It was thus decided to study in detail one isolate in the archdiocese, preferably an island, to find out what were the historical, demographic, and cultural factors influencing its inbreeding coefficient

AN ISOLATE STUDY

Objectives

As stated above, a clearer understanding of social, cultural, and demographic factors influencing the rate of consanguinity and inbreeding was necessary. An isolate study could also provide the necessary information for calculating the true inbreeding of the population and permit the beginning of a study on the effects of inbreeding on the French Canadians.

Introduction

After the data on consanguinity in the Archdiocese of Quebec were obtained from the records of Church dispensations, an opportunity was sought to study the genetic structure of the French Canadian population. A rural isolate in this region seemed to offer the best opportunity for obtaining accurate details and clear understanding of the demographic features in that population. It was mandatory to find an isolate where the influences of urban environment were minimized, where the population stock was intact and homogeneous, where retrieval of genealogical information would be easy, and where the population was large enough for at least preliminary statistical studies of demographic and genetic interest.

According to Martin,[35] Isle-aux-Coudres is typical of such an isolate. It is fairly easily accessible to investigators, being only 70 miles from Quebec City. Its population—about 1700 in 1954—had been established on the island for about 250 years and was homogeneous. The socioeconomic status of the population is very close to that of the rest of rural Quebec. This geographical and demographic isolate was therefore selected for a detailed study.

Methods

A census of the island was completed in the summer of 1965, including information on the reproductive performance of all families established on the island having one parental member still alive. The collaboration of the influential priest of the parish of St. Louis and of the island physician contributed greatly to the success of the census: only five persons refused to reply to direct questioning. The census consisted of the usual demographic data and, in addition, contained detailed information on the outcome of every pregnancy of each couple and the health of every person investigated. A genealogy was drawn for each family, at least up to the fifth generation, from Church records and genealogical dictionaries.[17]

Results

Geography and History

Isle-aux-Coudres was discovered by Jacques Cartier on his second voyage to America on 6 September, 1535. He named it "isle es Couldres" because of the hazel trees he found there, whose fruits he found more delicious than the ones in France. The island is situated in the St. Lawrence River about 60 miles downstream from Quebec City and 1½ miles from the north shore of the St. Lawrence. It is 2.75 miles wide at its maximum and 6.5 miles long along the orientation of the river, its total surface being about 12.2 square miles. It is fairly flat, the highest point being 300 ft above the water line. The north shore of the island is the highest, and the terrain drops toward the south shore, where landing is difficult at low tide. However, the island can easily be approached by boat from the north.

On the north shore of the St. Lawrence, there are steep cliffs up to a height of 1300 ft. The only recess on the shoreline is at Baie St.-Paul, where two small rivers open up on a small, fertile valley. The original settlers of this region converted the land to agriculture around 1675, but the Baie St.-Paul valley soon became crowded for good farming; and demographic pressure brought the first settlers to the fertile lands of the Isle-aux-Coudres about 1720.

At first, the island was used mainly as a stopover for ships coming up the river to, Quebec and Montreal and as a pilot exchange point. In 1677, Etienne de Lessart obtained the island by concession from Frontenac but failed to settle it. In 1687, because of failure of Lessart to comply with his contract, the concession changed hands and became the possession of the seminary priests who at the time owned also the whole north shore of the river in this area as a gift from Monseigneur de Laval. The priests did not start any settlement there before the eighteenth century. By 1710, the inhabitants of Baie St.-Paul and Petite-Riviere St. François (neighboring parish) asked Intendant Raudot for concession of lands on the island. This was finally granted, and the first ten land titles were awarded in 1728. But according to tradition the first inhabitant of the island was a certain Joseph Savard, established as a squatter with his family in 1720. (The name Savard disappeared from the island after 1831.)

Population

Martin[35] divides the island's demographic history into three periods: a period of settlement, 1728–1795; a stable period, 1795–1875; and a period of expansion, 1875–1954.

Period of Settlement, 1728–1795. From 1728 to 1765, when Canada came under British rule, the increase in population was due mainly to immigration. The census of 1765 shows 41 families living on the island, with a population of 213. The island was evacuated and the inhabitants were relocated by military authorities in 1759–1760 because of Wolfe's invasion of Quebec. The move had little effect on family life, and afterward the people returned to their homes on the island.

From 1765 to 1795, the population doubled to 556 through natural increase. By 1790, all available land on the island had been appropriated and consequently the population size was stabilized. The birth rate reflects this very well, as it was 60 per 1000 from 1761 to 1770, 56.5 per 1000 from 1771 to 1790, and 30.4 per 1000 from 1781 to 1790.

At the end of this period, the economy of the island was based mainly on agriculture with exportation of potatoes. There was also a trade in porpoise oil (*marsouin*) and the establishment of two flour mills. The population was fairly prosperous.

Stable Period, 1795–1875. The stable demographic period was characterized by very slow increase in population size, although the natural increase was always around 20 per 1000. There was now strong emigration, inhabitants leaving the island around the age of 20–25 years. In 1844, the proportion of the class 0–20 years old was 54.7%.

Mailloux[33] states that from 1790 to 1868 the population surplus emigrated almost totally to parishes near the island on the north shore. From there they later emigrated to Lac St.-Jean and became the founding fathers of the Chicoutimi region. Migration continued later and is a main characteristic of the population of the island. Genetically as well as anthropologically, the important point here is that this population soon became an "old" population in the sense that early in its history it became a "founding" population, a rare situation for a "young" population such as the French Canadians (in comparison with Europeans).

As in the period of settlement, agriculture and porpoise fishing were the main staples of economy on the island, and the standard of living was still relatively good.

Up to 1824, communication with urban centers was maintained by canoes and schooners until a road from Quebec to Baie St.-Paul along the cliffs and mountains of the north shore became practicable. Communication with the mainland still depended on big canoes; no ferry operated regularly between the island and the mainland at that time.

In this period there was no increase in the amount of arable land. By 1801, a road went around the island, and there were four county schools with 169 pupils.

Period of Expansion, 1875–1954. From 1871 to 1951, the population of the island increased by 296% from 566 to 1676 inhabitants. The number of families in 1954 had more than tripled since 1868, mainly because many families had established their sons on the island either by dividing the original land or by allowing their sons to build houses to live in while working outside the island on seasonal work.

This demographic change in living conditions could also have changed the homogeneity of the population by permitting outside marriages, but this has not been the case, probably because of the great isolation a stranger would feel in living on the island and not being a part of the cultural group.

By 1930, a ferryboat came in use between the mainland and the island and today it has been replaced by an all-weather metal ferryboat which makes daily trips even during winter through the ice. Telephone and electricity came to the island in 1954.

In the first half of the twentieth century, migration goals changed, the inhabitants going to cities following the trend of rural–urban migration. Most of the emigrants went to Montreal, where their knowledge of small boats permitted them to dominate completely the low freight handling on the docks by 1954.

By 1954, the island had become, for many, a place to live while working outside. As a consequence, the economy of the island has changed: agriculture is still a principal feature, but a great part of the economy now depends on salaried jobs on the outside, mainly in the field of merchandise handling and maritime jobs. The tourist trade has increased but is still a seasonal affair, resorts being open during the summer.

Population in 1965. The island in 1965 had not changed much from 1954 except for an increase in the tourist trade and the introduction of television. To show that the population of the island is fairly homogeneous, a list of family names found on the island in different years is given in Table IV. It can be seen that the number of names has stayed around 20 since 1762 but that the proportion of some has changed drastically.

Endogamy can be suspected by looking at the eight commonest family names in the 1965 census, where they represent 83% of the families living on the island as compared to only 40% in 1762. On the other hand, of the five commonest names, which in 1762 represented 55%, two have now completely disappeared from the island.

Even if this method does not measure endogamy directly, it can be seen if a name stood for 2.5% of the population in 1762 and 200 years later it is carried by 24.3% of the population's heads of family, the genetic potential of these ancestors should be represented in good

TABLE IV. Family Names (%) on Isle-aux-Coudres, 1762–1965

Family name	1965 (N = 255)[a]	1954 (N = 256)	1868 (N = 70)	1831 (N = 69)	1762 (N = 40)
Dufour	24.3	24.2	10.0	5.8	2.5
Harvey	18.0	17.6	7.1	4.3	7.5
Degagne	10.2	9.0	17.1	8.7	2.5
Tremblay	8.6	9.0	20.0	20.3	17.5
Bouchard	7.8	8.2	8.6	4.3	7.5
Boudreault	5.5	4.7	4.3	1.4	0.0
Perron	5.5	5.5	7.1	5.8	2.5
Gagnon	3.1	3.1	2.8	5.8	0.0
Pedneault	2.7	4.7	1.4	1.4	0.0
Bergeron	2.3	2.3	2.8	4.3	2.5
Castonguay	2.3	1.9	0.0	0.0	0.0
Demeule	2.3	2.3	1.4	2.9	2.5
Lajoie	2.3	2.7	1.4	5.8	2.5
Mailloux	2.3	1.9	2.8	4.3	0.0
Leclerc	0.8	0.8	2.8	2.9	0.0
Boivin	0.4	0.4	0.0	1.4	2.5
LaForest	0.4	0.4	1.4	1.4	0.0
Porlier	0.4	0.0	0.0	0.0	0.0
Aube	0.0	0.4	0.0	0.0	0.0
Desbiens	0.0	0.4	2.8	2.9	10.0
LaPierre	0.0	0.4	0.0	0.0	0.0
LaPointe	0.0	0.0	2.8	5.8	0.0
Savard	0.0	0.0	0.0	1.4	0.0
Others	0.8	0.1	3.4	9.1	40.0
Number of family names	18	20	19	24	23

[a] N = number of families.

proportion in the present population. This method also gives an idea of the isolation to which the population on Isle-aux-Coudres has been subjected.

As a consequence of its high birth rate, the island has always maintained a "young" type of population pyramid. An important reason for this shape is known from sociological studies[35] to be migration outside the island at the time of marriage. In Table V, beginning in 1951, a diminution is evident in the 0–20 years of age class that is already affecting the pyramid shape in 1965. All other causes of

TABLE V. Percentages of the Population by Age
Groups

Year	Age group (years)		
	0–20	20–65	65+
1844	57.4		
1931	53.3	41.8	4.9
1941	49.2	46.0	4.8
1951	50.5	44.7	4.8
1965	47.4	48.3	4.3

mortality being equal in that class, this means that a lowering of the birth rate has been taking place on the the island in recent years.

In order to make comparisons between generations and to see any evolution that might have taken place from one generation to another, families from the census were divided into completed and incompleted families. Completed families were those in which the mother was 45 years old or older at the time of the census (July 1965), one parent had died before the mother was 45, or the mother had had a hysterectomy and/or bilateral ovariectomy before the age of 45. All other families were considered uncompleted. There were 143 completed and 107 uncompleted families in the 1965 census. This shows the demographic limits reached on the island and the important role that migration must play in maintaining the equilibrium between two succeeding generations.

Age at First Marriage. All data available have been used to study the distributions of age at first marriage for both completed and uncompleted families. For completed families, males marry on the average at 26.7 years of age (standard deviation 4.7 years) and females marry at 23.4 (standard deviation 4.59). For uncompleted families, the average age at first marriage is 26.9 for males (standard deviation 3.88) and 23.4 for females (standard deviation 3.52). The mean values show some accordance with those given by Henripin[25] for the early eighteenth-century Canadian population: 26.8 years of age for males and 21.9 for females marrying for the first time another single person.

Geographical Location of Marriage Partners. Immigration is not an important factor in this population, only 17 persons having come from outside the island, five males and 12 females. Of these, seven came from Charlevoix County and can be considered, for genealogical purposes, as having come from the same population as the island. This leaves ten out of 514 persons (1.9%) coming from what may be considered a stranger ancestral group. Of these ten persons, only one male and two females belong to completed families, a fact which renders this group homogeneous for genetic studies.

Consanguinity

Inbreeding on the island has been studied by three methods: (1) from requests for Church dispensations, (2) from genealogies of partners up to five generation, and (3) by the isonymy method of Crow and Mange.[10]

Church dispensations for 255 marriages give a mean coefficient of inbreeding, F_w, equal to 0.005251, which is a little lower than that for second-and-a-half cousins.

If inbreeding coefficients are calculated from genealogical information on these same families, going back five generations to include third and third-and-a-half cousins, a mean value of F_w of 0.011790 is obtained. This is a little lower than that for second cousins and represents an increase of 0.006539 over the previous estimate. Mange[34] also found in his study that inclusion of two more generations doubled the estimate of F_w.

At this rate of increase, 0.003319 per generation, after ten generations the F_w will be roughly 0.028484. Given a generation time of 25 years years, this would trace ancestors of these families back to 1715, when most of their ancestors were in fact established in Canada. Whether this arbitrarily chosen increase is acceptable remains to be seen and can be judged only on complete genealogical data of all the families of the island.

Figure 2 shows the pedigree of one randomly selected family from the 1965 census, tracing all the ancestors of the married partners to the time when they came to Canada. The F_w value for the total pedigree is 0.019496. Whether the immigrant ancestors were related is not known. The contribution of different generations included in the pedigree of Fig. 2 is given in Table VI.

If we now take the average inbreeding coefficient for the

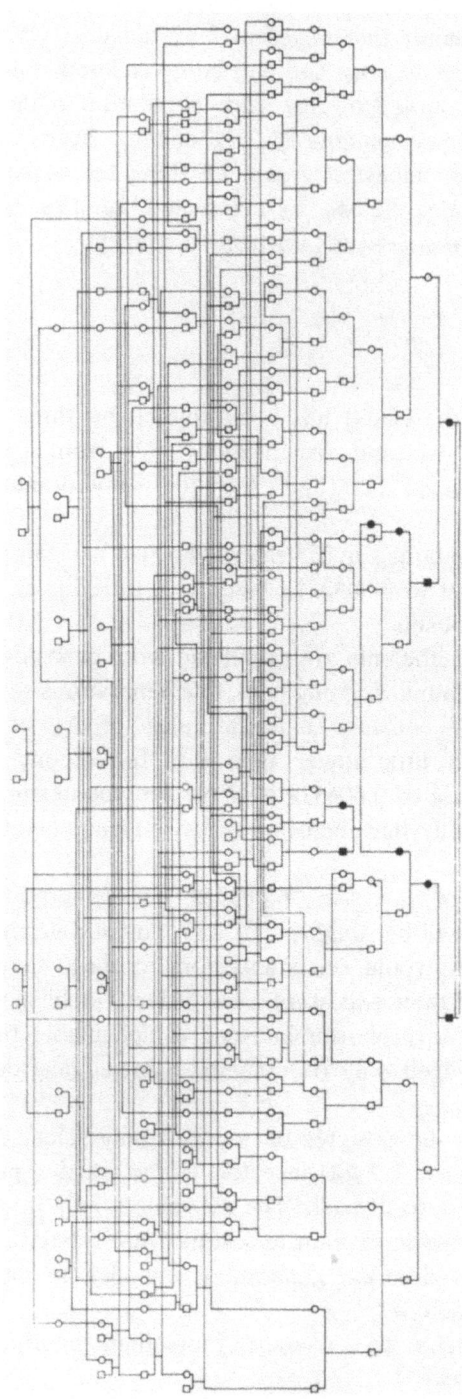

Fig. 2. Pedigree of a family on Isle-aux-Coudres with all ancestors back to the time they immigrated to Canada.

TABLE VI. Contributions of Different Links in the Pedigree of Fig. 2 to
the Total Inbreeding Coefficient F_w

Number of ancestors in a link	Number of links	Value of F_w	Percent of total F_w
9 (4 generations)	1	0.0078125	40.0
14 (7 generations)	13	0.00317383	31.3
15	24	0.00292969	
16 (8 generations)	37	0.00225830	17.6
17	39	0.00119018	
18 (9 generations)	68	0.00103760	9.0
19	93	0.00070958	
20 (10 generations)	84	0.00032036	2.0
21	32	0.00005204	
22 (11 generations)	11	0.00001049	0.1
23	3	0.00000143	
24 (12 generations)	1	0.00000024	
25	1	0.00000012	
26 (13 generations)	1	0.00000006	0
Total		0.01949641	

population calculated over five genealogical generations, or 0.011790, and if we assume a distribution of F_w identical for each generation to that of the pedigree of Fig. 2, we get 0.012602 as a mean coefficient of inbreeding for the population, which corresponds roughly to estimates by other methods.

The completeness of pedigrees for five generations was 97.05% and to have obtained the same accuracy for 10 to 12 generations would have been time consuming because marriages before 1800 are difficult to trace. It was felt, however, that we had enough material to test the applicability of Crow and Mange's[10] isonymy method.

Depending on the transmission pattern of family names in a population, the frequency of marriages between two partners with the same family name could be used in measuring inbreeding. This method assumes that there are no known changes in these names, that there were no unrelated ancestors with the same name, that cousin marriages of the different types and subtypes occur at random, and that the maximal value of F_w is not 1 but 0.25 because the method does not apply to marriages in which one partner is a direct descendant of the other or in which the partners are sibs. In theory, the proportion of marriages between persons of the same family name should always

TABLE VII. Results of the Isonymy Method on Two Populations on
Isle-aux-Coudres in 1831 and 1965

	1965	1831
F_t	0.018627	0.003623
F_r	0.027057	0.016192
F_n	−0.008667	−0.012776
Number of families	255	69
P	19/255 = 0.0745	1/69 = 0.014492
Genetic drift in 134 years	$F_r' = 0.011045$	

reflect the same amount of inbreeding in the population, there always being one-fourth of the cousin marriages of all types between persons of the same family names. Despite all these drawbacks, the method may have some usefulness in giving at least a range of inbreeding that can be compared to other methods.

Without going into the details of the method, inbreeding coefficients were calculated for the population at two intervals. F_t is the total inbreeding coefficient of the population, F_r that for the inbreeding from random matings, and F_n that from nonrandom marriages. These are related according to Wright[49] and Crow and Mange[10] in the following manner[1]:

$$F_t = F_n + (1 - F_n)F_r$$

It should be noted that if both F_t and F_r are necessarily positive, F_n can be either positive or negative. It could well be negative if consanguineous marriages were avoided.

In Table VII, results are given for two censuses as well as an extension measuring the degree of random genetic drift taking place in 134 years.

The random component of inbreeding is probably very close to the total inbreeding in any well-defined human isolate.[2] The formula for F_r is then a good estimator of this inbreeding if the preliminary conditions are met, as they are in our population. We have an estimate of $F_r = 0.026489$ for 1965. From extension of the five-generation population average we had 0.028484 and from the pedigree in Fig. 2 we had 0.023602, estimates which agree well with the isonymy method.

We can also see the avoidance of close consanguinity in this population by the negative values of F_n. Genetic drift has increased the inbreeding by 45.45% over the last 135 years accoring to the isonymy method. This method can be used here as a reflection of genetic drift if names are viewed as alleles at the same locus. Name have a probability of loss at each generation of 0.5; thus a name carried by a male in a population has the same probability of irrevocable loss in the next generation (through females) as does a single gene.[1]

The situation found on the island is probably the same in all rural areas of the province because emigration and the homogeneity of the population remaining maintain a high degree of random inbreeding. If we consider the French Canadians as a whole and remember the relatively small number of ancestors of this 4.8 million population (6000–8000) more than 300 years ago, we can also say that they can be considered an isolate with an appreciable amount of random inbreeding, although perhaps to a lesser degree than Isle-aux-Coudres. In addition to the limited number of ancestors, the reproductive performances of some of these ancestors should be considered. It was calculated around 1950 that Pierre Tremblay, who came over from France and married in Quebec in October 1657, had about 90,000 descendants of the same name. This is just one example of the possible contribution of one ancestor to the gene pool of the present French Canadian population.

For these reasons, the estimates of F_w in the study of the Archdiocese of Quebec in the preceding discussion should probably be multiplied by a factor of 4, especially for rural estimates.

Genetic Load

The genetic load data were calculated from completed families at the time of the 1965 census according to the minimum χ^2 method of Schull and Neel.[41,42] According to these authors, their exponent model gives identical results as the maximum likelihood method of Morton *et al.*[36]

Using the exponential model proposed by Morton *et al.*,[36] the solution of the minimum χ^2 regression of mortality on F classes is given by simultaneously solving for α and β iteratively in the following equations:

$$\sum N_i P_i / \hat{P}_i = \sum N_i \tag{1}$$

$$\sum N_i P_i F_i / \hat{P}_i = \sum N_i F_i \tag{2}$$

TABLE VIII. Mortality Rates According to Inbreeding Groups and Consanguinity Classes

Inbreeding from Church records

		Coefficients			
		0.0 (1)	0.1562 (2)	0.0312 (3)	0.0625 (4)
Fetal wastage (miscarriages and abortions)	Families	95	23	8	2
	Rates	57/849	23/217	10/83	1/29
		0.06714	0.10599	0.12048	0.03448
Perinatal deaths (stillbirths and neonatal)	Families	91	23	8	2
	Rates	56/792	9/194	6/73	1/29
		0.07070	0.04639	0.08219	0.03448
Infantile and juvenile deaths (1 month to 15 years of age)	Families	90	22	7	2
	Rates	65/737	9/185	5/67	5/27
		0.08820	0.04865	0.07463	0.18519
Total mortality (conception to 15 years of age)	Families	95	23	8	2
	Rates	177/849	41/217	21/83	7/29
		0.20848	0.18894	0.25301	0.24138

Inbreeding from genealogies

		Coefficients				
		0.0 (1)	0.00542 (2)	0.01207 (3)	0.02301 (4)	0.04277 (5)
Fetal wastage (miscarriages and abortions)	Families	22	47	22	25	11
	Rates	12/207	32/442	22/182	15/230	11/118
		0.05797	0.07240	0.12088	0.06522	0.09322
Perinatal deaths (stillbirths and neonatal)	Families	21	47	19	26	11
	Rates	12/197	32/410	8/146	13/229	7/107
		0.06091	0.07805	0.05479	0.05677	0.6542
Infantile and juvenile deaths (1 month to 15 years of age)	Families	21	46	19	25	10
	Rates	15/183	35/378	7/138	17/216	10/100
		0.08197	0.09259	0.05072	0.07870	0.10000
Total mortality (conception to 15 years of age)	Families	22	47	22	26	11
	Rates	39/207	99/442	51/182	45/230	28/118
		0.18841	0.22398	0.28022	0.19565	0.23729

where N_i, P_i, and F_i are, respectively, the number of observations in the ith inbred class characterized by the observed proportion of deaths P_i and the inbreeding coefficient F_i.

The data available from completed families on which genetic loads were calculated are given for two methods of calculating inbreeding in Table VIII, from Church records of dispensations, and from genealogies for five generations.

Equations (1) and (2) were first solved by trial and error. Subsequently, the calculations were checked and given more accuracy by the iterative method for fitting a weighted regression model published in Fortran II by MacCluer et al.[31]

Table IX gives the values of genetic loads calculated by the method of minimum χ^2 for two inbreeding groups, one calculated from Church records and the second from five genealogical generations. The genetic loads correspond to the observed rates of mortality given in Table VIII.

Table IX is presented in the same manner as those in Schull and Neel's book[41] by giving the expected values of mortality according to the regression model for each consanguinity class which can be compared with observed values of Table VIII. When analysis is based on all classes of study, its values are given under $F \geq 0$; when only inbred classes were used, the values are given under $F > 0$. Significances at the 5% level and 1% level are given χ^2 values according to their degrees of freedom.

The test of the model consists of χ^2 values for internal consistency of the data. The value h is a variable proposed by Schull and Neel[41] which is normally distributed with zero mean and unit variance. If improbably large, either positively or negatively, it demonstrates an internal inconsistency in the data.

The value of α represents the mortality in the noninbred class due to environmental and genetic causes, while β represents the mortality brought about by consanguinity at a value of complete inbreeding of 1 by genetic causes alone.

Given certain assumptions such as an equilibrium population, nonsynergistic gene action, or epistasis, the Morton et al. argument asserts that the ratio β/α will be great if the majority of loci are of the classical type (mutational), if there is a balance between mutation and selection, and that the "optimum" genotype is the homozygote. On the other hand, this ratio will be small if genetic variability is maintained

TABLE IX. Genetic Loads Calculated from Exponit Model According to Inbreeding Groups

Inbreeding from Church records		Estimated values				Estimates of		Test of model (χ^2)			
		P_1	P_2	P_3	P_4	α	β	Regression	Residual	Total	h
Fetal wastage	$F \geq 0$	0.07239	0.07249	0.07260	0.07281	0.0751	0.0072	0.00	7.45[a]	7.45	
	$F > 0$	0.09140	0.11270	0.08990	0.04265	0.1449	−1.6209	3.09	0.66	3.76	0.39
Perinatal deaths	$F \geq 0$	0.7229	0.06206	0.05171	0.03068	0.0750	−0.7019	2.16	1.50	3.66	
	$F > 0$	0.4997	0.05096	0.04925	0.04581	0.0541	−0.1155	0.02	1.81	1.82	−0.05
Infantile and juvenile deaths	$F \geq 0$	0.08045	0.07251	0.06450	0.04827	0.0839	−0.5503	0.85	9.38[b]	10.23[a]	
	$F > 0$	0.05723	0.04679	0.08635	0.16040	0.0056	2.7121	6.67[b]	0.39	7.07[a]	−0.40
Total mortality	$F \geq 0$	0.20493	0.21177	0.21856	0.23196	0.2293	0.5535	0.21	1.42	1.64	
	$F > 0$	0.20557	0.19495	0.22067	0.26967	0.1844	2.0777	0.89	0.76	1.65	−0.27

Inbreeding from genealogies		Estimated values					Estimates of		Test of model (χ^2)			
		P_1	P_2	P_3	P_4	P_5	α	β	Regression	Residual	Total	h
Fetal wastage	$F \geq 0$	0.06798	0.07064	0.07389	0.07921	0.08845	0.0704	0.5266	0.59	6.82	7.42	
	$F > 0$	0.07820	0.07654	0.07770	0.07960	0.08291	0.0786	0.1884	0.06	5.65	5.70	0.05
Perinatal deaths	$F \geq 0$	0.06781	0.06653	0.06499	0.06240	0.05783	0.0702	−0.2525	0.17	1.53	1.69	
	$F > 0$	0.06559	0.07023	0.06748	0.06282	0.05456	0.0753	−0.4549	0.43	1.09	1.53	0.06
Infantile and juvenile deaths	$F \geq 0$	0.07798	0.07853	0.07922	0.08037	0.08237	0.0812	0.1131	0.02	3.03	3.05	
	$F > 0$	0.07871	0.07668	0.07804	0.08034	0.08432	0.0786	0.2252	0.07	3.03	3.10	−0.02
Total mortality	$F \geq 0$	0.21095	0.20564	0.19910	0.18778	0.16849	0.2369	−1.2421	1.27	15.54[b]	16.81[b]	
	$F > 0$	0.19967	0.21798	0.20732	0.18871	0.15662	0.2570	−2.0528	2.84	12.92[b]	15.76[b]	0.10

[a] Significant at the 5% level.
[b] Significant at the 1% level.

primarily through a balance of opposing selective forces or if the nongenetic contribution to mortality is appreciably larger than the genetic one.

Lethal equivalents are groups of genes of such numbers that if dispersed in different individuals they would cause on the average one death. Because of the smallness of the population studied and the small range of F_w on which the estimates are made, estimates of β when extrapolated to $F_w = 1$ will have great variability.

The values obtained for lethal equivalents when not negative are not very high and compare well with those reported by Schull and Neel[41,42] for Japan.

Calculating inbreeding coefficients from genealogies has the effect of decreasing the control noninbred group as more of these now become "consanguineous." Even then, there do not seem to be marked changes in the number of lethal equivalents carried by the individual. One reason for this might be that the contribution of environmental causes of death to the calculation of α is very large; a second one could be that the population is relatively homogeneous because of continuing isolation and that control groups with minimal effects of inbreeding cannot be obtained; a third is the possibility that the sedentary population of the island is more "fit" than the emigrant population that leaves the island. This last point would be very unusual but interesting to study in the population originating from Isle-aux-Coudres and now living in Montreal.

In conclusion, the interpretation of genetic load determinations in a small (less than 2000) and old isolate is difficult because of homogeneity and lack of control groups and because of a large environmental contribution to α, giving a small β/α ratio which is uninterpretable.

Disease

From information volunteered by people visited during the census, we found one family with muscular dystrophy (orofacioscapulohumeral type), three families with Charcot–Marie–Tooth disease, one family with oculopharyngeal muscular dystrophy, one family with myotonia dystrophica, two families each with one child affected with Wilm's tumor, and one family with children showing congenital absence of nails.

Even though the population is in general hospitable, they have a tendency to hide their mental defectives and those suffering from disabling disease.

No studies of blood groups and serum proteins or screening procedures were done at this time because of fear of antagonizing the population.

Conclusions and Decisions

A better understanding of historical and demographic data was obtained from this study as it related to inbreeding. In the French Canadians, the inbreeding level would be at least four times that calculated from Church records and isolates remaining in rural areas would be homogeneous, even though close consanguinity was avoided. The basis of studies related to genetic drift and founder effect was well established.

The lack of clear positive effects of inbreeding on genetic load prompted the decision to study consanguineous couples from a larger geographical area, comparing them to no consanguineous controls. The hypothesis to be tested was that, aside from regional or isolate peculiarities, the homogeneity of the population could be so great as to prevent such studies, mainly because of the impossibility of defining a nonconsanguineous group, everybody being related.

It was also decided to pursue studies in a regional disease (hereditary tyrosinemia) in order to establish its epidemiology, its genetics, and the importance of genetic drift of the "founder effect" type.

Therefore, both an inbreeding effect study and a regional disease study were initiated.

AN INBREEDING STUDY

Objectives

The precise objective of the inbreeding study was to compare consanguineous and nonconsanguineous couples in the whole eastern part of province and to try to avoid isolate factors which could influence results. The effect of inbreeding on social, cultural, developmental, and demographic data was also to be studied.

Material

All consanguineous marriages between 1953 and 1957 inclusive were determined for eastern Quebec. Then each marriage was verified at the Demography Office for Quebec, and two control marriages from the same place, in the same year, and with a woman of the same quinquennial age bracket were chosen sequentially for each consanguineous one.

An alphabetical list was made and the latest address available (1969–1970) from the service of family allowances of the province was searched for. If these couples had any children, their names would be necessarily found and a request for participation in the survey was sent to them.

Of 1200 families found, 660 accepted and were visited in 1969–1970 by the same nurses and allied health personnel engaged full time for the study. The survey consisted of demographic and reproductive family data and our individual health histories for each member. A modified Denver developmental test and the Raven Colored Matrices were administered to most children. A total of 195 consanguineous families and 465 control families participated.

Results

Of all the available data, only those that show social, cultural, or health-related differences will be presented in this chapter. They should help characterize the population for further genetic background necessary for family and/or regional studies.

There were no differences between the groups as far as number of persons living in the house, their marital status, type of housing, number of rooms in the house, year of birth of fathers and mothers, sibship size of fathers and mothers, and necessarily, because of the sampling procedure, year of marriage. Looking at the localization of the families in 1969–1970, we find that 75% of controls live in urban areas compared to 60% for consanguineous couples, especially in cities of more than 25,000 inhabitants. This is unexpected since the sampling

TABLE X. Reproductive Data for Each Group of Families

		Controls	Consanguineous
Pregnancies	Mean	4.26	4.74
	Variance	4.14	6.11
Live births	Mean	3.74	4.03
	Variance	3.16	3.95
Living children	Mean	3.63	3.81
	Variance	3.03	3.27

method was to get controls from the same place as the consanguineous couples and it reflects the fact that being inbred favors less migration. We cannot find in the study the reason for this sedentary phenomenon.

Economic status also shows a differential income of about $2000 annually in favor of controls. Occupations reflect the expected difference between rural and urban job opportunities.

Father's education lacks considerably in consanguineous couples compared to controls, as 70% have less than 7 years' schooling compared to 48% for controls. There are no such differences among the mothers.

If we ask fathers about consanguinity in their parents, 11.8% of the consanguineous group as compared to 3.4% of controls had consanguineous parents. For mothers, there were 7.6% and 4.0%, respectively. This is another unexpected finding, as if consanguineous couples constituted a subisolate where some remote system of consanguineous mating took place.

The sample of consanguineous couples for the study was comparable to the distribution found in the study of the Archdiocese of Quebec for 1950, being 67.7% second cousins, 12.8% first-and-a-half cousins, and 16.9% first cousins.

There are no apparent differences between the two groups as far as mean number of pregnancies, live births, and living children at the time of survey, as shown in Table X.

The data were reexamined after separation into four classes: urban and rural controls, urban and rural cousin.

The difference in economics is visible only between rural controls and cousins while there is no difference in the cities. The same applies for father's education, where the difference is most visible in rural

TABLE XI. Percentages of Consanguineous Marriages among Parents of Couples Sampled for the Survey

	Father's parents	Mother's parents
Urban controls	3.4	4.4
Urban cousins	6.7	10.7
Rural controls	4.8	5.2
Rural cousins	16.5	9.1

areas where consanguineous fathers have less than 7 years' schooling in 75% of cases compared to 59% for rural controls. There is the same differential in mothers but to a lesser extent.

Table XI shows a significant difference in rural areas between consanguinity in parents of fathers. Consanguineous mothers show this differential also in the cities. This table provides further data for the hypothesis that a rural system of consanguineous mating seems to exist. The importance of such phenomenon would be to help increase random inbreeding in rural isolates at a faster rate than expected, thus compounding the genetic drift phenomenon in relation to regional genetic markers.

The only constant finding in Table XII seems to be a differential of one more pregnancy in rural areas as compared to urban ones. There are certainly no broad differences between cousins and controls.

TABLE XII. Reproductive Data According to Consanguinity and Area

		Rural		Urban	
		Control	Cousins	Control	Cousins
Number of families		217	121	248	74
Pregnancies	Mean	4.7	5.1	3.9	4.2
	Variance	4.08	6.65	3.88	4.71
Live births	Mean	4.1	4.3	3.4	3.6
	Variance	2.91	4.25	3.10	3.16
Living children	Mean	4.0	4.	3.3	3.5
	Variance	2.81	3.42	2.98	3.84

When looking at individual records for children, it was found that there were no differences between consanguineous and control families in the four subgroups for sex, multiple births, complications of pregnancy, type of birth and presentation, birth weight, maturity, congenital malformations, neonatal jaundice, or neonatal convulsions.

The distribution of scores for the modified Denver developmental scale and the Raven Colored Matrices did not show any differences between cousins and controls when compared within urban or rural areas.

Discussion

This long and complicated study has been very disappointing in terms of effects of inbreeding and has not answered the questions proposed at the beginning in terms of fertility differentials.

However, a better understanding of the sociocultural background of. consanguinity was gained and the foundations of genetic drift were better understood. If consanguineous couples, for many reasons, are less prone to migration and if there exists a secondary inbred system of mating among these families, the rapidity of genetic drift for a given regional gene can be better understood.

Conclusions and Decisions

It was thus decided to abandon for the time being population studies of consanguinity and spend our efforts on studying regional genetic diseases in order to intervene eventually by treatment and counseling in the populations at risk.

Consanguinity studies were relegated to the time when all civil records for the whole French Canadian population become available in computer format and when inbreeding levels and mortality can be studied over 12 generations, re-creating the conditions prevailing at the founding and the breakup of the many isolates that constitute the population history of Quebec.

A REGIONAL GENETIC DISEASE

Objectives

The main objective of the regional study was to determine the genetic causes of regionalization of a disease. Hereditary tyrosinemia is now well known in French Canadians and was chosen because of its apparent distribution in an isolate in Quebec.

Introduction

The population studies were done in 1968, and more epidemiological information on the disease in the whole province has come out of recent work in newborn screening.[4]

Around 1964, a group of physicians in Chicoutimi became aware of an increased incidence of lethal infantile cirrhosis in their region of the Province of Quebec. In 1965, Larochell et al.[28] reported 29 such cases, 14 of which were familial.

Some of these cases were studied by Scriver et al.[43] and Sass-Kortsak et al.[39] and reported as cases of hereditary tyrosinemia at a symposium in 1966.

Cases of hereditary "tyrosinosis" were also reported from Scandinavia by Zetterstrom[50] in 1963, by Vestermark et al.[47] in 1964, by Gentz et al.[14] in 1965, and by Halvorsen et al.[22] in 1966.

The Disease

There are two clinical forms of hereditary tyrosinemia: One form begins with acute hepatic failure in early infancy and is the form presented by affected children in this study. The other form appears in patients who survive the acute liver failure and is characterized by chronic hepatic and renal disease. This second form has been called "Baber's syndrome" by Scriver et al.[43]

The clinical manifestations in the French Canadian patients have been reviewed by Larochelle et al.[29] on the basis of 37 cases.

The babies are products of full-term normal pregnancies and normal deliveries. The first signs and symptoms appear usually between the second and fourth months of life, and if not treated the child usually dies in the same month that the disease is discovered.

Clinically, infants are irritable and feverish. Hepatomegaly and edema are very frequent and the infant becomes lethargic and comatose. Anorexia, vomiting, diarrhea, and abdominal distension are present. A hemorrhagic syndrome secondary to hepatic failure occurs early. A peculiar odor is also present from an early stage if blood methionine is elevated.

Hematological studies reveal a normocytic anemia with leukocytosis. Bleeding and coagulation times are normal. The prothrombin time is increased. Hypoglycemia is very severe, and the glucagon test is negative. Hepatic functions are abnormal, reflecting cellular damage.

Biochemically, plasma amino acid analysis reveals mainly an increase in phenylalanine, tyrosine, and methionine. Belanger et al.[3] have reported that all patients showed a marked increase in α-feto-protein. Urine samples show generalized aminoaciduria, and δ-aminolevulinic acid excretion.[16]

At autopsy,[37] findings are limited to the liver, kidneys, and pancreas. Loose and diffuse fibrosis with severe distortion of lobules is found in the liver. There are zones of early nodular regeneration. The kidneys are enlarged and show interstitial edema and marked dilatation of the tubules with vacuolar and granular degeneration. The islets of Langerhans are hyperplastic in about half the cases.

Liver specimens show absence or greatly reduced activity of p-HPPA oxidase[27] as well as reduced activity of methionine-activating enzyme and cystathionine synthase.[13]

Dietary management of hereditary tyrosinemia is available[15,23,29,40] but is not quite satisfactory to normalize the biochemistry, at least in French Canadian patients.

The Isolate

The Lake St. John–Chicoutimi area is an isolated geographical region where the population is clustered around Lake St. John and the Saguenay River. The only means of communication with the rest of the province are to the west by a single road to Quebec City, which goes through about 125 miles of wild forests and a provincial fish and game park, and to the south by another road along the Saguenay River to Charlevoix County.

Medical resources in the region consist of regional hospitals and a large university hospital where serious or difficult cases of infantile cirrhosis are referred to the pediatric service. This explains the alertness of the physicians of Chicoutimi, manifested around 1964, to the problem of infantile cirrhosis.

The history of the settlement of this region dates from the 1840s, when 50 families from Charlevoix County migrated to Lake St. John. Most of the population living there now is descended from this group.

The Pedigree

Figure 3 presents the pertinent simplified portions of a pedigree which related 29 families having children affected with hereditary tyrosinemia to one common ancestral pair.

The complete pedigree, including all links between the 58 parents of the 29 sibships and the ancestral pair, Louis Gagné and Marie Michel, contains 1650 individuals. All could not be drawn in a comprehensible pedigree, but all links were used to calculate the coefficients of relevant consanguinity (F') for each family as they related to the common ancestral pair. These figures do not represent total inbreeding of the children of these families, since each parental pair is also related through many other ancestors. Since there is only one ancestral pair common to all 29 families, F' represents the consanguinity derived from it.

The average coefficient of relevant consanguinity (F') for all 29 families is 0.001693 (Table XIII), which is the equivalent of parents being related on the average as about third-and-a-half cousins. The average number of relationships of parents to the ancestral pair is 26.5.

If it is assumed that there are at least ten common ancestral couples for each parental pair, the mean coefficient of inbreeding of these families for all their common ancestors is probably about second cousins, which correlated well with other isolates from the same ancestral stock, namely, Isle-aux Coudre Charlevoix.

There is no doubt that the ancestors in the common paths to the ancestral pair involved in the transmission of the gene came from Charlevoix.

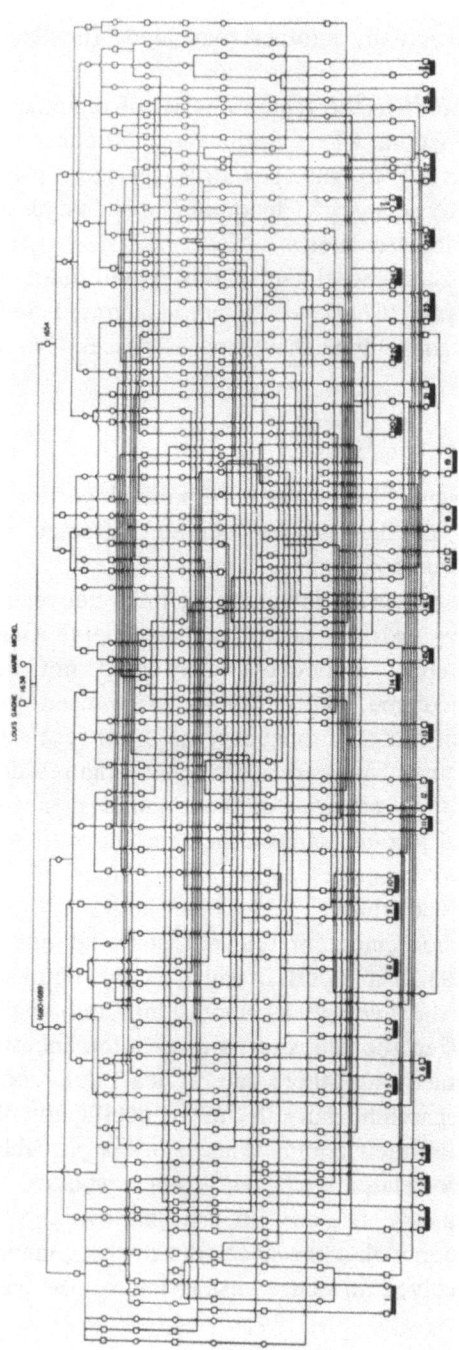

Fig. 3. Pedigree of family with tryosinemia.

TABLE XIII. Coefficients of Relevant Consanguinity (F') for 29 Families Affected with Hereditary Tyrosinemia to One Common Ancestral Pair

Family	Pedigree number	F'	Number of relationships of parents to the ancestral pair
O. Lar.	1	0.000572	27
A. Lab.	2	0.001299	34
A. Tre.	3	0.000291	28
N. Bra.	4	0.001209	31
R. Gag.	5	0.000108	18
R. Pot.	6	0.000512	26
L. Gil.	7	0.002821	28
M. Mar.	8	0.008103	21
G. Cla.	9	0.000065	15
H. Lap.	10	0.000254	16
R. Plo.	11	0.000067	14
Y. Sim.	12	0.000200	31
L. Vil.	13	0.000194	18
G. Dem.	14	0.000151	18
M. Har.	15	0.000548	30
R. Lal.	16	0.000307	24
B. Bil.	17	0.000332	31
C. Mur.	18	0.000052	20
E. Lap.	19	0.001017	39
P. Gag.	20	0.000341	23
R. Mar.	21	0.000398	18
G. Gag.	22	0.000341	23
M. Gue.	23	0.000369	44
A. Duc.	24	0.000123	14
G. Les.	25	0.000515	29
G. Gir.	26	0.001016	37
M.-A. Cot.	27	0.024343	36
G. Sim.	28	0.001046	48
R. Tre.	29	0.002515	28
Average		0.001693	26.5

The Ancestors

The ancestral pair shared in common by the 58 parents of the 29 sibships studied are Louis Gagné and his wife Marie Michel, married in France around 1638. Son of Louis and Marie Launay of Igé (Orne) in

Normandy, Louis Gagné migrated to Canada around 1644, followed by his elder brother Pierre in 1653.

Louis Gagné was born at Igé in 1612. Marie Michel was the daughter of Pierre and Louise Gory of St.-Martin-du-Vieux-Bellème (Orne). By 1644, they were in Quebec. In 1650, Louis Gagné was given a concession of land at Ste.-Anne-de-Beaupré, near Quebec. Louis died around 1661 at the age of about 50, having had nine children. In 1666, Marie Michel married Paul de Rainville.

Two of the children, Louise and Ignace, are important to the pedigree. Louise was born at Igé (Orne, France) in 1642 and was married at Beaupré (Canada) in 1654 to Claude Bouchard, founding ancestor of Charlevoix. Ignace was born in Quebec City in 1656 and married Barbe Dodier at Ste.-Anne-de-Beaupré in 1680. After her death, he married Louise Tremblay at Ange-Gardien in 1689. One daughter, Louise, in 1703 married Robert Dufour, who was one of the first settlers of Isle-aux-Coudres.

The Genetics

Formal segregation studies done on these 29 families revealed that the disease is inherited as an autosomal recessive trait.

A high carrier rate is suggested by the absence of first cousin marriages in the 29 families studied. Using Dahlberg's formula ($k = c/16q$) and assuming a frequency of first cousin marriages (c) of 0.75% (much higher than the observed frequency of 0.55% and 0.37% since 1945 for the neighboring Diocese of Quebec), we have an expected frequency of first cousin marriages (k) of 2.4–3.8% or 0.5–0.8 first cousin marriages among the 21 families used in segregation analysis. These estimates agree well with the absence of such marriages in the 29 families studied and reflect a high frequency of the gene for hereditary tyrosinemia in this population.

Prevalence at Birth and Regional Distribution

Using results from the newborn screening in the province (10 October 1970 to 30 September 1972), 14 newborns were eventually identified as suffering from hereditary tyrosinemia.

Eleven cases came from the Lake St. John–Chicoutimi region: four of these had familial antecedents for hereditary tyrosinemia. Pregnancies were uneventful and all newborns weighed more than 2900 g at birth. However, survival was very poor, with 11 affected infants dying before 1 year of age. One survivor has reached the age of 2 years.

From the total number of live births in the Province of Quebec, the proportion of newborns tested by the screening method of blood tyrosine determination was 81.6%. This percentage varied from a low of 61.2% in the Outaouais region to a high of 99.1% in the Eastern Townships. Evidence of tyrosinemia from the first blood specimen was found in 0.82% of all tested newborns; expected from the finding that tyrosinemia is a common entity in infants with low birth weight,[27] about 51.1% of newborns with initial tyrosinemia were premature by weight criteria (2500 g or less).

The proportion of initial positive results showed little variation from one region to another. The present study reports a minimal prevalence of 14 cases per 168,727 live births in the Province of Quebec and confirms an exceptional prevalence of 14.6 cases per 10,000 live births; one in 685 live births in the French Canadian geographical isolate of the Lake St. John–Chicoutimi region.

In a partially inbred population, the frequency of individuals homozygous for a particular gene is given by $Fp + (1 - F)p^2$ and the frequency of heterozygous individuals by $2(1 - F)pq$, where p is the frequency of the particular gene, q is $1 - p$, and F is the coefficient of consanguinity. This can be applied to the population of the above isolate. As $Fp + (1 - F)p^2$ is 0.001462 and F ranges from 0.000475 to 0.001899, p will vary from 0.037981 to 0.037306 and the frequency of carriers from 0.073077 to 0.071828 or one in 14 persons. This high frequency of the gene for hereditary tyrosinemia in the Lake St. John–Chicoutimi region is related to the "founder effect" coming from Charlevoix by the migration to the area in the 1850s.

Conclusions and Decisions

Hereditary tyrosinemia is a good example of a regional disease where the frequency of carriers is quite elevated secondary to random inbreeding and genetic drift.

For a problem of such epidemiological magnitude, efforts at coordinating research and development of screening at birth and improved treatment were necessary. The reduced effort in population genetics research in the province prompted a practical application in the development of genetic services for inherited diseases present in the population and led to the creation of a Provincial Network of Genetic Medicine.

A GENETIC CARE DELIVERY SYSTEM

Introduction

The Quebec Network of Genetic Medicine provides screening and diagnosis, genetic counseling, and treatment for over 30 hereditary conditions. It is operated by four university medical centers for the Ministry of Social Affairs. The budget for the Network is provided by the ministry.

The network observed two dominant working principles:

1. Integrated communication between its regional centers, the central laboratories, and the patients.
2. The use of mandatory pilot studies prior to implementation of a new service.

The work cited in this section is reported in a collaborative effort by myself and C. R. Scriver, C. L. Clow, and D. Dufour of the Network.[26]

History

Genetic screening was initiated by the province in 1969 on the recommendation of the heads of the pediatric departments at the four provincial medical schools (Laval, McGill, Montreal, and Sherbrooke). A pilot study[6] had demonstrated the feasibility of screening for purposes of medical intervention in the province. The initial working committee was composed of two representatives from each university and appropriate representation from the ministry.

The first task of the working committee was to organize screening for neonatal hyperphenylalanemia; this program began in February 1970. The committee designed the subsequent Network program by delegating separate tasks to its four different centers and by integrating the existing regional systems for follow-up, diagnosis, counseling, and treatment of patients with genetic disease.

The committee selected two problems for initial emphasis: one hereditary tyrosinemia; the other, the evaluation of ambulatory care of hereditary metabolic disease by allied health personnel.[5,7] The ministry agreed that operational research for purposes of disease prevention was in its own best interest at a time when a universal prepaid Medicare system was being inaugurated. The committee found the formalized relationship between research and service a stimulating opportunity, and research and development has remained a cornerstone of the Network program.

In 1972, the Network of Genetic Medicine was created to encompass a range of interrelated activities. The objective was to coordinate applied medical genetics in the province, related to disease prevention. The responsibility of the operation of the Network was invested with the universities, while financial support and final approval of the programs resided with government.

Services Offered by the Network

Mass Screening

Blood. In the mass screening program, capillary blood from the heel is collected on filter paper at 5–7 days of age. Phenylalanine is estimated in the material by the automated fluorometric method of McCaman and Robins[30]; tyrosine is measured simultaneously by Hochella's method of Grenier and Laberge.[20] Most recently, thyroxine (T_4) determination by the method of Dussault and Laberge[12] has been added to the repertoire of tests applied to whole blood spots received on the filter paper kits.

Urine. A urine sample is collected from the infant on filter at 14 days by the parents in home. Chemical tests for reducing substances, cystine, and keto acids are performed on eluted material, and after spotting by a semiautomatic device[44] amino acids are determined by one-dimensional partition chromatography on thin layer; the uric acid–creatinine ratio is also measured on the eluted sample by an automated method.[32]

High-Risk Screening

The following tests are provided under the appropriate circumstances: cytogenetic screening of referred patients; modified assay for serum hexosaminidases A and B[11] and two-test discrimination of heterozygotes[18] in the Ashkenazi community; prenatal diagnosis at two centers in the Network for selected indications[24]; chemical and chromatographic screening for aminoacidopathies and other disorders; assays of hexosaminidase, arylsulfatase, β-galactosidase, sphingomyelinase, and acid phosphatase on leukocytes, cultured skin fibroblasts, and cultured amniotic fluid fibroblasts.

Confirmatory Diagnosis

Initial positive screening tests are verified on a second sample. Confirmatory diagnosis is then pursued at one of the regional centers.

Counseling Services

Genetic counseling is provided for all patients identified in the newborn screening program; counseling for reproductive options is offered in reference to prenatal diagnosis, and for presumptive heterozygotes identified in the Tay–Sachs testing program; continuous counseling is provided in the treatment programs. The counselors are professional medical geneticists, pediatricians with expertise in the relevant care, and allied health personnel trained for the role.

Treatment

Treatment resources include diets and medication, continuous monitoring of treatment effect, and evaluation of clinical progress. Ambulatory methods are emphasized, and in-home care is provided for patients with hereditary metabolic diseases.

Repositories

The Network maintains two repositories: one for screening and demographic data, the other for cultured skin fibroblasts.[19]

Research and Development in the Network

Applied research for purposes of helping the patient with genetic disease has been a consistent theme of the Network.[8] Many developments in the laboratory have since been incorporated into the regular service activities of the Network. Ongoing pilot studies embrace screening for thalassemia minor in the Montreal Greek community, blood lipid analysis in children, and a "food bank" to facilitate the use of semisynthetic diets for treatment of patients with hereditary metabolic disease.[9] A series of publications describes new methods for diagnosis, counseling, and treatment and reports the results of clinical investigation sponsored by the Network.

Cost of Network

The provincial government provided $3–4 per live birth (birth rate 1.38 per 1000 population) to support the service functions of the Network and another $1–1.50 per birth for research and development. The Network has been fortunate to capitalize on existing facilities including laboratories, medical services, and medical genetics programs within the Quebec Medicare system. It also benefits from university-derived support of several committee members, and from the academic programs in genetics. The budget of the Network therefore represents an amount added to the existing costs of medical service and education within the province.

The cost of the Network can be evaluated in terms of the benefits it brings to an integrated prepaid system of health care delivery. For example, there has been a reduction in the prevalence of mental retardation and morbidity due to phenylketonuria, homocystinuria, and maple syrup urine disease. Admission rates of patients to institutions for the retarded have fallen, and no patient with phenylketonuria is known to have been missed in the screening program. The Tay–Sachs testing program, coupled with the prenatal diagnosis service, has prevented the birth of four Tay–Sachs infants in 2 years and will thus eliminate the burden for their care had they been born. The treatment program has kept patients in the home and at school and has significantly reduced the cost required for in-hospital and outpatient care.

Results of Screening

Compliance rate in the blood testing program is 92% of live births; compliance in the 14-day urine testing program is better than 80%. Ninety-seven percent of hospitals with obstetrical services participate in the voluntary program.

The incidence of phenylketonuria in Quebec Province in 1:23,000 live births, which is similar to the incidence of nonphenylketonuric hyperphenylalaninemia. Among the French Canadians in the province, the incidence of phenylketonuria is about 1:35,000 births and of hyperphenylalanemia 1:24,000 births, conforming to the relative frequencies for these traits in continental France, from where French Canadians have emigrated. Hereditary tyrosinemia affects 1:8000 live births in the province. Nearly all of these patients are born in the Lake St. John district, where the frequency of the disease is 1:650 live births. The screening program as it pertains to tyrosinemia serves several purposes:

1. To enumerate the relative frequencies of hereditary tyrosinemia and neonatal tyrosinemia.
2. To introduce genetic counseling into the region at high risk for hereditary tyrosinemia.
3. To facilitate research on the disease and to evaluate mechanisms.
4. To stimulate research into the causes for a relatively high rate (1%) of neonatal tyrosinemia in the French Canadian population.

Galactosemia caused by uridyltransferase deficiency (1:120,000) and galactokinase deficiency (1:120,000) have been detected in the blood screening program. The urine screening program has identified persons with histidinemia, cystinuria, isolated glutamicaciduria, renal iminoglycinuria, maple syrup urine disease, Fanconi's syndrome, and argininosuccinicaciduria.

Communications

Role of the Network

Two central laboratories are responsible for all communication related to mass screening of the newborn population (blood screening at Laval, urine screening at Sherbrooke). Each center is responsible for communication in his special projects, such as Tay–Sachs heterozygote detection, prenatal diagnosis, cytogenetics, or high–risk urine screening on hospitalized patients.

Normal test results are computerized in a data bank. Trimestrial printouts are returned to the 135 hospitals participating in newborn screening. Since almost all births in the province take place in hospitals (96%), the ministry fulfills its obligation to retain the patients' data while obviating the burden of mailing and filing a large volume of normal test results. When abnormal test results of technically unsatisfactory samples are identified, the Network contacts the parents directly for a second sample. Only when a positive test result has been confirmed is the patient's physician involved directly. Studies performed in 1972 revealed that compliance rates for follow-up samples improved greatly when the parent instead of the physician was asked to obtain the repeat test. The Quebec Corporation of Physicians has agreed that direct communication between the Network and the patient is in the best interest of all concerned. As a result, the average elapsed time between birth and initiation of treatment of patients with phenylketonuria is only 17 days (range 13–20 days) in the provincewide program and as low as 12 days at one center with a largely urban referral region. When the diagnosis is established, the Network plays a consultative role to the physicians. The latter assumes charge of the patient's health care; the Network center supervises only the management of the particular genetic disease.

Consent for participation in the program is invested with the client, who complies voluntarily with screening, counseling, and treatment. Since the Network is operated as a public health program within

Medicare, the onus is on the client if he chooses not to participate. A survey of mothers at the time of delivery revealed virtual unanimity in favor of preventive screening, the purpose of the Network program, and the need for them as parents to participate in the urine testing program. This opinion was offered even though only 10% of parents were previously aware of the scope and existence of the program.

Role of the Physician

The physician receives help in the care of his patient from his regional center, where the responsibility for follow-up and confirmatory diagnosis has been invested. In Quebec Province, the physician is a resource person for the patients in quest of medical services. It is assumed that most practicing physicians at present have little experience with the diagnosis, counseling, and treatment of the majority of genetic diseases. Consequently, centralization of special resources and regionalization of the influence of centers at which expertise for rare diseases exists can aid the physician and his patient. Regional centers for management of genetic disease comply with current recommendations of the World Health Organization.[48]

Conclusions and Decisions

The Quebec Network for Genetic Medicine is a voluntary program operated by four university-based genetic centers within the Quebec Medicare system. Its purpose is to apply its knowledge to the patient with genetic disease and its major effort at present is through the provision of screening and diagnosis for a broad spectrum of Mendelian inborn errors of metabolism, with special emphasis on regional and/or ethnic genetic disease.

Research and development, based on the genetic epidemiology of the population, is an important activity in the Network program. All services to date have originated from the pilot research project components of the program.

The program utilizes the four genetic centers, each situated at a university medical center, to centralize its activities and to regionalize its influence. The Network relies heavily on the patients (and parents) as the primary respondent(s) for compliance. Consent for participation is a function of the Medicare system. Physicians assume responsibility for the general health care of patients with genetic disease. The regional genetic centers assist the physician in a consultative capacity and provide resources for detailed counseling, monitoring, and treatment.

Decisions on future involvement in the genetics of French Canadians will be channeled through the Network, the emphasis being to identify and search for etiology and treatment of additional regional diseases. Population approaches will be more oriented toward the organization of genetic services for these specific problems and toward heterozygote detection than toward usual population genetics studies.

Better understanding of genetic forces at work in this population will continue to be a goal, but methodology will be more oriented toward epidemiological and historical findings.

It becomes clear that the Network is a good operational system to influence and direct comprehensive genetic services delivery to the population. Other fields of services that will be affected by genetic input in the near future will be cytogenetics, prenatal diagnosis, and counseling services.

SUMMARY

This chapter has been an attempt from someone involved in the genetics of French Canadians to outline the path followed since 1968 in human genetics through different approaches to this isolated population using different methods of research.

The description has been intended to be naive and practical in order to share with others the evolution from human genetics to daily involvement in genetic medicine. From classical studies of consanguinity, to demographic analysis of an isolate, to a broad inbreeding study, to, finally, the identification of a prominent regional genetic disease, the background has been set for a collaboration and rewarding association of genetic centers obligated to deliver the best knowledge to patients suffering from genetic disease. The author is aware that methodology might have been more sophisticated, but the voluntary goals of all these research projects have been to accumulate enough genetic information on the French Canadian population to justify his becoming involved in applied research profitable to his population.

ACKNOWLEDGMENTS

The goals of the investigations described herein were attained with the help of many people but especially through the admirable cooperation of C. R. Scriver, L. Dallaire, and B. Lemieux as well as J. Gelinas and C. Castonguay.

This work was supported by Grants NIH-GM 00795 and GM 10189; NHW 604-7-617; CAC (Killam 4875); MRC MA-4294 and MAS demonstration D-5.

BIBLIOGRAPHY

1. Allen, G., Random and non-random inbreeding. *Eugen. Quart.* **12**:181. (1965).
2. Allen, G., On the estimation of random inbreeding. *Eugen. Quart.* **13**:67 (1966).
3. Belanger, L., Belanger, M., and Larochelle, J., Une cirrhose infantile associée à la néoproduction d'alpha-l-foetoproteine, *Nouv. Presse Med.* **1**:1503 (1972).
4. Bergeron, P., Laberge, C., and Grenier, A., Hereditary tyrosinemia in the province of Quebec: Prevalence at birth and geographic distribution, *Clin. Genet.* **5**:157 (1974).
5. Clow, C. L., and Scriver, C. R., Ambulatory care of hereditary metabolic disease, *in: Ambulatory Pediatrics* (M. Green and R. J. Haggerty, eds.), pp. 650–659, Saunders, Philadelphia (1968).
6. Clow, C. L., Scriver, C. R., and Davies, E., Results of mass screening for hyperaminoacidemias in the newborn infant, *Am. J. Dis. Child.* **117**:48 (1969).
7. Clow, C., Reade, T., and Scriver, C. R., Management of hereditary metabolic disease: The role of allied health personnel, *New Engl. J. Med.* **284**:1292 (1971).
8. Clow, C. L., Fraser, F. C., Laberge, C., and Scriver, C. R., On the application of knowledge to the patient with genetic disease, *Prog. Med. Genet.* **9**:159 (1973).
9. Clow, C. L., Ishmael, H., Scriver, C. R., Murray, K., Campeau, H., Long, D., and Steinberg, H. A., The national food distribution centre for Management of patients with hereditary metabolic disease, *Bull. Genet. Soc. Can.*, **6**:29–31 (1975).
10. Crow, J. F., and Mange, A. P., Measurement of inbreeding from the frequency of marriages between persons of the same surname, *Eugen. Quart.* **12**:199 (1965).
11. Delvin, E. E., Scriver, C. R., Pottier, A., Clow, C. L., and Goldman, H., Maladie de Tay-Sachs: Dépistage et diagnostic prénatal, *Union Med. Can.* **101**:683 (1972).
12. Dussault, J. H., and Laberge, C., Dosage de la thyroxine (T⁴) par méthode radioimmunologique dans létat de sang séché: Nouvell méthode de dépistage de l'hypothyroidie congénitale? *Union Med. Can.* **102**:2062 (1973).
13. Gaull, G. E., Rarsin, D. K., Solomon, G. E., Harris, R. C., and Sturarran, J. A., Biochemical observations on so-called hereditary tyrosinemia, *Pediat. Res.* **4**:337 (1970).
14. Gentz, J., Jagenburg, R., and Zetterstrom, R., Tyrosinemia, *J. Pediat.* **66**:670 (1965).
15. Gentz, J., Linbald, B., Lindstedt, S., Levy, L., Shasteen, W., and Zetterstrom, R., Dietary treatment of tyrosinemia (tyrosinosis), *Am. J. Dis. Child.* **113**:31 (1967).

16. Gentz, J., Johansson, S., Undblad, B., Lindstedt, S., and Zetterstrom, R., Excretion of δ-aminolevulinic acid in hereditary tyrosinemia, *Clin. Chim. Acta* **23**:257 (1969).

17. Gerard, Fr. E., *Receuil de Genealogies des Comtés de Charlevoix et Saguenay,* 575 pp., La Malbaie (1941).

18. Gold, R. J. M., Maag, U. R., Neal, J. L., and Scriver, C. R., The use of biochemical data in screening for mutant alleles and in genetic counselling, *Ann. Hum. Genet.* **37**:315 (1973).

19. Goldman, H., The repository for mutant human cell strains, *MRC Prenatal Diagnosis Newsletter* **1**:5 (1972).

20. Grenier, A., and Laberge, C., Rapid method for screening for galactosemia and galactokinase deficiency by measuring galactose in whole blood spotted on paper, *Clin. Chem.* **19**:463 (1973).

21. Grenier, A., and Laberge, C., A modified automated fluorimetric method for tyrosine in blood spotted on paper: A mass screening procedure for tyrosinemia, *Clin. Chim. Acta* **57**:71 (1974).

22. Halvorsen, S., Pande, H., Loken, A. C., and Cjessing, L. R., Tyrosinosis: A study of 6 cases, *Arch. Dis. Child.* **41**:238 (1966).

23. Halvorsen, S., Dietary treatment of tyrosinosis, *Am. J. Dis. Child.* **113**:38 (1967).

24. Hamerton, J. L., The medical research council working group on prenatal diagnosis of genetic disease, *MRC Prenatal Diagnosis Newsletter* **(1)**:2 (1972).

25. Henripin, J., La population canadienne-française au début du XVIII siécle, *Cahiers de Travaux et Documents de l'INED*, No. 22, 118. pp. (1954).

26. Laberge, C., Scriver, C. R., Clow, C. L., and DuFour, D., Le réseau de médecine génétique du Québec: Un programme intégré de diagnostic, conseil et traitement des maladies métaboliques héréditaires, *Union Med. Can.*, **104**(3):428–431 (1975).

27. LaDu, B. N., and Gjessing, L. R., Tyrosinosis and tyrosinemia, in: (J. B. Stanbury, J. B. Wyngaarden, and D. S. Frederickson, eds.), Chapter XII, 296–307. McGraw-Hill, (1972).

28. Larochelle, J., Privé, L., and Mortezai, A., Study of 29 cases of cirrhosis in the infant of which 14 were familial, Presented at the 42nd Annual Meeting of the Canadian Paediatrics Society, Ottawa, June 28–30. (1965).

29. Larochelle, J., Mortezai, A., Bélanger, M., Tremblay, M., Claveau, J. C., and Aubin, G., Experience with 37 infants with tyrosinemia, *Can. Med. Assoc. J.* **97**:1051. (1967).

30. McCaman, M. W., and Robins, E., Fluorometric method for the determination of phenylalanine in serum, *J. Lab. Clin. Med.* **59**:885. (1962).

31. MacCluer, J. W., Griffith, R., Sring, C. F., and Schull, W. J., Some genetic programs to supplement self-instruction in FORTRAN, *Am. J. Hum. Genet.* **19**:189 (1967).

32. McInnes, R., Lamm, P., Clow, C. L., and Scriver, C. R., A filter paper sampling method for the uric acid:creatinine ratio in urine, *Pediatrics* **49**:80. (1971).

33. Mailloux, A., *Promenade Autour de l'Ile-aux-Coudres: Ste Anne Pocatière,* 130 pp., F. H. Proulx, (1880).

34. Mange, A. P., Growth and inbreeding of a human isolate, *Hum. Biol.* **36**:104. (1964).

35. Martin, Y., Isle-aux-Coudres: A socio-economic study, manuscript. (1956).

36. Morton, N. E., Crow, J. F., and Muller, H. J., An estimate of the mutational damage in man from date on consanguineous marriages, *Proc. Natl. Acad. Sci. U.S.A.* **42**:855. (1956).

37. Privé, L., Pathological findings in patients with tyrosinemia, *Can. M. Assoc. J.* **97**:1073. (1967).

38. Rious, M., and Martin, Y., *French Canadian Society,* Vol. I, McClelland and Stewart, Toronto (1964).
39. Sass-Kortsak, A., Ficici, S., Paunier, L., Kooh, S. W., Fraser, D., and Jackson, S. H., Clinical and biochemical study of three patients with tyrosyluria, *Can. Med. Assoc. J.* **97**:1056. (1967).
40. Sass-Kortsak, A., Ficici, S., Paunier, L., Kooh, S. W., Fraser, D., and Jackson, S. N., Observations on treatment in patients with tyrosyluria, *Can. Med. Assoc. J.* **97**:1089. (1967).
41. Schull, W. J., and Neel, J. V., *The Effects of Inbreeding on Japanese Children,* Harper and Row, New York: (1965).
42. Schull, W. J., and Neel, J. V., Some further observations on the effect of inbreeding on mortality in Kure, Japan, *hum. Genet.* **18**:144. (1966).
43. Scriver, C. R., Silverberg, M., and Clow, C. L., Hereditary tyrosinemia and tyrosyluria: Clinical report of four patients, *Can. Med. Assoc. J.* **97**:1047. (1967).
44. Shapcott, D., Lemieux, B., and Sahapoghi, A., A semi-automatic device for multiple sample application to thin-layer chromatography plates, *J. Chromatog.* **70**:174. (1972).
45. Stern, C., Consanguinity, in: *Principles of Human Genetics, p. 395,* Greenman, San Francisco (1960).
46. Sutter, J., and Goux, J. M., L'aspect demographique des problèmes de l'isolat, *Population* **16**:447. (1961).
47. Vestermark, S., Wulf, H. L. G., and Zachanchristiensen, B., Familial hepatic cirrhosis in infancy, *Danish Med. Bull.* **11**:46. (1964).
48. World Health Organization, *Genetic Disdorders: Prevention, Treatment and Rehabilitation,* Series No. 497, Geneva. (1972).
49. Wright, S., Coefficients of inbreeding and Relationship, *Am. Naturalist* **56**:330. (1922).
50. Zetterstrom, R., Tyrosinosis, *Ann. N. Y. Acad. Sci.* **111**:220. (1963).

Index